STUDIES IN ANCIENT TECHNOLOGY

VOLUME III

STUDIES IN ANCIENT TECHNOLOGY

BY

R.J. FORBES

VOLUME III

WITH 46 FIGURES AND 24 TABLES

THIRD EDITION

E.J. BRILL
LEIDEN • NEW YORK • KÖLN
1993

This volume is a reprint of the second edition 1965.

The paper in this book meets the guidelines for permanence and durability of the Committee on Production Guidelines for Book Longevity of the Council on Library Resources.

Library of Congress Cataloging-in-Publication Data

Forbes, R. J. (Robert James), 1900-
Studies in ancient technology / by R. J. Forbes.—3rd ed.
p. cm.
Includes bibliographical references and indexes.
ISBN 9004006214 (v. 1: cloth).—ISBN 9004006222 (v. 2: cloth).
— ISBN 9004006230 (v. 3: cloth)
1. Technology—History. I. Title.
T16.F67 1993
609—dc20 92-39555
CIP

ISBN 90 04 00623 0

PRINTED IN MALTA BY INTERPRINT LIMITED

CONTENTS

CHAPTER ONE

COSMETICS AND PERFUMES IN ANTIQUITY

Introduction

The use of perfumes and cosmetics is nor was confined to civilisation. Even now they belong to the parcel of strange customs adopted by primitive people, both men and women, to decorate and beautify themselves. Even now African warriors will stain their skin purple with henna, their hair blue with indigo and pencil their eyelids. Butter and dung are used to plaster their hair and the perfumes and cosmetics used change practically every mile. In Australian the male aborigines have monopolized cosmetics and carry compacts containing yellow, red and white paints, the women being allowed to decorate their faces on certain specified occasions only. In the New Hebrides both braves and medicine-men have make-up boxes containing yellow ochre, white coral lime and purple ashes made by burning coconut-shells. The new pigments introduced by European traders two centuries ago were readily sold and even proved the most important trade-objects in demand. American Indians use iron salts in conjunction with vegetable extracts applied on a base of bear grease or deer grease. Animal fat is generally used as a cold cream.

These customs are on a par with tattooing, that is introducing blue paint made from ashes of coconut with water into punctures of the skin, the filing of teeth, the decoration of the body with artificial scars, the extending of lips or ear-lobes. They are all part of the social pattern and mostly have a magico-religious background.

It has been said that "six thousand years are nothing when a woman wants to paint her face" (1). However, more probably men were the first to adopt paints when going to war or to woo. Prehistoric graves have revealed thin layers of red ochre spread over the body which represent either war paint or ochre spread over the dead body after death. Unfortunately very few traces of perfumes and ointments dating back to prehistory have been reported. We are on safer grounds when we reach the preclassical civilisations of the Ancient Near East, though even there the manufacture of cosmetics and perfumes can not properly be substantiated by the analyses of finds from the excavations. The complex character of these concoctions and their extreme age enhances the difficulties that already beset the analyst of modern samples of cosmetics. Though their complexity, their variety and the skill of their makers show that the art of the unguent-cooker certainly goes back to prehistory many modern identifications of ingredients such as published by REUTTER are very doubtful, to say the least. The story of perfumes and cosmetics will have to be made up mainly of data culled from written texts, philological evidence and the representations on ancient monuments of their manufacture and application.

THE ANCIENT NEAR EAST

Even in the earliest historical periods the use of cosmetics is fully developed in ancient Egypt. Unguents, creams, pommades, rouges, powders, eye-paint and nail-paint are commonly used. We moderns use cosmetics for strictly materialistic purposes such as cleansening the skin, allaying skin troubles and imperfections, protecting it against cold and generally beautifying body and face.

Their use in ancient Egypt was both hygienic and magico-religious. The human skin is not only open to the influence of weather but also to that of dirt, sweat and bacteria. The natural thin layer of fat is insufficient in extreme weather conditions. Hence the use of cosmetics or oils to protect the skin against the blistering heat of the summer sun was essential in the Near East. They formed part of the general hygiene of the ancient Egyptians who bathed very frequently and followed this up by rubbing the body with oils and creams. The oils kept the skin supple and the unguents gave the skin its necessary elasticity in the dessicating heat of the Egyptian sun. They were perfumed with the strong scents the Egyptian loved.

Therefore ointments and aromatic oils were a necessity of life for all classes of society. As the texts have it "Oil is the remedy of the body." PTAH-HOTEP, the author of the earliest precepts of life so dear to the Egyptians, says: "If thou art a man of standing, thou shouldst found thy household and love thy wife at home as is fitting. Fill her belly; clothe her back. Ointment is the prescription of her body." (2450 B.C.). We find an "apportioner of ointment" in the reign of King Amenhotep III. The papyrus Harris states that "no future vizier shall make any requisition upon any prophet of these temples for ointment....", leaving the priests to distribute it themselves. King Seti I increases the army's rations of ointment. They formed such an important item in the pattern of life, that the ancient Egyptians even went on strike to get them. Thus during the reign of King Ramses III the workers of the Theban necropolis came out for supplies of food were short and of bad quality, also "we have no ointments". Therefore ointments figure largely in medical recipes of all kinds and of all ages in Egyptian history.

Incidentally the general use of ointments gave rise to the manufacture of the many beautiful receptacles which grace our museum collections. Many of them are made of alabaster, a material also preferred by the ancient Greeks and Romans, who give an explanation for it (see page 33). In Egypt and Mesopotamia a substitute was found in the less costly small glass jars and bottles, made by moulding hot plastic glass rods of different colours onto a sand core and then heating them afterwards to fusion. These were the forerunners of the classical blown glass containers which still imitate the original alabaster forms.

In the Semitic world the magico-religious aspect of cosmetics is much more prominent. It is true that the cosmetics contained the "oil of life which makes the joints more supple" (2), and that "ointment and perfume rejoice the heart" (3). The use of ointments was sufficiently common to make Jesus say "when thou fastest, anoint thy head and wash thy face" (4) if he wants the believer to keep a spiritual fast rather than its outward signs. In the days of Ahaz the captives were released and they "arrayed them and shod them and gave them to eat and to drink and anointed them" (5). But even though Jews, Sumerians and Assyrians used "precious ointment on the head, that ran down upon the beard, that went down to the skirts of his garment" (6) they were far less clean than the Egyptians. Such things as bathtubs were used by the rich only. The Mesopotamians seem to have washed their entire body only on festive occasions. Purity with them was a spiritual concept rather than a hygienic one.

This ritualistic aspect of the use of ointments is far more important than the medical one even in ancient Egypt. Philological evidence discloses that this religious use of unguents and perfumes was extremely old and it explains the great variety of costly ingredients required by ancient ritual for the gods and only much later applied by the worshipper to his own body. In the Petersburg Papyrus the snake-goddess is promised aromatic offerings and the nine holy oils to anoint her statue. In the Gilgamesh Epic (7): "The gods smelled the savor, the gods smelt the sweet savor, the gods gathered like flies over the sacrificer." This ritual application of perfumed unguents to the statues of the gods, the worshippers and the dead is a frequent theme in ancient religious literature. The manufacture of these "holy oils" was an intricate mixture of techniques and ritual. The ancient Egyptian "unguent of the gods took 93 days to prepare, the heken oil 365 days" before it was suitable for the service of the gods.

The ancient Egyptians had two general words denoting cosmetics. The first word for "perfume, unguent, incense" is connected with a root meaning "agreable, pleasant" [1]. The second one "liquid" [2] goes back to the term for the little jars in which perfumes and cosmetics were stored. There are many other more specific terms for cosmetics, four of which go back to the oldest texts. The first [3] denotes the application of cosmetics and it is connected with the aromatic oil, which is the main compound of the nine "holy oils" and which also appears in the many medical recipes for unguents which combine the magical and the medical aspects of ancient medicine.

The second term [4] may be derived from the name of the country just north of the Second Cataract (8) bordering on Nubia "whence aromatic incense came". This term is connected with that for the offering of unguents and the ritual that went with it and even with a word for "unguent-maker" which occurs in late-Ptolemaic texts only.

The third term [5] was originally a medical term, but then we must remember that medicine and religion were intimately amalgamated in those days. It is also used for wound-balsams. It gave rise to later terms denoting the unguent-kitchen and the unguent-cooker, which latter term also occurs as an epithet of the god of unguents, Šsmw. The fourth term denotes medical anointing and is also applied to the preparation of balsams [6].

In Middle Kingdom texts (about 2000 B.C.) two new terms appear. The first one [7] has definitely a medical meaning, it occurs in many Old Kingdom titles of physicians already such as "chief physician". It shows that the magical anointing and preparation of balsams were part of their stock of trade, though embalming was of course a separate branch but closely related. This term also denotes the anointing of head and body at festivities, and in Ptolemaic texts even the anointing of the statues of the gods. The second term [8] denotes the purely worldly cosmetic skin treatment.

As the centuries flow by this beautifying with cosmetics begins to figure more largely. We find a term for anointing at festivities and dinners [9] which gives rise to a word for unguent-maker and to a term "anointing of lamps" meaning filling them with the usual vegetable oils and fats. Other terms for anointing [10] or adorning [11] (whence a term for unguent-kitchen) also stress this purely practical use of cosmetics.

This secularisation of the originally religious, magical and medical aspects of cosmetics is also obvious from the terminology of the many types of unguents and cosmetics mentioned in Egyptian texts. Most of these 35 specific unguents can no longer be identified accurately. Out of this total 22 cosmetics are mentioned in Middle Kingdom or older texts, that is they belong to the days before 1600 B.C. No less than ten of these are purely pharmaceutical as they do not occur in religious texts, the others have a ritual function and when applied in medicine may have been used largely because of their magical importance. Among the 13 later terms only one has a definitely pharmaceutical use only, all the others are exclusively used to beautify the human body or face.

In Mesopotamia too we find this close relation between religion, magic and medicine on one hand and cosmetics and incense on the other. The word for aromatic herbs in general [12] also denotes all substances oozing or filtering forth from the plants, hence resins and gums (incidentally this term is a Greek word of Egyptian origin [13]), which is related to those words denoting simplicia or medical herbs and unguents or pastes. The craftsmen using these herbs are the perfumer, the exorcist and the barber. It should be remembered that the priest supervising embalming in ancient Egypt has a name [14] which is connected with the knowledge of herbs too. The perfumer plays the same part in life in ancient Mesopotamia as the barber does in ours, witness the expression "slander circulates in the perfumer's shop" for our modern "business as usual". The use of pomades, careful barbering and perfuming the beard were characteristic of the Assyrian and Babylonian gentleman indeed; the Greek poet ALEXIS (fourth cy. B.C.) and the philosopher POSEIDONIUS (first cy. B.C.) speak of "Babylonian unguents" and the "Assyrian perfumes" figure in the classical poems by HORACE and TIBULLUS. Ointments also play a large part in the records of feasts in the palace and tributes exacted from conquered countries. HERODOTUS mentions that "the Babylonians anointed their whole body" (I.175).

The Akkadian word for ointment is closely connected with the name of the priests who concocted the offerings of incense [15] and with the word for anointing oil and the vase that held it or the spatula that distributed it.

In ancient Palestine we find perfumed oils used in the consecration of the tabernacle of the congregation and the ark of the testimony (9). Olive oils is specifically excluded as an ingredient (10) but unguents are used to anoint Christ's body (11) and the elected māsīaḥ or king. The bereaved should refrain from anointing themselves (12). Unguents were kept in an alabaster box (13).

THE PREPARATION OF PRE-CLASSICAL COSMETICS

The data discussed prove that Eiffert's contention that priests were the compounders and perfumers in ancient Egypt is only true in the sense that they had to recite the proper incantations and to bless the unguents made by the unguent-makers of ancient Egypt.

It would be virtually impossible to enumerate all the ingredients the ancients used to compound their cosmetics, for many terms mentioned in ancient recipes still remain unidentified. Analysis of the finds in ancient temples and cemeteries hardly ever yield useful data as even the analysis of modern compounds is an exceedingly difficult task. Still it is possible to obtain a general idea of the main ingredients, oils, fats and perfumes used.

We have tabulated the more common oils mentioned by classical authors discussing preclassical medicine and pharmacy, in those cases where identification is possible the name has been given (Table I). Castor-oil was the typical vegetable oil of the poor apart from olive-oil but it was more suitable for unguents; ben-oil (myrobalan or moringa oil from the Moringa nuts) and radish oil, colocynth oil and sesame oil are also common in recipes. Balanos oil from Egypt (the behen-oil so dear to the classical unguent-cookers and expressed from kernels of the Balanites Aegyptiaca) was not used by the ancient Egyptians, nor does linseed oil occur in their recipes. HERODOTUS, DIODORUS and STRABO describe the pre-classical production of these oils and their qualities. The ancient recipes demonstrate their use in the kitchens and unguent-laboratories. Most of these oils were also burnt in lamps. The ancient Egyptians denote them with a general term for vegetable oil or fat [16], the inhabitants of ancient Mesopotamia had a similar term which gave rise to a special word [17], denoting the producers of sesame-oil which is thus shown to be their principal product and which according to HERODOTUS (14) was obtained with a yield of nearly $^1/_3$.

All the fats at the disposal of the ancient perfumer were animal. Though the ancient Egyptians had a pharmaceutical term denoting the fat in plant or animal [18], we hear practically of none but animal fats. Butter fat and cheese were hardly suitable for cosmetics, but ox fat, sheep fat and goose fat are mentioned in very early texts and there was a special term for fat of sacrificial animals [19] often mentioned in medical texts. Fish oil was known both in Egypt and Mesopotamia [20] but it is doubtful whether it played any part in cosmetics. Many

TABLE 1

Vegetable oils of the ancient Near East

IL	OBTAINED FROM	EGYPTIAN	ACCADIAN
ond oil	Amygdalis communis v. Sative	?	(^{šam}šiqdu matqu)
nos oil	Balanites Aegyptiaca	×	?
oil	Moringa oleifera	×	×
:or oil	Ricinus communis	dgm (V.500.14)	^{šam}AG-PAR, šagabigalzu
cynth oil	Colocynthis vulgaris	šnj-tȝ (IV.502.11)	×
brathum oil	Cinnamomum Malabrathum	×	(Imported from India)
uce oil	Lactuca sativa	ibsȝ (I.64.14)?	^{šam}ḪI-IṢ-ŠAR, ḫassu
ed oil	Linum us tassimum	dšrt (V.493.2)?	(^{iṣ}KAT, kitû, pištu)
: oil	Olea Europaea	bȝḳ (I.424.2)	(Imported from North)
sh oil	Raphanus sativus	×	(^{šam}ŠÁ-GI, puglu)
lower oil	Carthamus tinctorius	ḳnnj (V.54.21)?	?
ame oil	Sesamum orientale indicum D.C.	×	ŠE-GIŠ-NI, šamaššammu

Evidence of use but terms for plant or oil still undetermined

No direct evidence of knowledge or use of plant and oil

s given in brackets denote name of botanical species, when specific term for oil is still unknown.

of the oils mentioned in ancient texts are really the perfumed oils extracted from certain plants, especially the "seven (ten) holy oils" so frequently mentioned in religious texts. Hence our table shows practically all the fats and oils available to the ancient perfumer.

Such animal perfumes as musk, ambergris, civet and castor were not available to the perfumers as they were extracted from animals beyond the pale of ancient Near Eastern trade. It would, however, be impossible to tabulate all the vegetable perfumes available to and used by them. Hence we have tabulated those natural perfumes from ancient Egyptian and Mesopotamian texts which still occur in our range of perfumes. Recent studies of ancient medical texts and lexicographical studies (20a) have greatly facilitated their identification. Apart from these classical authors mention many others such as henna flowers, the root of the iris, wine and many other ingredients now no longer in use (Table II).

TABLE II

Natural perfumes used since Antiquity

LATIN	ENGLISH	PARTS USED	EGYPTIAN	SUMERIAN	ACCADIAN
Amygdalis communis L.	bitter almonds	seeds	?	—	^{iṣ}sirdu
Pimpinella anisum L.	anise	seeds	mśt (I.88.9)	—	^{šam}šamrânu
Acorus calamus L.	calamus	rhizomes	mbj.t (II.243.15)	GI-DÙG	qanû ṭabu
Cassia tora	cassia	flowers bark	kd.t (V. 79.9) ḳḳtj (V. 71.13)	—	^{šam}qulqullânu ^{šam}kisat ṣiri
Cedrus Libani Barr.	cedar	wood	mš'-ib (?)	^{riq}ERIN	erinu
Abies cilicia Ant. et Ky.	cedar	wood	š (I.228.1)	^{iṣ}Ù-KU	ašuḫu
Laurus Cinnamonium Andr.	cinnamon	bark	tj.šps (V 243.7)	—	?
Citrus medica L.	citron	fruit	ϭITPE	^{šam}A-AM	ildaqqu, adaru
Zingiber officinale Roscoe	ginger	rhizome	?	—	^{šam}kurkanû ša šadî
Heliotropaeum Europaeum Benth.	heliotrope	flowers	?	^{šam}ŠI-ŠI	imḫur-pâni
Acacia Nilotica L.	"mimosa"	flowers	šnj.t3 (V 498.1)	^{iṣ}ḪAR	kiškanû
Mentha piperita L.	peppermint	flowers leaves	'3gj.t (I. 368.10)	^{šam}BÙR-DA	urnû
Rosa sanctus Rich.	rose	flowers	w3rtw	SILA-ŠAR	kasî
Rosmarinus officinalis L.	rosemary	flowers leaves	nkpt (II.346.3)	—	^{šam}MÁ-ereš-MÁ-RA
Cyperus rotundus L.	rushes	flowers	šbn (V.442.1) šbt (IV. 82.4)	GI-ŠUL-ŠÁR	qân šalali
Cyperus esculentus L.	rushes	flowers	gj.w (V. 157.3)	—	^{šam}kunqu
Santalum album L.	sandel	wood	?	—	^{iṣ}Elammaku
Cymbopogon Schoenantus	gingergrass	roots	?	^{šam}DUG-GA	lardu

The religious nature of perfumes is clear from the ancient Egyptian nomenclature. Though the Egyptians had a term for "smell" they always refer to perfumes as the "fragrance of the Gods" [21]. This indicates that perfumes were originally used for offerings and that this religious aspect was never forgotten. There was a special term indicating the offering of perfumes [22] and a special priest was in charge of this ritual. Also we find a special term for the fragrance of incense [23]. More general terms for fragrance are of later date, they are connected with the word for nostril [24] or derived from the name of the carob tree (St. John's bread tree, Ceratoria siliqua) and its sweet smelling fruit [25]. In Mesopotamia too perfumes and incense were primarily used for purification, ritual cleansening and offering making the worshipper acceptable to the gods to whom these perfumes were agreeable. Hence LUCAS' suggestion that perfumes were introduced to cover up the rancidity of the unguents or their oils does not seem adequate.

In many cases the ancients used vegetable oils with a natural perfume but they also had to extract essential oils from some base materials. Unfortunately our knowledge of their techniques is far from complete, and classical authors like PLINY mention the base materials and the oils isolated but tell us little about the techniques used in preclassical days (15). We are certain that the modern ecuelle method in which fruit is rolled in hollow vessels fitted with spikes or the sponge process in which peels of citrus fruit (after the removal of the pulp) are steeped in water, squeezed over sponges, which when saturated are themselves expressed, were unknown in Antiquity. Nor did the ancients dispose of modern solvent extraction and distillation methods using live steam or boiling with water. Some primitive form of distillation method may have been used. It is reported (16) that primitive peoples near the sources of the Nile macerate herbs in water, cover the vessel with strips of cloth steeped in grease or fat and boil the contents of the vessel until all the perfumes have evaporated fixing them in the fat or grease, which can then be scraped off the cloth. This may be a very ancient method.

This leaves us with three processes for producing perfumes from flowers, fruits and seeds. The first of these was enfleurage, the saturation of layers of fat with perfumes by steeping flowers into the fat and replacing them as soon as their perfume had penetrated into the fat. Using animal fats, as we do, the ancients could easily make the pomade so popular in their days. We see these pomades in the form of perfumed balls or cones [26] attached to the heads of the gaily decorated merry-makers at festivities and they form part of the regular make-up of an Egyptian lady. We are reminded of the "precious ointment upon the head, that ran down the beard, even Aaron's beard, that went down the skirts of his garment" (17).

The second process was maceration, that is dipping flowers, etc. into hot fats or oils at about 65° C (150° F). This is the process most popular in ancient recipes where the perfumer is told to heat his herbs in oil and to strain the mixture while hot. This process was quite feasible using the apparatus which the kitchens of the Ancient East had used from times immemorial. Indeed we find that the pharmacists and perfumers draw heavily on cooking techniques and kitchen utensils for their craft. Thus they, together with the smith and the cook, have greatly influenced the rise of early laboratory apparatus in the first centuries of our era.

Thirdly there was the possibility of expressing the flowers or seeds. Here the manufacture of essential oils and perfumes leaned heavily on the techniques of producing oils and wine. Hence though few Egyptian reliefs show the expressing of perfumes from flowers, we have ample knowledge of the development of such presses from Egyptian viticulture and oil manufacture. The oldest form of this press was treading the base material in some form of tub or basin, a scene often depicted from the oldest times onwards. The first real press is also shown on such monuments. It consisted of a linen cloth enclosing the grapes or seed, then folded together in such a way that the two corners on each side enfolded a stick. By torsion of the two sticks in opposite directions pressure could be exerted on the contents of the linen bag. This scene is often depicted in a rather puzzling way by the artist, but is meant to show two men on each side twisting their sticks and a fifth man who tries to keep these sticks apart as they tend to converge when the cloth is compressed by torsion.

As early as the Third Dynasty (2700 B.C.) a further improvement is shown. One of the sticks is replaced by a nooze attached to one of the two uprights of a frame carrying the bag-press. The other end still has the stick that is twisted by a set of workmen, whilst an inspector is usually shown as he is testing the cloth with his hand for possible holes or cracks. This is the last stage of mechanisation of the press before the classical world invented the beam-press and the screw-press (18).

Incidentally, the few reliefs depicting the manufacture of perfumes show the earliest form of the bag-press only, though certainly the improved form was used. However, essential oils do not seem to have made by expression very often for the recipes usually specify a direct incorporation of the perfume of herbs and flowers into the carrier oil or fat by maceration or enfleurage.

Apart from perfumes and oils the ancient unguents and beauty preparations often contain milk, honey, salts and such aromatic gum-resins and oleo-resins as were also used in manufacturing incense. In fact the ancient East like the classical world and the modern East went in for strong scents. Table III gives these "resins", as they are usually wrongly called, as far as their identification from the ancient texts is possible. Some of these ingredients must have acted as fixators, depressing the evaporation of the essential oils. We will find that the classical authors were well aware of this principle and may be inherited it from their pre-classical ancestors. However, much analytical work

TABLE III

Gum and gum-resins of the ancient Near East

GUM OBTAINED FROM	ENGLISH	EGYPTIAN	SUMERIAN	ACCADIAN
—	substances oozing or filtering forth from plants gums, resins	ḳmjt (V.393) κωμι (κόμμι, gum)	ŠEM-ŠIM	rîqu, riqqu
Myrtis communis L.	myrtle	?	GIR	^{riq}âsu
Amyris Gileadensis	Mecca balsam	inḥ3 s" - sńn (IV.166.13)	—	^{šam}arganu, marguṣu
Ferula Gobbaniflua Boiss	galbanum	ꜣps (?) (III.366.1) 3WJŠ3 (I.6)	^{riq}HAL	baluḫḫu
Styrax officinalis L.	storax, liquid amber	mn wr (II.79.6); ḥdw (III.212.11)	^{riq}BAL, ^{riq}MUK	balukku
Ferula Persica Willd.	sagapenum	—	—	^{šam}barirati
Pinus pinea L.	pine	wśt nr mrw (II.109.1)	^{riq}LI	burašu
Juniperus drupacea Labill	juniper	dḳr (?) (V.496.3)	^{riq}DUP-RA-AN	daprânu
	prach-gum	—	—	darrugu
Cedrus Libanif Barr.	cedar cedar-pitch	mš' ib (?) wḥm, tj-irsšwj	^{riq}ERIN —	erinu —
Cupressus semperviriens L.	cypress of the cemetries	sr.w (III 463.5)	—	^{riq}imdu
Pinus Halepensis Mill.	fir - gum	śf pr m w'n (I.255.20)	^{riq}RIM, ŠEM-LAGAB	ṭuri, ṭiru
Boswellia sp. Oli banum	opopanax (frankincense)	s'ntr (IV.180.7) (qsr-nw'n)	^{riq}GIG	kanaktu
Pinus Halipensis	gum from pine-conis	prt. w'n (I.285.18)	ŠE-LI-PAR	kirkiran burași
	fir (terebinth)	w'n (I.285.16)	^{riq}GAM-GAM	kukru
Balsamadendron myrrha Nees	myrrh	'ntw (II.283.1)	^{riq}ŠIŠ	murru
Euphorbia Antiquorum L.	male and female gum, liquid amber	'ntw ꜣdm	^{riq}AN-BAR ŠEM ^{d}NINURTA	nigibti
Artemisia Judaica L.	worm wood	—	—	^{šam}sîḫu
Sambucus nigra L.	elder	—	^{riq}MAN-DU	suadu
Nerium odorum L.	"nérion"	—	^{riq}GAM-MA	ṣumlalû
Buxus longifolia Boiss.	box	?	^{riq}ŠIM-ŠAL	šimmeššalu
Cypressus (general)	cypress	sr.w (?) (II.463.5)	^{is}ŠUR-MAN	šurmênu
Retana Ractum Forsk.	broom	—	^{šam}TIL-LA	urṭu
Cistus spec.	ladanum (from Damascus)	ibr (I.63.10)	—	ladanu
Balsamodendrum africanum Arn.	bdellium (Indian myrrh)	?	—	budulḫu
	stacte (from myrrh)	mḏt (II.85.13) bš (š)	—	—
Styrax benzoin	benzoin	šhm, nmt (I.119.4)	—	—
Ferula orientalis	ammoniakon	nht, ms' ms	—	—

on ancient perfumes remains to be done before we can decide on such niceties.

The laboratory operations mentioned in the recipes for such cosmetics were quite simple. The most frequent terms have been given in Table IV. Most of these were taken from the kitchen and therefore indicate originally some operation for the preparation of food. They were then borrowed by different craftsmen and applied to similar operations of the unguent-cooker, the miner and metallurgist or the dyer together with the kitchen apparatus transferred to these new uses and finally appear in the earliest alchemical texts.

Illustrations from the unguent-cooker's craft are not infrequent in Egyptian art. We have pictures of the oil-merchants carrying their products (classified by such qualifications as "clear", "fresh", "yellowish red") in animal skins. They also carry funnels for pouring them

TABLE IV

Laboratory operations in the ancient Near East

ENGLISH	EGYPTIAN	ACCADIAN
Drying	śšwj (IV. 281.12)	puṣṣû
Cutting up	n'g (II. 210.2)	kaṣâṣu (GÚM)
Triturating	šbn (V. 440.5)	kapâru, ḫamāšu (ḪUM)
Pulverizing	sn'' (IV. 156.13)	ḫašâlu, zâku (SÚD)
Grind together	tmtm (V. 309.10), tštš (V. 330.5)	qamû
Peeling	hf (II. 489.13), ḳḳ (V. 71.12)	—
Expressing	'tḫ (I. 237.1), 'rf (I. 211.3)	magâgu, mašâdu, ṣaḫâtu
Strain, screen	nḳr (II. 344.9)	parâsu
Decanting	b3k (I. 424.13)	ṣurrupu
Filling	mḥ (II. 116.6)	salâḫu tabâku
Shaking	nh (II. 282.5)	—
Mixing	šbj (V. 436.4)	balâlu, labâku
Kneading	šbn (IV. 440.7)	mazû
Stirring	nḏ (II. 369.13)	sapâḫu
Heating	irj srf (IV. 196.6)	sekêru
Boiling	3fr (I. 9.19)	bašâlu
Roasting	'wg (I. 173.8)	ša'û

into pottery or stone vessels and are shown in the act of mixing different oils. Women are depicted expressing the essential oils (shown as light-blue) from a kind of lilly, which was the heraldic flower of Upper-Egypt. Possibly this essential oil may, therefore, have had some extra magical potency in Egypt. However, the actual representaton of the preparation of the unguents is rare.

Still we have a fairly complete picture of an unguent-cooker's workshop (19). A table carries a flat shallow bowl, such as we often find, filled with unguents, on the dinner table. Two assistents are engaged in pounding dried herbs or fruit with pestles in mortars. Both mortars and saddle-querns were used in Egypt and Mesopotamia for desintegrating operations and may be small handmills too. Such small rotary mills [27] were certainly known in ancient Mesopotamia and used for pigments and flour. Akkadian texts mention the use of pestle and mortar to crush beans, corn, herbs and fir-gum. The Egyptians do not seem to have used the rotary mill at all.

Returning to our picture we see a third artisan kneeling, having crushed something on a saddle-quern. A fourth person mixes the

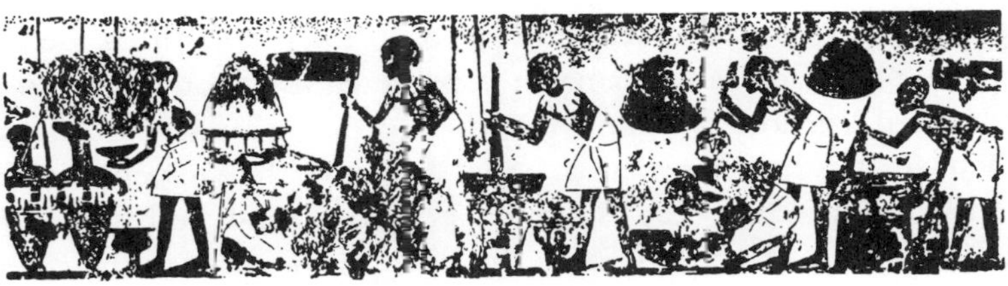

Fig. 1. Egyptian unguent-cooker's workshop
(After WRESZINSKY)

ingredients crushed on this quern and the oils with his pestle or a large spatula in a large bowl. The mixtures must then have been added to the contents of the bowl full of oil or molten fat which the fifth assistent is stirring on the fire. A further assistent takes something from one of the three decorated pottery jars and throws it onto a sieve from which the liquid drops into a vessel below. This may be wine or oil aromatised by the addition of herbs. The overseer or perfumer proper sits on a small stool overlooking the scene and shaping something with an adze. The workmen all wear curious collars, which seem to

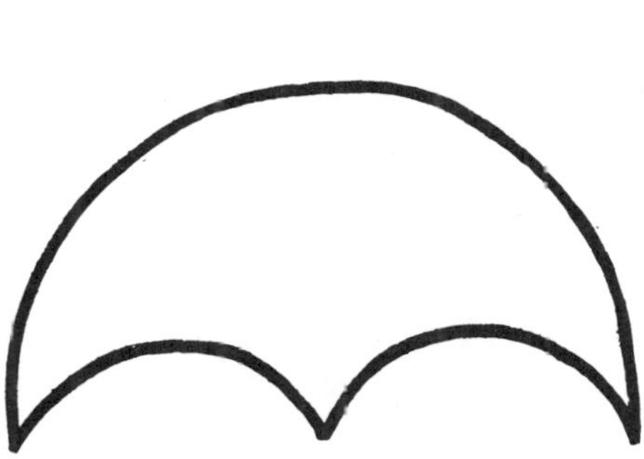

Fig. 2. Unguent-cooker's knife

indicate that they are busy preparing some "holy oil" for such collars are also worn by priests officiating.

The unguent, solidifying after cooling, was shaped into balls or cones. We know the name of a metal tool [28] used for this purpose, which seems connected with the words for mould and ball. It is a crescent-shaped knife, the inner rim being formed by two semi-circles, but its precise use is unknown.

In ancient Egypt these unguent-cockers were separate artisans closely related with the barbers, the pharmacists and physicians and with the priests, who used their products in the temple ritual and who may have guided their operations with incantations and recipes. This pertains to ancient Mesopotamia too. The "compounder of unguents" [29] is often mentioned in the Bible, he is often identical with the pharmacist and his name is rendered as "apothecary" in the Authorized Version. We know that they formed a guild in the days of Nehemiah and that there was a special "street of the unguent-makers" in ancient Jerusalem (20). They cooked roots and herbs in water, poured oil onto it and decanted the oil. Others crushed their herbs directly in the (heated) oil and sieved the contents of the vessel after thorough mixing. Though it has sometimes been suggested that their work was later carried on by female slaves in the household, the passage quoted (21): "And he will take your daughters to be perfumers and to be cooks and to be bakers" merely shows that unguents were sometimes prepared in the household, a custom that we still find in the classical world and much later. Early texts (22) distinguish between the compounding of "holy oils" and cosmetics. We are also given a comparison between the art of the physician (iatros) and the pharmacist-perfumer (myrepsos). The physician prescribes certain herbs to his patients, and "of such doth the apothecary make a confection; and of his works there is no end; and from him is peace over all the earth", however "he that sinneth before his Maker, let him fall into the hand of the physician" (23). In the days of Christ we find the preparation of ointments heriditary in the Abtinas family. Rabbi Juda carried on the trade of perfumer as a side-line and the Talmud remarks that "the world can not exist without a perfumer or a tanner" (24). Certain recipes from Palestine seem to have been as famous as the "balm of Gilead" for a late book (25) still mentions an "Ointment of King Agrippa of Judaea". In fact in classical times many eastern unguents imported by Greek or Asiatic "pharmaci" or "pharmacopolae" seem to have been made by Syrian or Jewish "unguentarii" (26).

We have a few recipes of ointments and beauty preparations which are worth quoting as they are typical of the many others, which are less complete. Some of these recipes were found written on the back of the famous Edwin Smith Surgical Papyrus (27) which goes back to the sixteenth century B.C., but the original of which may even be a thousand years earlier. The recipes noted down on its back, however, are probably contemporary with the sixteenth century B.C. version of the papyrus. The most important recipe in this collection reads thus (XXI.9):

"Beginning of the Book of Transforming an Old Man into a Youth. Let there be brought a large quantity of fenugreek fruit [30] about two khar. It should be bruised and placed in the sun. Then when it is entirely dry let it be husked as grain is husked and it should be winnowed until only the fruit thereof remains. Everything that comes therefrom shall be measured and let the husks be sifted after the manner of the treshing floor with sieves. Measure likewise everything that comes from these fruits and make them into two portions. One consisting of these fruits and the other of the husks. Treat one like the other (e.g. make them alike).

Let the whole be set aside mixed with water. Make into a soft (pasty) mass and let it be placed in a new jar over the fire and cooked very thoroughly, making sure that they boil, evaporating the juice thereof and drying them until it is like dry, without moisture therein. Let it be removed from the fire. Now when it is cool let it be put into another jar in order to wash it in the river. Let it be washed thoroughly, making sure that they are washed by testing the taste of this water that is in the jar until there is no bitterness at all therein. It should be placed in the sun, spread on the launderer's (bleached) linen.

Now when it is dry, it should be ground upon the grinding quern. Let it be mixed with water. Make like a soft (pasty) mass and let it be placed in a jar over the fire and cooked thoroughly, making sure that it boils, that little drops of oil may go forth therefrom. A man shall dip out the oil that has come of it with a dipper. Put into a hin-jar after having coated the interior with clay. Knead and make thick its (the day's) consistency. Dip out this oil and pour upon a linen sieve into the top of this hin-jar. Now afterwards it should be placed into a vase of costly stone (albaster).

Directions for use (XXII.7—10)

Anoint a man therewith. It is the remover of wrinkles from the head. When the flesh is smeared therewith, it becomes a beautifier of the skin, a remover of blemishes, of all disfigurements, of all signs of age, of all weaknesses which are in the flesh. Found effective myriads of times."

This recipe should be compared with the oatmeal or almond meal mixed with water used by the modern beauty operator to remove wrinkles (28). The Smith Papyrus also mentions the two following recipes:

"Two recipes for the complexion (XXI, 3—8).

(XXI, 3—6) Recipe for transforming the skin: Honey 1, red natron 1, northern salt 1. Triturate together and anoint therewith.

(XXI, 6—8). Another recipe for beautifying the face: Alabaster grains 1, natron kernels 1, northern salt 1, honey 1. Mix together and anoint therewith."

Honey and milk were favourite mediums in Antiquity for mixing solid materials to treat the skin. Hence these two recipes should be compared with modern recipes for "skin toning lotions" which may contain alcohol, glycerine, lactic acid (35%), water and perfume.

A chapter of the Ebers Papyrus (29) of the early sixteenth century B.C. repeats the two latter ones from the Edwin Smith Papyrus but adds several of its own:

"LXXXVII. Recipes to improve the skin.

Remedy to expel dandruff on the head: Powder of ground and roasted barley 5 ro, powder of roasted bran 5 ro, soft grease 5 ro, are mixed together and it is anointed therewith; but if the scurf comes off his head then his crown shall be turned to the ground without applying any remedy to it. Now after his crown gets done with the anointing with this remedy, it shall be anointed with fishoil on the second day, anointed with fat of hippopotamus on the third day, and anointed with ladanum on the fourth day; if anointed with unguent [31] of sour wheatened bread; it is applied to his crown every day."

(Dandruff is now usually treated with mixes containing soft greases such as beeswax, lanolin, petrolatum, olive oil or liquid petrolatum to dissolve the dry cuticle. We also hear of a "scalp oil" [32], used for the massage of the scalp. Curiously enough the term "anointing with oil" is also used metaphorically to denote the glazing of pottery.)

Next follow a set of recipes for the removal of wrinkles, starting with the two from the Edwin Smith Papyrus and continuing with:

"Another to expell wrinkles from the face: Gum of frankincense 1, wax 1, fresh balanites oil 1, rush-nut 1, are ground fine, put in viscous fluid and applied every day. Make it and thou shalt see."

(This may find its modern counterpart in a cold cream consisting of white wax, almond oil, borax and stronger rose water.)

"Another to let the face be stretched (freed from wrinkles): powder of gum with water of the fruit of the padew tree [33]; now after she has washed her face every day, she shall anoint her face therewith.

Another: Gall of ox, gum, powder of ostrich-egg, germinated spelt [34], are mixed, made into dough and pounded with viscous fluid, and the face is washed therewith every day.

Another: Turpentine, honey, germinated spelt, are made into a dough and pounded with viscous fluid and the face washed therewith very often.

Another: Water of the kebew plant [35], powder of alabaster, gum, green frit are mixed with honey, made into a dough and pounded with woman's milk and the face anointed therewith."

(These compare with the longer recipe given in the Edwin Smith Papyrus and their modern oatmeal equivalents.)

"Another to expell spots in the face: Interior of the fruit of the kesbet tree [36] is mixed with red ochre and applied to the face very often."

The natron used in these recipes find its equivalent in the sodium sesquicarbonate, sodium carbonate and sodium chloride of modern bath salts, for the ancient "natron" was a natural sodium carbonate found in the oases of the Western desert.

Preclassical eye-paints, rouges and powders

The use of eye-paints goes for back into prehistoric times. Beautifully decorated stone palettes used for grinding of the ingredients for eye-paints were found in some of the earliest prehistoric Egyptian graves. The name of this palette [37] is probably connected with the word "to protect". This protection was twofold, for not only were these eye-paints used to avoid the terrible eye-diseases still a scourge of the East, but they certainly had a magico-religious meaning too. Eye-paints or their ingredients are offered to the gods, their statues are painted with them and they are often mentioned in connection with the "Eye of the God Horus" which the evil god Seth tore from him and which he recovered in a battle that plays a prominent part in the religious texts.

The mineral ingredients used for eye-paints were generally carried in small linen or leather pouches, shells, hollow reeds or wrapped up in leaves. In such containers we find them in the graves too and so we can identify them analytically. The general term for eye-paint is "liquid" [38] but we also find terms derived from the ingredients. The more common term is later used for the mineral stibnite [39] and also for the metal antimony (in the cases when small statues of the gods are fashioned from it) but originally it seems to mean galena or lead sulphide. This is corroborated by the analyses of samples of eye-paints from the tombs. This galena also occurs in medical recipes against eye-diseases and in list of offerings it is constantly mentioned together with the green eye-paint which we will discuss.

Upto the later stages of Egyptian history it was customary to paint the upper eye-lid black with galena and the lower one green. Hence in all texts the black galena is coupled with the green malachite [40]. This copper compound is used as an eye-paint apart from its more common use as an ore, as a green pigment and as an ingredient for medical recipes [41]. It is found in the early Tasian graves of prehistory upto the nineteenth dynasty (about 1400 B.C.). The finds of galena eye-paint go back to the Badarian period and continue until the Coptic period. Both ingredients were found locally in Egypt, but we also hear of imports "from the Asiatics", from Western Asia, "Punt" (Somaliland?) or Coptos.

The Mesopotamian equivalent [42] is usually translated "stibium powder", but here again analyses of archaeological finds and records of the mines confirm the use of stibnite or galena. Accadian texts also mention the occasional use of orpiment or realgar [43], the "yellow eye-paint" which is contrasted with red ochre [44], that was more rarely used. The Accadian term for galena gave birth to the Arabic kohl which from a specific eye-paint came to mean a "finely divided powder", then "a subtle spirit" and being thus applied to very volatile substances gave birth to our word alcohol.

We can trace the gradual change of these eye-paints from a real remedy and defence against eye-diseases and the flies transmitting them to means of beautifying the eye. The older double and quadruple tubes in which the eye-paints were stored still bear the qualifications "good for the sight" or "to stop bleeding". Later such expressions as "to lay on the lid and the lashes" become more frequent. Then the toxic properties of the ingredients become less important and the colour ranks first. Hence burnt almond shells, soot or manganese dioxyde begin to oust the galena and malachite, which latter ingredient

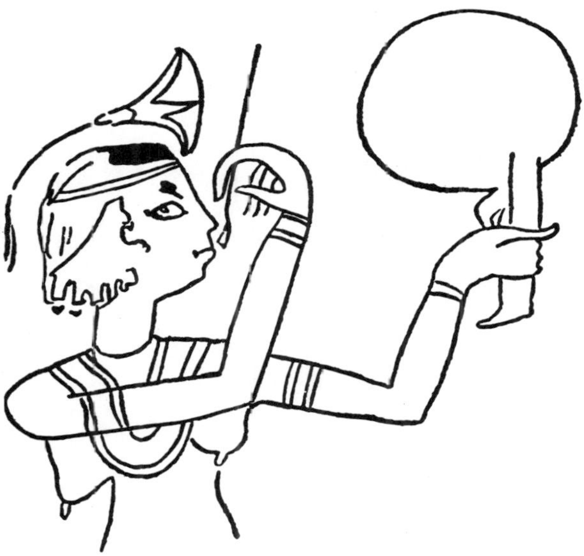

Fig. 3. Lady using lipstick
(After ERMAN-RANKE, *Aegypten*, p. 258)

is often replaced in later periods by the green resin from conifera [45], which was also used as an ingredient of incense and unguents. Soot later became the most popular ingredient and it still figures in modern mascara recipes mentioning lampblack, paraffin and petrolatum.

The manufacture of eye-paint was very simple. Fats or oils were not used in their manufacture. The mineral ingredient was ground on the well-known palettes or on a small flat stone. The finely ground powder was then made up into a paste with water or with a solution of some water-soluble gum, such as the "gum" of the Accadians [46] and the "gum-water" of the ancient Egyptians, which was also used for the preparation of inks. Resins do not figure in the recipes for eye-paints.

The paste or suspension is then applied to the eye-lid with the finger or with the pear-shaped end of the kohl-stick, a bone, wooden or ivory rod found in many excavations. This instrument is also depicted in the rare sign for "make-up artists" [47], the pronounciation of which is unknown. It shows an eye-paint rod immersed in a small spherical bowl. Some kind of small spatula or scalpel seems to have been used to judging from the signs used in a later word for eye-paint [48].

In Egypt lips and cheeks were coloured red with red ochre, often with a lip-stick consisting of a reed holding a small piece of ochre at one end. The red colour often applied to the palms of the hand, the soles of the feet, nails and hair was derived from henna (Lawsonia

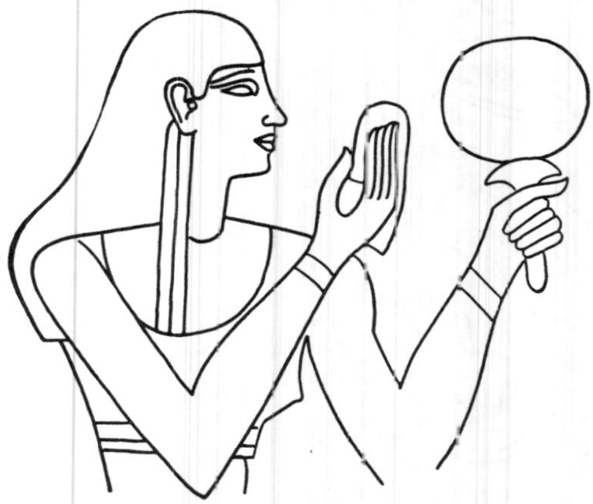

Fig. 4. Egyptian lady using powder-puff

inermis) made into an unguent or paste with oil or fat. The inhabitants of Mesopotamia used red ochre and henna or Asa foetida [49], but their ancestors, the Sumerians seem to have preferred yellow ochre as a face powder, which is sometimes called "golden clay" (50) or also "face bloom" [51]. The Egyptians were less liberal with their face powders but pictures show that the ladies of ancient Egypt knew how to use a powder-puff.

We know practically nothing about the dental, shaving and bath preparations used by the ancients, but in Mesopotamia pumice stone is generally used as a depilatory and referred to as the "barbers' stone" [52].

Though we have mentioned a late term for "make-up artists", this occupation was originally combined with that of perfumer and barber. We have much evidence on the minute regulations which made the king's life in Egypt a succession of rites which can be compared with that of Louis XIV at Versailles, except that the ancient Egyptian king had to go through these ceremonies as a part of his religious functions in the state. The state department controlling these functions and organizing them was the House of the Morning (30), its functionaries noblemen and royal princes. They bore titles like Keeper of the Kilt, Keeper of the Diadem or Director of the Royal Hairdressers and Manicurists. Of course they were no owners of beauty parlors but overseers of the royal hairdressers and slaves who looked after the toilet of the king. Though the religious aspects of these ceremonies

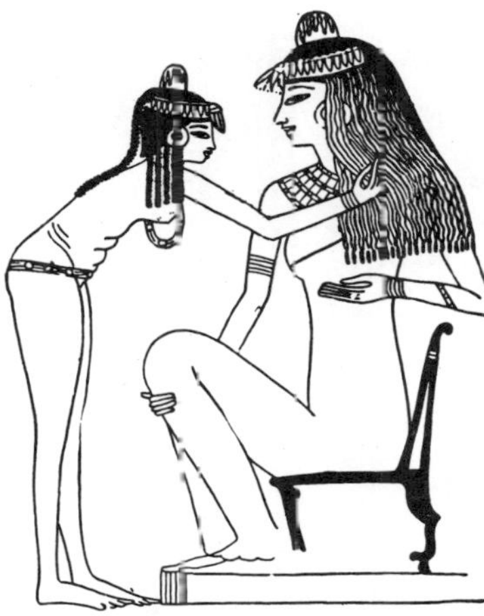

Fig. 5. Lady and Servant with Ointment Cones

were lost after the sixth Dynasty (about 2300 B.C.), the different operations were still carried out by slaves and artisans attached to the royal household.

These "doers-of-hair" [53] were hairdresser, hair-maker and wig-maker as well as make-up-artists. They were skilled servants attending their master's toilet, also making and arranging the hair and the wigs, which were either worn as toupees or for ceremonial occasions at early times. One of the earliest female hairdresser, Innu, is shown on an eleventh dynasty relief (31), dating about 2000 B.C., dressing the hair of Queen Kawit (fig. 6). The wigs were mostly made of human hair, padded in the case of the large ceremonial ones with vegetable fibre (32). Only a small proportion of the wigs of later date are made entirely of vegetable fibre, but never of animal hair (horsehair, wool). Many of these wigs have been found in excavations and tombs (33). It is probable from classical reports, that the different functions combined in the earlier palaces were later left to specialists such as we find in great number in Greek times in Egypt and the East.

Incense

The gum-resins and oleo-resins mentioned in Table III were not only produced by the perfumer but they were the ingredients too of

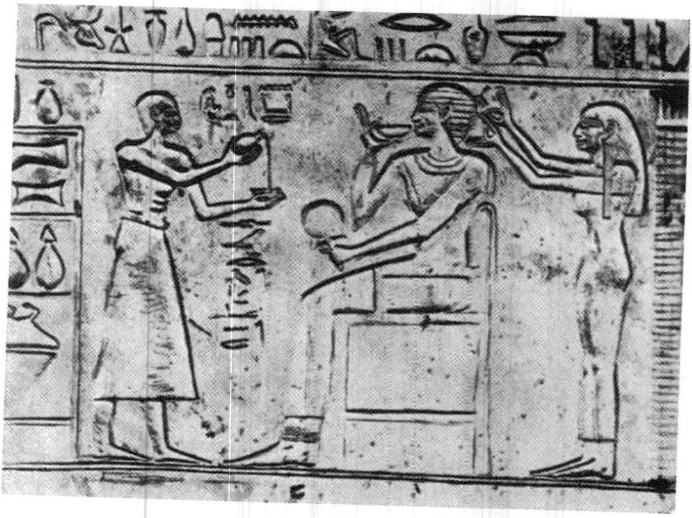

Fig. 6. The toilet of Queen Kawit
(After sarcophagus in Cairo Museum)

the incense-maker. In Egypt the use of incense goes back to the Pyramid Age, incense-burners of the period have been found. Some of these were vessels but we also have long spoon-shaped incense burners with long handles which feature in the reliefs showing the worshippers offering incense to their patron-god.

Incense performed the function of "pleasing the nostrils of the gods" by burning, many have no natural fragrance but give off sweet smelling fumes when burnt [54]. The identification of all the aromatic substances and oleo-resins used in the ancient Near East is very difficult though remains of incense date back to about 1500 B.C. in Egypt. Many of the ancient terms must needs remain unidentified (34).

There is no doubt that such products played an important part in the trade in ancient Syria and Mesopotamia. Many towns, temples or palaces had rooms for storing them, e.g. the palace of Mari, and they were often imported from the mountainous regions of the eastern and north-eastern coastal districts of the Mediterranean (34a).

Unfortunately we have little information how such oleo-resins were extracted. Possibly such techniques as used in the rubber industry in

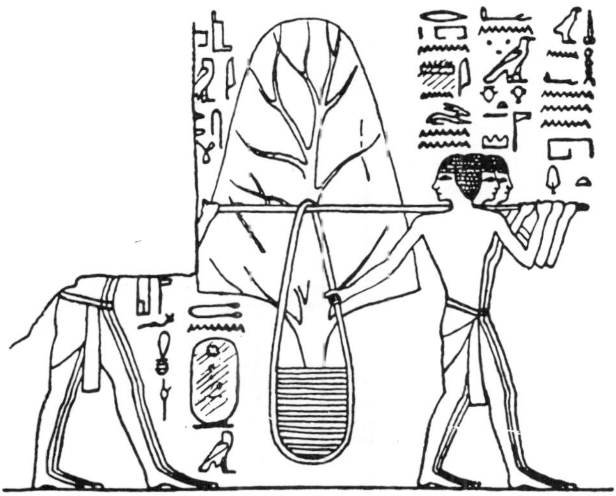

Fig. 7. Incense trees imported from Punt
(NAVILLE, *Deir el Bahari*, pl. 79)

the Far East and in the resin industry of the southern part of the Landes (France) were applied: "A vertical cut was made in the tree and a small container attached to its lower end collects the resin which oozes forth from the wounded tree." In some cases such resins may have been the by-product of the charcoal industry as described by Pliny (Nat. Hist. XVI.52—56) who tells us that the first product obtained when heating billets of wood in a charcoal furnace may be resin or light tar, the consistency of which depends largely on the rate of heating and the temperature obtained. Some were clearly liquid like the 120 Litres of riqqu, packed in a nabalu mentioned in a text from Mari, but others seem to have been of a more or less solid consistency.

This might explain the occurrence of different kinds in Mesopotamia, characterized by the words for oil (ì, *šamnu*), resin (or gum) (šim, *riqqu*) and perhaps also wood (giš, *isu*) in instances where it is listed by weight. Some were measured by measures of weight, others by measures of capacity, evidently dependent on their solidity or fluidity. For example *asu* (myrtle) and gi-dùg-ga (sweet reed) were measured by talents and minas (VS XVI 36 and TCL X 81), *kukru* and *burašu* by kurs and sutu's (CT XXIX 13 = VAB VI 226 and TCL X 81). With regard to *erinnu* (cedar) and *šurmenu* (cypress), the main distinction was between giš (wood) and ì (oil), the former measured by talents and minas, the latter by *sutu* and *qa* (cf. TCL X 72, 81 and 82). Also if these

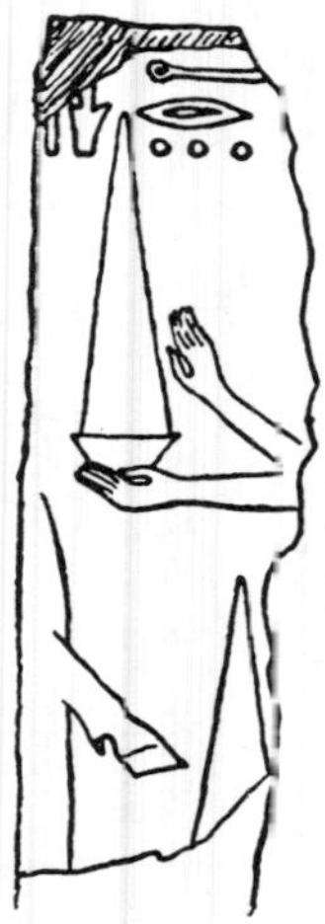

Fig. 8. Cone of incense
(NAVILLE, *Deir el Bahari*, pl. 70)

articles were preceded by the determinative giš they must have been some kind of extracts. In any case, it is clear that a distinction was made between the gums and resins in different forms—myrtle, e.g., is found as giš, šim and ì in the texts mentioned already—and this distinction may be of interest as throwing light on both their use and their preparation, about which, however, except in medicine, little is known.

The Egyptians obtained their incense from "Punt", now generally accepted to be Somaliland (in some cases Southern Arabia), from the coastal range of the Lebanon [55] and Asia Minor in general, and from Palestine, Syria and Nubia. It was imported in the form of heaps of small grains ("dry myrrh") or in the form of semi-liquid, plastic resins such as the "fragrant liquid myrrh".

The term for burning incense [56] had given its name to the frankincense from Punt. The word "fruit" denotes incense in the expression for incense "fruit of the Gods" [57]. A later term [58] is probably connected with the Egyptian word for "peace" or "happiness". In some cases Hebrew words [59] have become attached to certain types of imported incense.

The fragrant liquid components seem to have been expressed from the semi-liquid gums or oleo-resins in certain cases. Thus a fragrant liquid was produced from myrrh by compressing it. This liquid [60], the "stacte" of the Greeks, was added to certain cosmetics. A Ptolemaic text illustrates this technique. "The red myrrh is weak because of its liquid content, its fragrance is very sweet, if expressed in the bag (bag-press!) its content of liquid myrrh is one-fourth". The dry forms

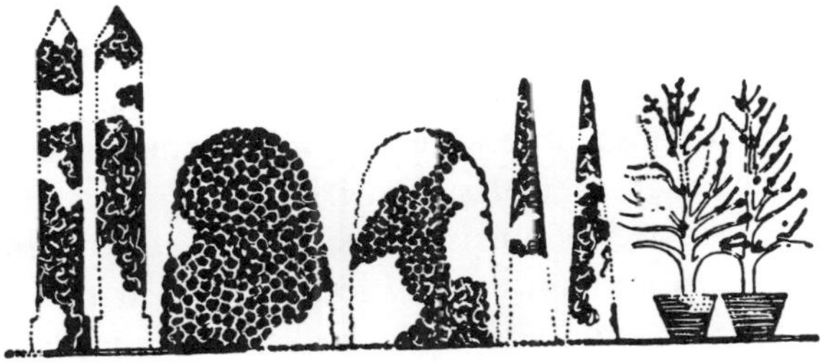

Fig. 9. Heaps and cones of incense
(After WRESZINSKY, pl. 348)

of incense seem to have been submitted to some kind of heat moulding. Incense was not only sold as small balls or grains [61] but the reliefs show us discs and cakes or lumps of incense [62]. This process had a special name and so had the "incense-shaper" [63]. A late text tells us that the "degree of compression of the mass was $^1/_2$", indicating that some kind of scale was used to characterize this.

By kneading or compression (in moulds?) the incense was also shaped into such special forms as the high cones, "white breads" [64] depicted on the walls of tombs and temples. The temple walls of Deir el Bahari illustrate the attempt of the ancient Egyptians to import the "incense trees" from Punt to grow them in their own country and thus grow independent of the supply by long and dangerous expeditions down the Red Sea. This experiment seems to have failed. The Ptolemaic period represents the zenith of the use of great varieties of incense. During the first centuries A.D. the more costly types of incense grew rare and were replaced by resins from coniferous trees or terebinth, which may also have been the original incense used before the Pyramid Age.

Incense was of course also used in the Far East and we will mention here but one curious application. During the T'ang dynasty (A.D. 618—907) incense sticks of standard size came to be used for time measurement and after 950 the incense stick was widely used as a timepiece (34b).

The Classical World

The Greek historians were well aware of the different customs of the barbarians and they often report the immoderate use of perfumes by the Assyrians, Babylonians and other Orientals or describe the strange customs of certain tribes. Thus Herodotus (35), after discussing the use of steambaths by the Scythians, says: "...the Scythians never wash their body. Their women make a mixture of cypress, cedar and frankincense wood which they pound into a paste with a rough piece of stone, adding a little water to it. With this substance which is of a thick consistency, they plaster their faces all over and indeed their whole bodies. A sweet odour is thereby imparted to them and when they take off the plaster on the day following their skin is clean and glossy." The modern and less expensive substitute in these regions is lye (water passed through wood-ash) used as tan-water in the bath.

We have ample proof that oil to protect the skin was used in very early times in Greece. In the Homeric poems Telemachus is anointed when he visits Nestor (36), ointments are stored in the house (37) and perfumes are used for clothes (38). The bathroom is often used for anointing (39). In the Greek army before Troy Machaon son of Asklepios makes pastes of bruished herbs (katapasta), concoctions from herbs (pista, pomata) and ointments (christa).

The classical authors are unanimous in proclaiming that the Greeks imported ointments and perfumes from the East. This is well expressed by Pliny (40) who tells us: "This is the degree to which forests are valuable in the matter of scents and their various products were not sufficiently remarkable by themselves and luxury took pleasure in mixing them all in combination: thus perfumes were invented. It is not recorded who first discovered them. In the days of the Trojan war they did not exist, and incense was not used when prayers were made to the gods: even in the rites of religion people knew only the scent of cedar and citrus wood, trees of their own country, or more truly the reek, as it rose in wreaths of smoke, though attar of roses had already been discovered (by the Persians), for it is also specified as an ingredient in commending olive oil.

Perfume ought by right to be accredited to the Persian race; they soak themselves in it, and quench the odour produced from dirt with its adventitious attraction. The first case I am able to discover was when a chest of perfumes was discovered by Alexander among the rest of the property of King Darius when his camp was taken. Afterwards the pleasure of perfume was also admitted by our fellow countrymen as well as among the most elegant and also the most honorable enjoyments of life, and even began to be an appropriate tribute to the dead."

XENOPHON (41) reports that the Persian grandees had "perfumers (kosmetai) to anoint them and rub them and make them beautiful" and adds that Persian queens squandered the tribute of entire towns on their ointments. ATHENAEUS reports that King Darius III Codomannos had 40 unguent-cookers in his train (42) and the recipe of the Royal Ointment so popular in the classical world came from Persia.

However, the introduction of perfumed unguents must have started in Homeric times. The Greeks loved the beauty of the human body, beauty was requested from the gods in prayers and girls entered beauty contests freely and even from a sense of public duty. Gradually the custom of assisting and correcting Nature must have crept in. Long before the Persian wars the custom of perfumes (and perhaps of pomades) had already spread throughout Greece. They are mentioned by such poets as ANACREON (43), ALKAIOS, SAPPHO and ARCHILOCHOS before the sixth century. The use of perfumes in the sixth century seems to have been such that in 594 B.C. SOLON thought it fit to forbid men to sell perfumes and ointments (44) and the unguent-cookers were banished from Sparta (45). On the other hand the physician PRODIKOS of Selimbria on the Propontis, the discoverer of hygenic gymnastics (iatroliptica), propagated the medication by means of unguents (420 B.C.) (46), and the use of the strigil and oil to clean the body of the athlete on the training grounds must have helped to spread the use of ointments and perfumes. Many famous Greek such as XENOPHANES (47), SOCRATES (48), ARISTOPHANES (49) and THUCIDYDES complain about the misuse of perfumes by men which entails the free use by the members of the fairer sex. However the Greeks of the classical period never showed the bad taste of the later Romans. THEOPHRASTUS (50) lists the principal substances used as perfumes among which fenugreek, the main ingredient of the "telinon" ointment, was most popular.

The Etruscans seem to have introduced Oriental perfumes in Italy, but a more systematic "ars unguentaria (myrobrecharia)" seems to have come from the Greek towns of Magna Grecia in Southern Italy such as Sybaris, which traded such products to Etruria and Campania in the north. The first mention of perfumes and slave-specialists in the art of adorning the human body is found in the works of Plautus and his generation (51). Of course this art was not always purely vanity but in some cases (such as the victor in his triumphal procession painting his face red with minium) there was a positive religious background. In the days of Plautus the custom had not yet generally spread but we know that the censors for the year 189 B.C. forbade the sale of "unguenta exotica" in the city of Rome (52). This was probably a sumptuary decree as the perfume industry was in the hands of the Capuans (as Plautus confirms), who were not yet Roman citizens A hundred years later the censors of 89 (53) set a maximum price on wine and forbade "unguenta exotica" as a war measure and a "buy Roman" campaign in the midst of the disastrous Social War of the first century B.C.

The more general use of these products in Rome seems to have dated from the first century B.C. but the art of the perfumer seems to have reached its perfection only in the days of Seneca, in the heydays of the Roman Empire. It is then that we find bitter complaints about the immoderate use of perfumes and unguents such as that of PLINY (54):

"Perfumes serve the purpose of the most superfluous of all forms of luxury. For pearls and jewels do nevertheless pass to the wearer's heirs and clothes last for some time, but unguents lose their scent at once and die in the very hour they are used. Their highest recommendation is that when a woman passes by her scent may attract the attention even of persons occupied in something else, and their cost is more than 400 denarii per pound. All that money is paid for a pleasure enjoyed by somebody else for a person carrying scent does not smell it himself.

Still, if even these matters have to be graded after a fashion, we find in the works left by Marcus Cicero that unguents that have an earthy scent are more agreable than those smelling of saffron inasmuch as even in a class of things where corruption is most rife nevertheless some degree of strictness in vice itself gives more enjoyment. But there are people who get most pleasure from unguents of more dense consistency which they call thick essence (spissum) and who enjoy smearing themselves with perfume and not merely pouring it over them.

We have even seen people put scent to the soles of their feet, a practice said to have been taught to the emperor Nero by Marcus Otho; pray, how could it be noticed or given pleasure from that part of the body? Moreover we have heard that somebody of private station gave orders for the walls of his bathroom to be sprinkled with scent and the emperor Caligula had the bathtub scented and so later did one of the slaves of Nero — so that this must not be considered a privilege of princes. Yet what is the most surprising is that this indulgence has found its way into the camp. At all events the eagles and standards, dusty as they are and bristling with sharp points, are anointed on holidays — and I only wish we were able to say who first introduced this custom! No doubt our eagles were bribed by this reward to conquer the world. We look to their patronage forsooth to sanction our vices so as to have this legitimation for using hair-oil under a helmet!

I could not readily say when the use of unguents first made its way to Rome.... But good heavens: nowadays some people actually put scent in their drinks, and it is worth the bitter flavour for their body to enjoy the lavish scent both inside and outside. It is a well-known fact that Lucius Plotius the brother of Lucius Plancus who was twice consul and censor, when proscribed by the Triumvirs, was given away in his hiding place in Salerno by the scent of the unguent he had been using, a disgrace that acquitted the entire proscription of guilt, for who would not consider that people of that sort deserved to die?"

The great Roman baths had special anointing rooms with heated floors and pictures on the walls (55) and even some private houses contained such rooms (56). Each part of the body had its own perfume (57) and some Romans even anointed themselves several times a day (58). Precious unguents were given away at dinner (59) or even sprayed on the guests from pipes installed for the purpose (60). Many poets such as HORACE (61) warn against this excessive use of perfumes and paints and JUVENAL notes that during the reign of Nero it was not "done" to go to battle without perfumes, cosmetics and looking glasses. The use of scents in wines takes up several chapters of THEOPHRASTUS' essay *On Odours* and APICIUS' cooking recipes (62) mention such "conditi mirabili". Even lampoil was perfumed (63). The enormous amounts of money spent on "the luxury that follows men even in death, and indeed that which enriched Arabia" trouble PLINY (64) who states: "A hundred million sesterces every year, that is the sum which our luxuries and our women cost us: for what fraction of these imports, I ask you, now goes to the gods or to the powers of the lower world?"

THE MANUFACTURE OF CLASSICAL COSMETICS

There are several essays by modern experts on classical perfumes (65) but few go down to the original texts like PLINY (66) and THEOPHRASTUS (67). The latter's essay is very much worth quoting in full. THEOPHRASTUS was a friend and disciple of ARISTOTLE and during his long lifetime (371—287 B.C.) wrote several works on botany and many essays such as his *Concerning Odours*. A short analysis of this work should be given by anyone who wishes to discuss ancient perfumes.

The first six paragraphs of THEOPHRASTUS' essay deal with odours in general and their classification, with the concepts of smell and taste with odours of plants. Here he more or less defines his ideas on odours and says: "1. Odours in general, like tastes are due to mixture; for anything which is uncompounded has no smell, just as it has no taste: therefore simple substances (he means elements) such as water, air and fire; on the other hand earth is the one elementary substance which has a smell, or at least it has one to a greater extent than the others, because it is of a more composite character than they." He then claims that every plant, animal or inanimate thing has some peculiar smell, which we may not be able to perceive and cites a few examples of the excellent olfactory sense of animals.

The chapters 7—13 deal with the manufacture of artificial odours in general and especially with the use of perfumes in wines, of which the first two are important for our subject: "7—8. Now even uncompounded substances have certain odours ... however, to speak generally, the result that is obtained, and accordingly such mixtures are of two things (or classes of things), a liquid and a solid.... For tastes and odours alike are derived from these two things. The method of the maker of spices and perfume powders (diapasmata) is to mix solid with solid, that of those who compound unguents or flavour wines is to mix liquid with liquid: but the third method which is the commonest is that of the perfumer, who mixes solid with liquid that begin the way in which all perfumes (myron, chrismatos) and ointments are compounded. Further one must know which odours will combine well with which, and what combination makes a good blend, just as in the case of taste; for there too those which make combinations, and as it were season their dishes, are aiming at the same object."

In the next chapters on the oils used as vehicles for perfumes (14—20), Theophrastus seems to propose a theory in which the viscosity and "porosity" of the oil is important for its application in perfumes: "Now the composition and preparation of perfumes aim entirely, one may say, at making the odours last. That is why men make the oil the vehicle of them since it keeps a long time and also it is most convenient for use [65]. By nature indeed oil is not at all well suited to take an odour, because of its close and greasy character, and of particular oils this is especially true of the most vicsous such as almond oil, while sesame-oil and olive-oil are the least receptive of all.

15. "The oil most used is that derived from the Egyptian or Syrian balanos, since this is the least viscous; the olive oil which is most used is that pressed from coarse olives in the raw state (omphacium) since this is thought to be the least greasy. Some say that for unguent the oil derived from bitter almonds is best: these are abundant in Cilicia where an unguent is made from them. It is said that this is suitable for choice perfumes like the oil of the Egyptian balanos: this is suitable in itself, however the shells of the fruit are thrown into the oil to give it a good odour: indeed they are also thrown into that which is made from bitter almonds."

"17. They use spices in the making of all perfumes; some to thicken the oil (that is render it less volatile), some in order to impart their odour. For in all cases they thicken the oil to some extent to make it take the odour better, just as they treat wool for dyeing (that is he compares the action of the spice with that of a mordant). The less powerful spices are used for the thickening and then at a later stage they put in the one whose odour they wish to secure. For that which is put in last always dominates." Theophrastus then goes on to propound a theory that the spices absorb the viscous part of the oil thus rendering it less viscous, and continues: "19. That oil which is most receptive, for instance that of the Egyptian balanos, will also keep longest, and for the same reason: namely that oil which is most receptive unites, more than others, into a single substance as it were with the spices."

The next chapters (21—26) discuss the spices used in making perfumes: "21. Almost all spices and sweet scents except flowers are dry, hot, astringent and mordant. Some also possess a certain bitterness, as we have said above, such as iris, myrrh, frankincense and perfumes in general....

2. All spices are given their astringent quality by exposure to fire,

but some of them assume their special odours even when cold and not exposed to fire; and it also appears that, just as with vegetable dyes some are applied hot and some cold, so it is with odours. But in all cases the cooking, whether to produce the astringent quality or to impart the odour proper, is done in vessels standing in water and not in actual contact with the fire: the reason being that the heating must be gentle, and there would be considerable waste if these were in actual contact with the flames; and further the perfume would smell of burning.

23. However there is less waste if the perfume obtains its proper odour by exposure to fire than when it does so in a cold state, since those perfumes which are subjected to fire are first steeped either in fragrant wine or in water: for they absorb less: while those which are treated in a cold state being dry, absorb more....

24. However the superior iris-perfume is made by using the root dry and not subjecting it to fire: for then the virtue asserts itself more completely than when it is steeped in a liquid or subjected to fire. It also comes to pass that, if the perfumes have been first steeped their virtues are, as it were, squeezed out of them to a greater extent, because they take in and absorb less: and so, when they are making them astringent, they do not leave the spices in the oil for long, but take them out, so that they should not absorb an excessive amount.

25. For making each perfume they put in the suitable spice. Thus to make kypros they put in cardamom and aspalathos having first steeped them into sweet wine. To make rose-perfume they put in ginger-grass, aspalathos and sweet-flag: and these are steeped as in the case of kypros. So too into each of the others they put the spices that suit them. Into rose-perfume moreover is put a quantity of salt: this treatment is peculiar to this perfume and involves a great deal of waste, 23 gallons of salt being put into eight gallons and a half of perfume.

26. The manufacture of kypros resembles that of rose-perfume, except that unless one takes out the flowers and squeezes them out, decay sets in and ruins the perfume by giving it a disagreeable smell, since they cause decay as they get soaked. Similar is also the manufacture of quince-perfume: the oil is first made astringent, and is cold when the quinces are put into it: then they take them out before they turn black removing each batch before the next is put in: for as they turn black, decay ensues because they get soaked through — just as in the case of kypros."

THEOPHRASTUS then discusses the parts of various plants used for perfumes (27—31) and the composition of notable perfumes. His recipes are not very complete, nor are those of PLINY (68) and DIOSCORIDES (69), but the latter have been compiled in Table V, which shows the slight differences in composition and the preference which PLINY shows for omphacium, where DIOSCORIDES uses olive oil. THEOPHRASTUS then inserts a small paragraph on the colouring of unguents and perfumes: "31. Some perfumes are made up colourless, some are given a colour. The dye used for colouring red perfumes is alkanet; the sweet marjoram perfume is dyed with the substance called khroma which is a root imported from Syria."

From the chapters 32—34 on the properties of various spices we quote: "32. It is thought that not only the smells of the perfumes contribute to a plesant taste (of the wine) but also the qualities of pungency and heat which are found in some of them.... 34. Now some spices when fresh have at first heavy and punguent qualities but in the course of time become sweet till they have reached their prime and then they loose their properties again", in the examples discussed this seems to vary from two to ten years.

After discussing the medical properties of certain perfumes (35—36) the rules for the mixture of spices and the storage of perfumes (37—41) are detailed in which chapters THEOPHRASTUS states that much depends on the season of collection, the time and the "ageing".

"40. All those made from flowers have little vigour, they are usually at their best after two months and deteriorate quickly after. Perfumes are ruined by a hot season or place or by being put in the sun. That is why perfumers seek upper rooms [66] which do not face the sun but which are shaded as much as possible.... This is why men put them into vessels of lead and try to secure phials of alabaster, a stone which has the required effect: for lead is cold and of close texture and stone has that same character, that being the best for keeping perfumes, which has it in the highest degree."

The properties of certain perfumes (42—50) and these of perfumed wines (51—56) are of less importance to us than the details on the making of perfume-powders and compound perfumes (57—60): "As to the mixing of solid substances to make powders and compound perfumes we do not find it here necessary to mix certain specified ingredients; the more numerous and the more various the perfumes are mixed the more distinguished and the more grateful the scent will be.... Again in perfumes of this class the aim and object is not to make the mixture smell of some one particular thing, but to produce a

TABLE V

The composition of classical perfumes according to Pliny and Dioscorides

P = Pliny Book XIII
D = Dioscorides Book I

Ingredients	Mendesion		Metopium	Cheap unguent	Malabrathum	Nardinum	Foliatum	Rhodinum		Krokinon		Sampsuchinon		Melinon		Susinum		Kuprinon		Telinum		Megalium		Kinnamominon		Myrtle-Laurel	Royal unguent	Illyrian iris	Amarakinon		Elatinon	Oinanthinon	Okiminon	Abrotominon	Anethimon	Narcissinon	Irinon	Gleucinon	Metopium	
	P9	D72	P9	P9	P14	D76	P18	P9	D56	P10	D64	P16	D58	P11	D56	P11	D62	P12	D65	P13	D57	P15	D69	P15	D74	P10	P18	P14	14	D68	D54	D5-	D50	D49	D61	D63	D66	D67	D72	Greek, Latin or Botanical Name
Balm																							x				x			x										Melissa officinalis
Allheal					x													x									x	x	x											panace, Ferula opoponax
Amomum						x	x							x									x				x			x										Amomum Subulatum, Cissus vitiginea
Balsam			x			x	x															x	x	x	x					x							x		x	Carpobalsam, Balsamodendron opobalsamum
Cat thyme																				x																				maron, Trifolium sipyleum
Cardamom			x														x	x	x		x																		x	Elettaria Cardamomum
Cassia		x											x	x								x				x														Cinnamomum iners Lawsonia
Cinnabar								x		x																														The plant "dragon's blood"
Cinnamon																x	x						x	x	x	x				x										Cinnamomum Cassia
Costus						x	x																x				x			x								x		Saussurea Lappa
Cyperus (oil)				x										x				x		x	x						x													Cyperus rotundus
Gladiolus																											x													
Fenugreek																				x	x					x														
Ladanum																											x													Rock rose, Cistus
Galbanum			x																																				x	
Lillies																x	x									x														
Majoram												x	x							x			x			x	x		x	x										sampsuchinos, Origanum Marjorana
Lotus																											x													
Mastic				x																																				
Melibt																				x																		x		Trifolium officinale
Myrrh	x	x	x		x	x					x		x			x	x	x	x				x	x	x					x						x	x		x	Balsamodendron myrrha
Narcissus																																				x				Narcissus poeticus
Myrtle-oil				x																						x														
Iris																											x	x									x			Iris germanica (florentina)
Nard						x	x																x			x				x								x		Nardostachys Jatamomsi
Pomegranate				x																																				
Quince														x	x																									Cydonia vulgaris
Oil of roses								x																																
Rush			x			x	x	x	x					x	x							x		x		x	x													Juncus acutus
Sweet-flag				x					x										x		x		x		x					x						x	x	x	x	Acorus calamus
Reed			x	x				x				x				x		x		x		x	x	x	x		x			x								x	x	Cymbopogon Schoenantus
Rose blossoms								x	x																															
Rosewood									x									x	x								x									x				aspalatum, Cytisus lanigerus
Malabrathum					x	x	x																				x													
Saffron (blossoms)								x			x					x	x																							Crocus sativus
Sisumbrion													x																											Stachys germanica
Saffron (oil)										x																	x													Krokinon
Southernwood													x	x				x																x						Artomesia Abrotanum
Laurel																										x														
Wood-balsam																					x	x	x	x	x															Xylobalsamum
Wild grape																											x					x						x		Oenanthe
Erupollos													x																											Thymus Sibthorpii
Elate															x											x											x	x		Phoinix elate
Dill																																			x					anethon, Anethum graveolus
Basil																																	x							okinon, Ocymum basilicum
Balanus oil	x	x				x	x									x	x					x	x	x	x		x			x										behen-nut oil
Olive oil									x		x		x		x					x	x					x					x		x	x	x	x				
Omphacium			x	x		x	x	x				x		x				x	x				x					x	x	x		x						x	x	oil or juice of unripe grapes and olive
Wine			x					x		x							x						x				x			x						x			x	
Sesame oil														x																										
Almond oil																																							x	
Resin	x	x																				x	x						x										x	
Honey			x	x				x	x							x	x			x			x	x	x		x	x		x							x			
Terebinth resin			x																																					
Alkanet								x	x	x																														
Flower of salt				x				x																				x	x											
Styrax gum																											x													

general scent derived from them all. This is why every day they open the vessel and remove each time that perfume whose scent is overpowering the other, adding at the same time smaller quantities of the less powerful scents, while some perfumes are added. When they make compound perfumes, they moisten spices with fragrant wine: and this certainly seems to be useful to produce a fragrance seeing that perfumers use it also. These compound perfumes last a long time. They are used to impart a pleasant odour to clothes, while the powders are used for bedding, so that they may come in contact with the skin: for this kind of preparation gets a better hold and is more lasting so that men use it thus instead of scenting their bodies directly. Some, before putting the powder in the bedding, soak it with fragrant wine, so that it may acquire its scent and some powders they moisten by mixing them with mead and wine or again simply with mead...."

The essay closes with a discussion of the characteristic smells of animals and on odours as compared with other sense-impressions (61—69). This careful study seems to have served as a base of PLINY's account, which like most of his work is anecdotic rather than scientific. However, he gives a useful summary of the manufacture of perfumes and unguents (70): "The recipe for making unguents [67] contains two ingredients, the juice and the solid part (succus and corpus), the former of which usually consists of various sorts of oils and the latter of scented substances, the oils being called "astringents" (stymmata) and the scents "sweetenings" (hedysmata). Together with these there is a third factor that many people neglect, that of colour, for the sake of which the dragon's blood plant and alkanet are added. A sprinkle of salt serves to preserve the properties of the oil, but to scents containing an admixture of alkanet salt is not added. Resin or gum are added to retain the scent in the solid part as it evaporates and disappears very quickly if these are not added.... What are called sprinkling powders (diapasmata) are made of dried scents, the dregs of unguents being termed magma. Among all scents employed the one added last is the most powerful."

PLINY himself enumerates the vegetable oils apart from the omphacium pressed from unripe olives or the seeds of grapes harvested in mid-summer, sweet almond oil, cyprus and balanos oil saying (71): "Oil is made from aspalathus, reed, balsam, iris, cardamom, melilet, Gallic nard (lavender?) all-heal, marjoram, helenium and cinnamon root by steeping all these plants in (olive-) oil and then pressing out the juice. In the same way rush-oil, rose-oil, henbane, lupine and narcissus-oil are made."

It will be observed that none of these perfumes or unguents contain fats, but that they are thickened by heating the oil and spices on a waterbath, adding resins and gums. The wine, perfumed wines, water or honey added also determine the final consistency. Only from PLINY's times onwards is lanolin (called "oesypon") mixed with honey and used as an unguent to remove spots from the face.

Great care should be taken in storing unguents and perfumes: "Unguents keep best in alabaster boxes, scents when mixed with oil.... Sunshine is detrimental to them; and the unguents improve with age. Therefore they are stored in the shade, in vessels made of lead. When. being tested they are put on the back of the hand, to avoid their being damaged by the warmth of the fleshy part." (72). Here again the alabaster receptacles, which had been in use for centuries, are preferred, the cold lead or stone were believed to have an excellent influence on the preservation of the qualities of the cosmetic as Theophrastus explained.

The olive-oil which is often used instead of the more expensive balanos-oil (often called "behen-oil" in the texts) comes from Achaia and Syconia, Sinope, Samos and later from Spanish Baetica too. Equally famous was the special quality of oil produced near the Italian centre of the manufacture of cosmetics, Capua, about which PLINY says (73): "Italy had won the highest rank in the world, particularly the district of Venafro and the part of it which produces the Licinian (olive-) oil, which causes the Licinian olive to be exceptionally famous. It is unguents that have given it its eminence because its scent is so well adapted to them, but it has also been awarded to it by the palate with its much more delicate judgment. Moreover no bird will touch the berries of the Licinian olive."

The classical texts already quoted give a wealth of information on the perfumes then used. PLINY correctly remarks that the fashion of perfumes changes rapidly, that the perfume from Delos had to make way for that of Mendes in Egypt, that of Corinth for that of Cyzicus and he mentions many more examples. As far as his data and those of DIOSCORIDES inform us on the composition of these perfumes and unguents they have been tabulated in Table V and hence there is no need to quote their texts on the "Mendesian scent, telinum, megalium, susinum, melinum, unguent of cypress" or whatever their name may be. PLINY, like the other classical authors, waxes lyrical over the "royal unguent, prepared for the Kings of Parthia", which closely ressembles the "oil of holy ointment" mentioned in the Old Testament (74), "and none of the components of this scent is grown in Italy, the conqueror of the world and indeed none in the whole of Europe excepting the iris in Illyria and the nard (lavender?) in Gaul". (75). The spices and oleo-resins commonly used were local brands but the ancient pre-classical types already discussed were still regarded as the very best in the classical world and they formed an important item of the trade with India and the East, much of which was concentrated in Alexandria.

The early Greeks were well aware of the fact that the "perfumes of Araby" came from the East. We have the delightful account by HERODOTUS (76): "Arabia is the last of inhabitated land and it is the only country which produces frankincense, myrrh, cassia, cinamon and ladanum. The Arabians do not get any of these, except the myrrh, without trouble. The frankincense they procure by means of the gum storax, which the Greeks obtain from the Phoenicians; this they burn and thereby obtain the spice." He then tells us the delightful stories of the winged snakes guarding the frankincense trees, the bats protecting the casia, the great birds bringing the cinnamom sticks and the beards of goats in which ladanum is collected as they graze. Later it was realised that many of these products did not hail from Arabia proper but came from India or even further east.

Alexandria was the big market for these gums and perfumes. There the Hammoniac gum (a type of elate-gum from the Oases of Ammon), frankincense from Yemen and Hadramaut and its brown variety from India, myrrh (from the Balsamodendron myrrha), cassia (the aromatic bark of the Laurus Cassia of S. India, hardly distinguishable from the brown powdered form of cinnamom), cinnamom (a closely allied bark from India,) ladanum (derived from a cistus or rock rose), malabrathum (the leaves of the Cinnamom Tamela [68]), opobalsmum (a second quality stacte), nardus or spikenard (Nardostychas Jatamansi Himalayan) and its Celtic variety (lavender or Saliunca Virg.), costus (the root of Saussurea Lappa from Kashmir), cardamom from northern India and galbanum (the gum resin from Ferula galbaniflua of Persia [69]) were imported.

Together with the local products and imports from Palestine, Syria and Asia Minor they were used for the blending and compounding of perfumes and unguents. This large scale manufacture is described by PLINY (77): "At Alexandria where frankincense is worked up for sale, good heavens!, no vigilance is sufficient to safeguard the factories (officinae). A seal is put upon the workmen's aprons, they have to wear a mask or a net with a close mesh on their heads, and before they are allowed to leave their premises they have to take off all their clothes: so much less honesty is displayed with regard to the produce with them as to the forests with the growers (where no such vigilance is kept)."

This manufacture, which was on a scale that must have called for considerable capital, was very much concentrated in the Canopus district of Alexandria (78). The many little fancy bottles and jars (lekythoi, bombyli, alabastra, aryballoi), which incidentally gave rise to a flourishing industry of stone and glass receptacles in Alexandria and other centres for the manufacture of perfumes, reveal a very wide trade by Alexandrian merchants who reaped a hundredfold profit, we are told (79).

This manufacture was definitely not a government monopoly (80). Seals marked "spices of Caesar" found in Roman Egypt may indicate that some kind of taxes in kind were levied in Upper Egypt which were then sold locally by the government to unguent-makers (81). In the third century the monopoly seems to have been replaced by a trade-tax. The sublease for manufacture and sale of unguents and perfumes is proved by papyri (82) of A.D. 161. In Oxyrhynchus, Egypt, there was a "street of the ointment-makers" and during the late third century A.D. a tax of 60 drachmae per month was paid by an "aromatopyles" (dealer in perfumes) and a "myropyles" (dealer in unguents) of Arsinoë (83).

In Africa we find few signs of a large trade in unguents and spices except for a single inscription in Madauros (84). Syria and Palestine were great producers of ingredients exported to Greece and Rome. The henna of Ascalon was greatly valued, like the balm of Gilead, already mentioned in the Old Testament (85), which was considered much better than that from Assyria or Petra and the groves of which were cut down in the Jewish War of 135 A.D. to prevent them from falling in the hands of the Romans. The attar of roses from Persia and Asia Minor and many other flowers and herbs are listed by our authors with Syrian styrax, nardus, silphion and other ingredients imported in Rome. There were several local centres for the manufacture of unguents and perfumes like Antiochia and Laodicea but none could compete with Alexandria. It seems that many inhabitants of Western Asia were engaged in the spice-trade like the former slave of King Mithridates and his friend, dealers in frankincense and ointments in Rome (86) or the nine ex-slaves of the Trebonii family who kept shops for the sale of incense (87) no doubt with the money invested by this Roman family like other patrons in the preparation of these imported products.

Greece too had its old centres for the manufacture of perfumes such as Corinth and Chaeroneia, famous for its "krinos-lilly unguent", a kind of cold-cream still made there in the days of Pausanias about

180 A.D. But these local centres were eclipsed by Alexandria and the new centre in Campania, south of Rome which competed with Alexandria for some time. We have already mentioned Pliny's report on the special type of olive-oil produced in that region and of the early days of Rome when Capua already made its "unguenta exotica".

Pliny tells us (88): "Yet in spring the Campanian fields having had an interval of rest produce a rose with a sweeter scent than the garden rose, so far is the earth never tired of giving birth, hence there is a common saying that the Campanians produce more scent than other people do oil." From this wild rose and many other local and imported ingredients the industry of Capua, located in the centre of the town called "Seplasia", made its products, not one firm but many producers. We have the names of several "unguentarii" and "thurarii" (88) who were all freedmen. Since we find no guild of unguent-makers it would seem that after all a large part of these shops were managed by a few large producers with an efficient organisation for the distribution of such products.

It would seem that there was some garden culture at Paestum for the Capuan perfume trade (89) and other ingredients came from the district below Praeneste and about Capua itself (90). The foreign spices needed could of course be bought at Rome, where Vespasian's Spice Market (91) was a centre of the trade. Though some local towns show their own manufacture of unguents such as the guild of unguentarii of Pompeii which left its traces on election posters (92), Capua seems to have outshone them and certainly to have captured a large amount of export trade. During the later Empire, however, adulteration of these products became rampant in Capua. Here Pliny has some interesting stories to tell.

We hear of a commercial magnate who tried to corner the market, "we have not forgotten Demetrius who was accused before the consuls by the whole Seplasia in the reign of Nero" (93) and of the use of the white drops interspecing the resin from pitch-pine "closely resembling frankincense that when mixed with it they are indistinguishable to the eye; hence the adulteration is practised in the Seplasia" (94). Worse, "now as often as the physicians turn to their books wishing to compound something from them, they put all their trust in the shops of the Seplasia which sophisticate and spoil all their wares. Ready-made plasters and salves are now on the market, and deteriorated goods and the deliberate falsifications of the Seplasia find their way into the mortar" (95).

This fraudulent policy cost Capua its chances in the western Mediterranean, slowly but surely Alexandria captured most of the trade of the west and the north which had formerly belonged to Capuan firms.

Classical make-up secrets

The descriptions left by classical authors of the make-up favoured by the Greek and Roman ladies make us wonder whether we would not consider it barbaric like the decorations which originally covered the marble statues now in our musea. The lack of proper mirrors and bad lighting have been blamed for this vivid make-up (96), but it would seem that this was merely a matter of ancient taste, for though indeed glass mirrors with a mercury back do only date from the fourteenth century, the ancient bronze polished mirrors were excellent. The preparations they disposed of were:

1) myra: balsams or unguents;
2) kerota, keromata: cerates;
3) acopa: painstilling unguents;
4) epichrismata: liquid unguents;
5) malagmata: unguents with vegetable powders;
6) parapasta: dusting powders;
7) diapasmata: cosmetic powders made by aspersion.

We have discussed the oils, perfumes and resins used for these preparations and should add that they also contained thaumaturgic or magical ingredients which had nothing to do with the actual recipe. Thus in ancient Rome the olive-oil mixed with dust and sweat which the gladiators and athletes scraped from their body with strigils was collected and sold as "rhypos" for the manufacture of unguents, believed to confer something of the energy of these fighters to the Roman ladies.

Greek ladies began to put on a face mask, mainly consisting of meal, which remained on all night and which washed off in the morning with milk. Such beauty masks were guaranteed to remove blemishes. Dioscorides recommends masks made of Chian or Selinan earth (mostly kaolin) mixed with equal parts of rosin and telinon of rose-unguents bleached by the sun. They were said to remove freckles and spots, sometimes honey, white of egg, bread crumbs or dough, traganth resins and asses' milk were added. Pompeiia, Nero's wife used masks made of fats, honey, flour or grated bread and unguents, which were washed off in the morning with asses' milk. Bean meal (lomentum) was also used.

The perfumes used were heavy from our point of view, sometimes they were different for each part of the body, but anyway personal taste in perfumes was appreciated. Though both men and women used perfumed ointments against colds, perfumes were generally abhorred in men.

After the beauty mask had been removed white lead powder was put on, then rouge, the eye-shadow and the eyebrows. Manicure and pedicure played a large part particularly as stockings were not worn

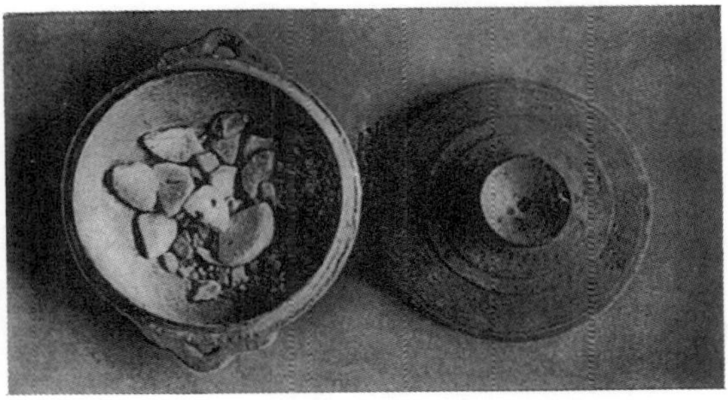

Fig. 10. Corinthian pyxis with lumps of psimythion (After SHEAR (98))

in antiquity. There was a belief that good ointment should be made with human spittle and hence certain cosmetics were chewed by slaves before application. This involved that these slaves had to keep their mouths clean by diet and by chewing certain aromatics. Incidentally the ancients favoured certain preparations to improve the breath, for instance they chewed "leaves of Malabar", the leaves from which malabrathum was made (Laurus Malabrathum L.) and Cosmus, the "parfumeur a la mode" in MARTIAL's days, sold pastilles for bad breath (97).

The women of Greece were the first to adopt white lead (lead carbonate) to whiten their faces (98). Although usually accompanied by unexplained cases of poisoning which often led to death of the individual, it remained popular for centuries. We only find warnings directed against old women who sought to recover youthful complexions in this way. This white lead was found in the form of round tablets in Athenian tombs of the third century B.C. The Roman ladies favoured white lead (99), earth of Chios or the white excrements of crocodiles.

In the toilet-box or pyx there was also the rouge, which in early Greece was made from vegetable extracts including seaweed, mulberry fucus (a lichen) and also from the "purple-snail". Later mineral substances like cinnabar were used, the Roman ladies always preferred them and used ruddle (red chalk), cinnabar, minium and vermillion. Henna was used as a nail-paint.

Eye-paints were still made of galena and stibnite, but soot, especially that made from date kernels, spikenard or rose leaves were much favoured. Greeks believed that eye-brows grown together were the sign of a hot temperament and therefore this was faked by painting. Patches were worn in Rome from the first century A.D., even by men.

Loss of hair was said to be prevented by a mixture of ladanum and myrrh (100), grey hair by frequent massage with bear grease or ointments made from worms. False hair was one of the affectations introduced in the Hellenistic period and not very common until the Roman Empire. Superfluous hair was removed with tweezers or by means of a depilatory such as the "halyconea" extracted from sea-swallows nests, introduced in the days of Ovid.

Hair was coloured black with several vegetable extracts or decomposed leeches. However, blonde hair was already most popular in ancient Greece, and the poet Menander gives us a recipe: "The rays of the sun are the best aid of making the hair fair and our own men know it. For after they have bathed their head copiously in a special ointment they sit in the sun, their heads uncovered and wait there for hours for their hair to turn, and it does!" We have not got the recipe for this hair-dye, but it may well be the recipe of the tenth century A.D., reported to go back to Antiquity: "Take dried cauls from the Orient, grind them to powder and mix in equal proportions with yolks of egg that have been boiled, then mix with wild honey. Rub on the hair in the evening and wrap the head in a kerchief. Wash the next morning with olive-oil and soap in fresh water. Be careful not to get a sun-stroke!" (101). The Romans also used a kind of crude soap imported from Gaul, called "sapo" to bleach their hair (102), it is sometimes claimed to give a reddish colour.

In Greece these beautification operations were carried out by household slaves and servants, but as these preparations grew more elaborate a whole staff of slave-specialists was required (103). Thus a Roman lady disposed of a whole army of "coscetriae (ornatrices)" skilled in the "ars ornatrix", which band consisted of "tractarices (tractatores)" for her massage after the bath, "unctoristes" to rub her skin with cosmetics, "dropecistes" (manicures and pedicures), "depilaristes", "pictrices" who brushed her hair, "ciniflones" or "calamistes" who combed, lustered (sometimes with gold dust!) and ondulated her hair with irons, "phialiges" and "stimmiges" who painted her brows and her hair, "psecacies" who perfumed and "ponceuses" who powdered her face, "catoptrices" who held her mirror, "flambaries" who held her fan, "appraciatrices" who directed them all, "loraries" who whipped wrong-doors and "cosmetes" in charge of the dresses. Ovid in the third book of his *Ars Amatoria* gives a good picture of the make-up of a Roman lady and MARTIAL in his epigrams laughs at Fabulla covered with chalk who is afraid of the rain, Sabella whose lead shrinks from the sun and Gellia who does not succeed in covering up her blemishes by perfumes better than would his dog (104).

In less lavish establishments the ordinary barbers (tonsores), were also concerned with the methods and means of beautification (105). They either concocted many of these cosmetics themselves or relied for supplies on the unguentarii or on the "rhizotonistes" (herbalists) who also made perfumes and cosmetics. JUVENAL mentions that the "barber of his youth now belongs to the new rich" (106).

ANCIENT LITERATURE ON COSMETICS

In view of this elaborate classical art of beautification there must have existed a large literature on cosmetics and the "ars ornatrix". The greater part of these have not been recovered, what is left, however, confirms us in our opinion.

The great physician HIPPOCRATES of Cos (about 450 B.C.) has given a few recipes for unguents (107) and his disciple PRODIKOS of Selymbria used them in his system of hygienic gymnastics. A hundred and fifty years later THEOPHRASTUS writes his essay *On Odours*. Then we have to wait until about 250 B.C. when HERAKLEIDES of Tarentum wrote on cosmetics, though GALEN who gave abstracts from this book says that this can no longer be regarded as medicine. Some fifty years later the Cypriote APOLLONIUS MYS wrote a book *On Unguents* and the physicians PHILONIDES and APOLLODORUS composed a lost *On Unguents and Garlands*, mentioned by GALEN.

The first feminine contribution is that of Queen CLEOPATRA VII, daughter of PTOLEMY XI Auletes who is said to have written a *Book on beautification* (50 B.C.), often quoted by Roman authors. It seems to have been a kind of formulary, called "Cleopatra gynaeciarum libri", which is quoted as late as the seventh century by PAULUS of Aegina.

In the early first century A.D. we find APICIUS' cookery book which also contains recipes for perfumes and perfumed wines, and PLINY's *Natural History* with its many scraps on cosmetics.

Roman poets like MARTIAL, JUVENAL and HORACE abound with scraps of information and LAIS of ELEPHANTIS, poetess of obscene literature, is said to have composed on *On things cosmetic*, meant for a special class of women. DIOSCORIDES' *Materia Medica* dates of about this same period, and by the end of the century the Syrian physician ARCHIGENES of Apamea wrote a book on cosmetics. This Archigenes and also KRITON, physician to the Empress Plotina, wife of Trajan, who wrote four books on cosmetics in Greek are quoted by GALEN (108). KRITON mentions 25 unguents, pomades, remedies against freckles and wrinkles, facewaters (nimmata), depilatories, perfumes for wash, clothes and beds, but his books are unfortunately lost.

Other fragments of CLEOPATRA's book can be recovered from the writings of AETIOS, who describes a "smegma of Cleopatra" in his *Iatrika*. It seems that many recipes have survived in the hands of the practical craftsmen such as pharmacists, unguent-makers and others to be collected much later by authors like NICOLAS MYREPSOS, physician to the Emperor Johannes Dukas Vatatzes in the thirteenth century. The systematic study of this and other recipe-books may reveal further evidence on the extensive literature on ancient cosmetics which no doubt existed.

It is doubtful whether any of the recipes helped on the long run for as the poet said of old (109): "You dye your hair, but you will never dye your old age, or smooth out the wrinkles of your cheeks. Then don't plaster all your face with white lead, so that you have not a face, but a mask; for it serves no purpose. Why are you out of your wits? Rouge and paste will never turn Hecuba into Helen!"

NOTES

[1] "ndm.śt" is derived from a root "nḏm" (II.381.16) (These figures refer to volume, page and line of ADOLF ERMAN and HERMANN GRAPOW's *Wörterbuch der Aegyptischen Sprache*, where the correct hieroglyphic notation of these words can be found)

[2] rḏw (II.469.14) from "ḏw" (V.549.24)

[3] "mrḥ.t" (II.111.1) from the root "wrḥ" (I.334.8)

[4] "mḏt" (II.185.13) may be connected with "mḏ3" (II.186.1) but gave rise to

the term for offering of unguents "irj.md̲t" and the ritual "ir.t dw md̲t" connected with it, hence "md̲t.j" (II.185.20) for unguent-cooker

[5] "nwd" (II.226.1) whence "nwd.t" (II.226.6) for woundbalsams, "is nwd" for unguent-kitchen and "nwd" (II.226.10) for unguent-cooker

[6] "sjn" (III.425.11) means "to anoint" and later "to rub, rub off"

[7] "gś" (V.201.12) whence "mr gś" (chief physician), "gś.w" (V.202.14) for magical anointing and embalming

[8] "sph3" (IV.105.18)

[9] "śgnn" (IV.332.9) personal anointing, whence "pś śgnn" (I.552.13) for unguent-maker

[10] "śwrḥ" (IV.71.3) anointing

[11] "ẖkr" (III.401.15) adorning, hence "is.ẖkr" (III.402.9), unguent kitchen

[12] The aromatic herbs, gums and resins are called ŠEM, riqqu, hence the terms:
úŠEM, urqûtu for simplicia and ŠEM-KU, damatu for unguents, pastes. The Ú, šamnu sign, meaning plant, herb, simple often preceeding such plant names. Hence the lúŠEM-MÚ, âšipu or exorcist, the lúŠEM, muraqqu or perfumer, and the lúŠU-I, gallabu or barber

[13] The Egyptian "ḳmjt" (V.39.3), hence the Greek koμμi, gum.

[14] The Egyptian "wt" (I.379.9)

[15] The verb "rîqu" is derived from "riqqu" mentioned above. ŠÉŠ, pašâšu is ointment, whence ŠUDÚG, pašîšu for unguent-cookers, Ì-BA, piššatu for anointing oil and gišDILIM-Ì-ŠŠÉ, napšaltu, jar for unguents or spatula

[16] " 'd" (I.139.23) whence the terms " 'd̲t" (I.240.4) and " 'nd̲t" (I.242.4), names of unidentified oils.

[17] "Ì, ÌA, šamnu", fat and "Ì-GIŠ, šamnu", vegetable oil, whence the name of the producers of sesame-oil "Ì-ŠUR, sâtitu"

[18] "d̲d3" (V.632.4), pharmaceutical fat

[19] "kn" (V.41.1) fat of sacrificial animals

[20] " 'h3" (I.217.5) or I-KIL, ikuku

[21] "śṯj-nṯr" (IV.350.2) from "śṯj" to smell

[22] "idt" (I.152.7)

[23] "śwḥ" (IV.72.15)

[24] "hmnw" (III.293.2)

[25] "nd̲m" (II.378.14), hence "nd̲m-śtj" (II.381.6), perfume, unguent, incense

[26] "ḥnb" (III.118.9)

[27] aHAR.SU, erû

[28] "bt" (I.483.12) connected with bd, mould for casting and bd̲, ball (I.488.9)

[29] The Bible mentions perfumed oils (šémen 'arēb) mixed by the "pattām" The Greek for unguent (myron) is usually given as bēsem (myrrh-oil?) in the Bible

[30] "hm3j.t" (III.94.6), salt, hence this fruit might be derived from one of the salicorna or soap-plants of the desert, more probably Trigonella Foenum-graecum L.

[31] The text of the papyrus Ebers has "ibt" which should be read "ib3t" (I.62.6), unguent

[32] "mrḥ.t iḥtj" (II.111.12)

[33] "p3dw" (I.501.7)
[34] "bdt" (I.487.8)
[35] "ḳb.w" (V.25.8)
[36] "kśbt" (V.141.1)
[37] "nḏ.t" (II.377.1) from "nḏ", to protect
[38] "rḏw" (II.469.14), liquid
[39] "mśdm.t" (II.153.8), Coptic CTHM, Greek stimmi, stibium. Hence the terms for eye-paint "śdm" (IV.370.9), "śdm.w" (IV.370.11) and "śmtj" (IV.144.15)
See also Fr. Jonckheere, *La mesdemet* (*Histoire de la médicine*, vol. II, 7,1952, pags. 1—12)
[40] "w3ḏw" (I.267.9)
[41] "tḥn.t" (V.391.20) for "unguents containing malachite"
[42] ŠEM-BI-ZI (-DA), egû, guḫlu, whence the Arabic koḥl
[43] ŠEM-SAHAR-GUŠKIN, šîpu, lêru
[44] IM-SA$_5$, šaršerru
[45] "ḫp3" (III.366.1)
[46] Accadian A-DAN, hilu; Egyptian "ḳmjt" (V.39.13)
[47] V.639.12
[48] "dśdś" (V.487.7)
[49] ᵘNU-LUH-HA, nuḫurtu, Asa foetida; IM-MAL-LI, kalû, yellow ochre
[50] IM-GUŠKIN, yellow ochre
[51] illur pâni, face bloom
[52] "aban alligi", barbers stone made of ᵃBALAG-GÁ, ᵃšû, pumice stone
[53] "ir.šnj", fem. "ir.t šnj", later nš.t (II.337.7)
[54] Latin "per-funum", perfume; "incendere", burning. The Egyptian equivalent is "śtj.ḥb", festival-perfume
[55] "ḫtjw" (III.349.9)
[56] "śnṯr" (IV.180.7); see also Fr. W. von Bissing, Versuch zur Bestimmung des Grundbedeutungs des Wortes NTR für Gott in Altägyptischen (SBAW phil.hist.Kl.1951, Heft 2)
[57] "dḳr nṯr" (V.496.3)
[58] "ḥtp" (III.196.4), "śḥtp" (IV.223.5)
[59] "ḳdrt"
[60] "mḏt", later called "bšš"
[61] "sr.w" (III.463.5)
[62] "mrrj.t" (II.110.14)
[63] "s3ḳ śnṯr" (IV.26.9)
[64] "t.hḏ" (V.210.7)
[65] This is misunderstood by Pliny in his *Nat. Hist.* XIII.19, where he says: "The fatter the oil is, as for instance oil of almonds, the better it helps to preserve unguents for a long time."
[66] "oikias hyperōous", mostly called "apotheca" (Gr. apodokion) that is store-room or wine-cupboard. The upper rooms of Greek houses were the woman-quarters or store-rooms.
[67] The Greek "myron", unguent is probably a Hebrew loanword
[68] the Hellenized Sanskrit word "tamālapaṭṭra"
[69] Hebrew "ḫelbenah"

Bibliography

(1) Eifert, V. S., *The Ancient Art of Beautification* (*Natural History* 1937, 663—674)
(2) Maqlu VII.31
(3) Prov. XXVII.9
(4) Matthew VI.17
(5) 2 Chron. XXVIII.15
(6) Psalms 133.2
(7) The Gilgamesh Epic. Tablet XI.159—161 (edit. Heidel, Chicago 1946)
(8) Gardiner, A. H., *Ancient Egyptian Onomastica* (London 1947, Vol. I, 37); L. Keimer, Notes prises chez les Bišarîn et les Nubiens d'Assouan (BIE, 34 1953, 329—449)
(9) Exod. 30.23—25; 37.29
(10) Deut. 28.40; 2 Chron. 28.15
(11) Luke 23.56; 24.1; John 19.40; Lev. 14.12
(12) 2. Sam. 12.20; 11.2
(13) Luke 7.37; 7.46
(14) Herodotus, I.193
(15) Pliny, *Nat.Hist.* XIII.2; XV.7; Athenaeus, *Deipnosoph.* I.66, III.124, XII.553; Theophrastus, *Concerning Odours* VI.28, IX,38, X,42, XI,55 But see M. Levey, *Perfumery in Ancient Babylonia* (*J. chem. Educ.* vol. 31, 1954, pags. 373—375)
(16) Barthoux, M. J., *Les Fard, Pommades et Colours dans l'Antiquité* (*XI Congres Int. de Géographie*, III-IV, Cairo 1925, 251—262)
(17) Psalms 133.2
(18) Forbes, R. J., *Man the Maker* (New York 1950, 65)
(19) Wresinsky, *Atlas zur altägyptischen Kulturgeschichte* (Leipzig 1923), Vol. I, plate 356
(20) Nehemiah 3.8; Pal. Joma 41 d.; Bab. Sota 22a
N. Shapiro, *Perfumery among the Jews in Antiquity* (Koroth II, 1958, 74—75)
(20[a]) J. R. Harris, *Lexicographical Studies in Ancient Egyptian Materials* (Berlin, 1961)
H. von Deines & W. Westendorf, *Wörterbuch der Medizinischen Texte* (Grundriss der Medizin der Alten Äegypter VII.2; Berlin, 1962)
(21) I. Sam. 8.13
(22) Exod. 31.25; 37.29
(23) Ecclesiasticus 38.1—5
(24) Kiddushin 82 b
(25) Nicolas Myrepsos, *Liber de compositione medicamentorum*, Ingolstadt 1541
(26) Esser, J., *Hautcremes einzt und jetzt* (*Pharmacia*, Juni 1937, No. 6, 179—181)
(27) Breasted, J. H., *The Edwin Smith Surgical Papyrus* (Chicago 1930, 492)

Loret, V., *Pour transformer un Viellard en jeune homme* (*Mem. Inst. Franc. Arch. Orient. Caire*, Vol. LXVI,2, 1935, 853—877)

(28) Dressel, H. F. and R. Hochberg, *The Dawn of Cosmetics* (*Drug and Cosmetic Industry*, Vol. II, 1941, 386—388, 393, 395)

Ch. Desroches de Noblecourt, *Fards et parures du visage au temps des Pharaons* (*L'Amour de l'Art*, Paris XXX, NS 49—51, 1951, 39—42)

E. Garetto, *L'acconciatura e le cosmesi della donna egizia nel Nuovo Impero* (*Aegyptus* 35, 1955, 63—85; 211—237)

W. S. Smith, *An Eighteenth Dynasty Egyptian Toilet Box* (BMFA 1952, 74—79)

(29) Ebbell, B., *The Papyrus Ebers* (Copenhagen 1937, 101—102)

(30) Blackman, A., *The House of the Morning* (*J. Egypt. Archaeol.*, Vol. V 1918, 148—165)

(31) Gauthier-Laurent, M., *Les scènes de coiffure feminine dans l'ancienne Egypte* (*Mem. Inst. Franc. Arch. Orient. Caire*, LXVI, 2, 1935, 674—696)

Riefstahl, E., *An ancient Egyptian hairdresser* (*Bull. Brooklyn Museum*, vol. 13, 1952, 7—16)

Capart, J., *l'Origine africaine des coiffures égyptiennes* (*Reflets du Monde* (Brux.) 1956, no. 8, 3—26)

Riefstahl, E., *Two hairdressers of the Eleventh Dynasty* (JNES 15, 1956, 10—17)

Wolf, G., *Geschichte der Frisur in alten Zeiten* (Darmstadt, 1952)

(32) Lucas, A., *Ancient Egyptian wigs* (*Ann. Serv. Ant. Egypte*, vol. 30 , 196

(33) Winlock, H. E., *Excavations at Deir el Bahari* (New York 1942,43),

(34) Lacau, P., *Deux magasins à encens du temple de Karnak* (ASAE 52, 1952, 185—198)

Steuer, R., *Myrrhe und Stakte* (Vienna 1933)

Steuer, R., *Über den wohlriechenden Natron* (Leiden 1937)

Steuer, R., *Stacte in Egyptian Antiquity* (*J. Amer. Orient. Soc.*, Vol. 63, 1943, 279—284)

Beek, G. W. van, *Frankincense and myrrh in ancient Southern Arabia* (JAOS LXXVIII, 1958, 141—152)

Ebbell, B., *Die ägyptischen aromatischen Harze der Tempelinschriften von Edfu* (*Acta Orientalia*, Vol. 17, 1939, 89—111)

(34) J. Bottéro, *Textes économiques et administratifs* (*Archives Royales de Mari* VII, 360 (Paris, 1957))

J. Bottéro, RA LII, 1958, 166

Labat, R., RA LIII, 1959, lff.

Leemans, W. F., *Foreign Trade in the Old Babylonian Period* (Leiden, 1960)

(34) Silvio A. Bedini, *The scent of time* (*Trans. Amer. Phil. Soc.*, N.S. vol. 53, 1963, part 5)

(35) Herodotus, IV. 175

(36) *Odyss.* III.466

(37) *Odyss.* II.339

(38) *Odyss.* V.264

(39) *Iliad* III.382, VI.288; *Odyss.* IV.121, XV.99

(40) Pliny, *Nat. Hist.* XII.1—3; Horace, *Odes* I.38.1

(41) Xenophon, *Cyropaedia* VIII.8.20
(42) Athenaeus, IV.129 A
(43) Anacreon, *Carmina* XXVIII.9
(44) Athenaeus, XV.687 A
(45) Athenaeus, XV.686 F
(46) Pliny, *Nat. Hist.* XXIX.2
(47) Athenaeus, XII.526 A
(48) Xenophon, *Conviv.* II.3; see also Martial, III.63.3
(49) Aristophanes, *Plutos* and 320 fragm. of *Thesmophoriazusen*
(50) Theophrastus, *Hist. Plant.* IX.4
(51) Plautus, *Rud.* 629—631; *Curculio* 90; *Most.* 42; *Trinummus* 252
(52) Pliny, *Nat. Hist.* XIII.25
(53) Pliny, *Nat. Hist.* XIII.24
(54) Pliny, *Nat. Hist.* XIII,20—25
(55) Pollux, VII.166; *Theophr. de sudore* 28
(56) Pliny, *Nat. Hist.* XXXV.5
(57) Athenaeus, XII.553 D
(58) Seneca, *Epist. mor.* 86.13
(59) Athenaeus, IV.129 A; Petronius, *Satyricon* cap. 60
(60) Plutarch, *Galba* 19; Suetonius, *Nero* 31.2
(61) Horace, *Odes* I.38; *Epod.* XIII,8,9
(62) Quintius Gavius Apicius, *de opsoniis et condimentis sive de re cullinaria libri decem*
(63) Martial, X.38.7
(64) Pliny, *Nat. Hist.* XII.84; VI.101
(65) Schmidt, A., *Drogen und Drogenhandel im Altertum* (2. Aufl., Leipzig 1927, 25—48)
Balsan, L., *L'industrie de la résine dans les Causses et son extension dans l'empire romain* (*Gallia* IX, 1951, 53—55)
Gattefossé, J., *La gomme d'euphorbe* (*Bull. Soc. Sci. Nat. et Phys. Maroc.* 34, 1954, 1129—133)
Rovesti, G., *Profumi, cosmetici ed essenze d'Italia attraverso i secoli* (*Riv. It. delle Essenzo e Profumi,* Vol. XIII, 1931, 355—378)
Rovesti, G., *Vergilio e le piante aromatiche* (*Riv. It. Ess. Prof.*, Vol. XII, 1930, 271—276)
Rovesti, G., *Perfumery in Etruscan and Roman Times* (*Chemist and Druggist, Spec. Issue,* June 25, 1932, 746—748)
Hausenstein, A., *Hautsalben und Hauptpflege im Altertum* (*Die Riechstoff industrie,* Vol. IV, 1929, 26—27, 46, 64—66, 88—89; Vol. V, 1930, 7—8, 22—23, 57, 71—72, 128—132; Vol. VI, 1931, 64—65, 79—80, 94—95, 113, 126—127, 179—180
Colin, J., *Luxe oriental et parfums masculins dans la Rome alexandrine* (*Revue Belge Phil.* XXXIII, 1955, 5—19)
(66) Pliny, *Nat. Hist.* XIII, 4—19
(67) Theophrastus, *Concerning Odours* (edit. A. Holt, Loeb Classical Library, London 1916)
(68) Pliny, *Nat. Hist.* XIII 5—18; XV, 28—31
(69) Dioscorides, *Materia Medica* I.52—76

(70) Pliny, *Nat. Hist.* XIII.7,19
(71) Pliny, *Nat. Hist.* XV.31
(72) Pliny, *Nat. Hist.* XIII.19
(73) Pliny, *Nat. Hist.* XV.8
(74) Exod. XXXI.23—25
(75) Pliny, *Nat. Hist.* XIII.18
(76) Herodotus, III.107—112
(77) Pliny, *Nat. Hist.* XII.59
(78) Lucian, *Nav.* 15
(79) Pliny, *Nat. Hist.* VI...101
(80) Clement, *Paed.* II.8
(81) *I.G.R.R.* 1375—1376
(82) *Pap. Fay.* 93
(83) BGU.9
(84) CIL VIII.16878
(85) Jer. 8.22; 46.11
(86) CIL I.1334
(87) CIL I.1398—1399
(88) CIL X.3966. 3968, 3974, 3975, 3979, 3982
(89) Martial, 12.31.3; 9.60.1
(90) Festus, 458 L; Petron., 76
(91) Loane, H. J., *Vespanian's Spice Market* (*Class. Philol.*, Vol.39, 1944, 10–21)
(92) CIL IV.609.2184
(93) Pliny, *Nat. Hist.* XXXIII.164
(94) Pliny, *Nat. Hist.* XVI.40
(95) Pliny, *Nat. Hist.* XXXIV.108
(96) Rhodes, G., *Beauty through the Ages* (*Chemist and Druggist*, *Special issue*, 25 June 1938, 735—741)
(97) Martial, *Epigr.* I.87
(98) Xenophon, *Oekon.* X
Leslie Shears, T., *Psimythion* (*Class. Studies presented to E. Capps*, Princeton 1937, pags. 314—316
Stevenson, L. G., *On the meaning of the word cerusa and psimithium* (*J. Hist. Medicine* X, 1955, 109—111)
(99) Martial, *Epigr.* I.72.5
(100) Dioscorides, I.128; Pliny, *Nat. Hist.* XII.76
(101) Badermann, *Die deutsche Parfümeriekunst in Mittelalter* (*Deutsche Parfumerie Ztg.*, Vol. V, 1919, 163—165, 175—177, 190—191)
(102) Pliny, *Nat. Hist.* XVIII.191; Martial, *Epigr.* XIV.27
(103) Cerbelaud, R., *Les parfums dans l'Antiquité* (*Aesculape*, janvier 1935, 12—19); Gobert, E. G., *Tunis et les parfums* (Revue africaine 1961; Libyca 9/10, 1961/2, 279—280)
(104) Martial, *In Maximinam* II, *In Gelliam* III
(105) Tanzer, H., *The common people of Pompeii* (Baltimore 1939, 54—55)
(106) Juvenal, I.24,25
(107) *Magni Hippocratis opera omnia*, Leipzig 1826, vol. II, 853
(108) Galen, XII.434
(109) Dio Chrysostom, VII.117 *Anth. Pal*, XI.408

CHAPTER TWO

FOOD, ALCOHOLIC BEVERAGES, VINEGAR

THE PREPARATION OF FOOD AND ITS TECHNIQUES

Food habits are not entirely dominated by materialistic considerations. It is true that the economics of obtaining foodstuffs, their availability in the climate and region inhabitated and man's conscious and subconscious knowledge of their biology and chemistry largely determine the choice of his diet. On the other hand the religious and social pattern of his life is a potent factor in his choice, the more so as we go back in history. The distrust of anything that tastes stranger or new is instinctive. Taboos for different classes and sexes strongly determine the diet. On the other hand the change of methods for preparing food meant the introduction of new criteria. Thus the introduction of cooked food meant a great change in diet. The evolution of methods for preserving food wiped out local differences in diet and in modern times the industrial production of foodstuffs and propaganda have materially influenced our diet (1).

The influence of the preparation of food on the evolution of technology should not be underestimated. In fact the kitchen is the birthplace of many technological terms, operations and apparatus (2). To it we owe the development of furnaces and ovens, grinding and crushing apparatus, the technology of fermentation and alcoholic beverages, methods for the preservation of perishable organic materials and the techniques of pressing fluids and liquids from seeds and fruit. Hence a summary of the evolution of diet (Table VI) will teach us the origin of many technological operations.

In the food-gathering stage of mankind food was consumed raw or roasted. Cooking came only when receptacles of some kind were invented, it came into its own only with pottery, that could stand heating. The post-war successes of Near Eastern archaeology and the excavation of such early sites as Jarmo have considerably enlarged our knowledge of the food consumed by the earliest inhabitants of this area. This stage can still be studied amongst such primitive people as the Eskimos (3) who eat most of their animal food fresh. Should they heat it, they resort either to roasting (keeping the inside rare) or to boiling, eating their food lukewarm or cold. Vegetable food was very plentiful, many of the plants then eaten are no longer used (4). Infusions or decoctions of vegetable foodstuffs were the basic forms of the Old Stone Age and lasted long into the New Stone Age. Roasting contributed but little to the development of kitchen utensils (Table VII). Heating of these sweet (natural) or acid soups was achieved by the immersion of pre-heated stones, not by direct heating.

TABLE VI

Evolution of diet

Procuring food	Preparing food
I Food gathering Wild grasses, bulbs, roots, rhizomes, fruit, nuts, berries. Wild animals and fish.	Natural, cooked or roasted food. Sweet (natural) or acid soups (infusions or decoctions) prepared by immersion of pre-heated stones. Porridges (?)
II Direct Food Production (Hoe agriculture) Einkorn, emmer, millet, maize, rice Leguminous plants, barley, buckwheat, oats Beginning of stock breeding Meat and Fish	Porridges made of cereals. Drying food Cooking on hot stones. First biscuits and flans made of cereals for food and for brewing. Thick soups and porridges leading to more stable pastes and doughs Decoctions fermented, alcoholic beverages Food contains sand and earth
III Industrial Food Production (Plough agriculture) Shift from emmer to barley Oats, barley, rye, wheat. Evolution of modern cereals: naked wheat, barley, spelt, rye. Decline of chase: Meat from domesticated animals and fish. Shift from barley to naked wheat. Contest between wheat and rye.	Crushed and sieved grains, manufacture of flour. Real bread (flans) Acid preservation of food (replacing dessication) Alcoholic fermentation used to soften dough. Use of leaven to make loaves of bread. Spices and condiments in bread Preparation of purer yeasts (beer yeast) Sand content rises to 2 %
IV Mechanized Food Production Age of White Bread	Condiments in bread disappear Renewed taste for country bread

The Upper-Palaeolithic hunter-fishers of Europe hunted above all the reindeer but also ate the meat of the wild horse, the bison and the hare. They caught Arctic willow-grouses and ptarmigans, salmon, pike, trout and bream. In Southern Europe game comprised the red deer, the roe deer, the wild pig and the aurochs. Limpets and mussels were eaten and honey was collected.

The mesolithic hunter-fishers lived almost exclusively on the land-mammals of the forest (red deer, aurochs, elk, roe deer, wild pig), sea birds, duck, geese and swans. Their principal fishery was concentrated on catching pike. On the sea coast they cut up and ate occasional stranded whales, they hunted seals, and caught cod, conger, haddock, crabs, bream, ray, skate and certain types of sharks. From the few remains of their plant-food we know that they ate hazelnuts, seeds of the water-lilly, wild pears and berries.

The New Stone Age with its acquisition of cultivated cereals, the earliest stockbreeding and its more developed pottery started cooking

TABLE VII

Lines of development of cooking

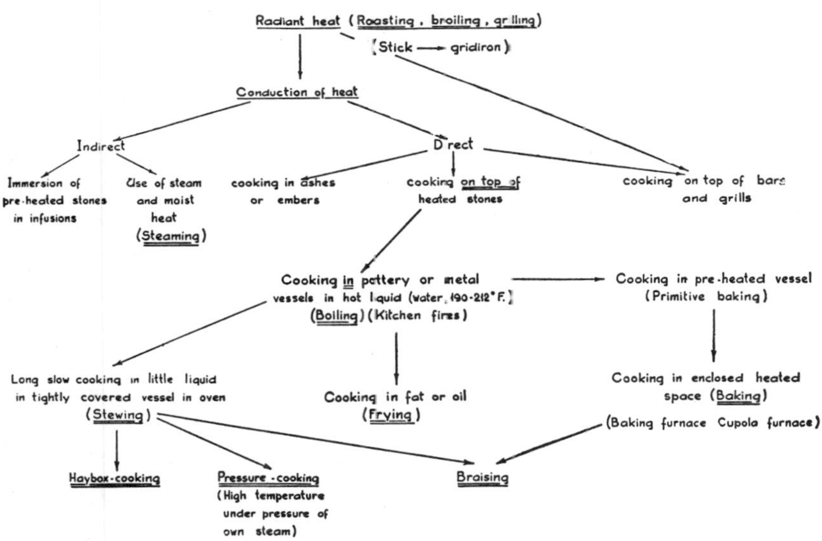

on its way as the major operation of the kitchen. Not only were cereals now dried for storage or efficient grinding bu the soups of older generations now become porridges cooked on top of stones heated directly. By the end of this period man had learned to prepare more stable pastes and doughs from these porridges. The first alcoholic beverages date from the end of this period. By that time flat biscuits and flans were prepared from cereals and used both as food and as a base material for brewing. Meat and fish formed an important part of the diet, wild animals still contributed a large percentage to the meat supply.

Venison consisted mainly of red deer but most of the meat consumes now came from the domesticated cow, pig and sheep. In some regions like Switzerland hunting remained more important until the end of the New Stone Age. Fowling still supplied oils used for lamps. Fishing also persisted as a means of feeding cattle and salmon, sturgeon and eels were caught in large numbers to be smoked or dried for winter use

Forest products were still collected in Neolithic Europe as a substitute for cereals in times of dearth such as acorns, beechnuts, hazelnuts, elderberries, strawberries and raspberries. Chestnut-flour was made into a kind of polenta. The root of Calla palustris, dried rhizomes of common reed and the bog bean, and the water-nut (trapa natans) were collected. Wild grass (Glyceria Fluitans) was harvested to make groats and flour.

The neolithic farmers of Europe grew mainly emmer and wheat, barley coming towards the end of the Bronze Age. Spelt, oats and rye too were late-comers. In the marginal areas of north-western Europe cereal crops were harvested before fully ripe Artificial drying had to make up for the shortage of sun-light to ripen the grain. This process of drying unripened grain is quite distinct from the old Mediterranean method of parching or roasting grain for storage or preparatory to milling. The latter was done to facilitate threshing and grinding and to impart a sweet flavour to the flour by part-conversion of the starch to dextrin. In both cases, however, heated floors or ovens were used, conical ovens dating from the early Iron Age.

The introduction of the plough and the cultivation of large tracts of irrigated and drained land shortly before the rise of the urban civilisations of the Ancient Near East start a new revolution in food habits. Grains were crushed and sieved, flour making was introduced and loaves or bread were baked alongside the older flat flans and cakes. Alcoholic fermentation was applied to the baking of these loaves. Spices and condiments were added to it. The rise of the modern cultivated cereals spelt a wider variety of cereal dishes. Meat was now mainly obtained from domesticated animals, the chase became the pastime of the rich, but fishing still supplied food for the masses.

With the coming of written documents we can supplement the data obtained from excavations in climates not always suitable for the preservation of the remains of food. We can now tabulate the foodstuffs used (Table VIII). Cereals form a substantial percentage of the food of the ancient Egyptians (5). The Papyrus Harris mentions more than thirty different forms of bread and cakes. Beans, peas and lentils were eaten though subject to certain taboos. Water melons, artichokes,

TABLE VIII

Principal food-plants of Antiquity

NGLISH	LATIN	EGYPTIAN	SUMERIAN	ACCADIAN	
n (general)	—		ŠE-PAD, ŠE	šeʿu	Hebr. zêrʿoîm
rn	Triticum monococcum	×	×	×	
er (husked)	Triticum dicoccum Schrank.	bd.t I.486.14	ZÍZ-A-AN(-NA) IM-GAGA	kunašu, buṭuttu, alapânnu	Hebr. kussèmeth
m wheat	Triticum durum Desf.	hrnt II.501.9 bd.t I.486.14	ŠE-IR-ZI	qutru	
e wheat (Rivet)	Triticum turgidum L.	×	?	?	
d wheat	Triticum vulgare	sw.t II.426	(DUGUD-BA), ŠE-GIG	kibtu	Hebr. ḥiṭṭā
wheat	Triticum compactum	—	—	—	
(Dinkel)	Triticum spelta	?	×	?	
ey	Hordeum vulgare L.	ʾit I.142.11 ʿnḫ.t I.205.10.	ŠE.BAR (-ŠE)	uṭṭaṭu	Hebr. śeʿôra. Arab. shaeir
owed barley	Hordeum hexastichon L.	šmʿj IV.476.8 šr.t IV.524.2	ŠE-IN-NU-ḪA	innunu	
- barley	—	—	BÚLUG	buqlu	
(Sorghum)	Andropogon Sorghum Brot. (Paniceum miliaceum L.)	×	ŠE	duḫnu, arzik	Hebr. dôḫen Arab. dúra, cuḫn
	Oryza sativa	—	^{šam}ŠE-LI-A	^{šam}kurangu	Hebr. ōrez
s	Ervum lens	ršr I.211.15	GÚG, KUKKA	kukku, ^{šam}andaḫšum	Hebr. ʾădâšîm Arab. adees
s	Vicia faba	iwrjt I.56.14 pr I.531.12	×	×	Hebr. pol Arab. túl
s	Phaseolus maximus Phaseolus vulgaris	× ×	— LU-ÚB-ŠAR	^{šam}amu(š)šu lubbu (luppu)	— maāsh — lūbā
	Pisum sativus L.	ϭⲁⲃϭⲁⲃ	?	?	— bisilah
ken peas	Cicer arietanum L	×	ZID-MAD-MAL	upuntu, maṣḫâti	— hûmmes
	Vicia nissoliana — Ervilia L.	? ?	— ^{šam}ŠE-ŠIŠ	kiššenu šêqušu	Hebr. kursenni Arab. kishné
s	Lapidium sativum L	(ḥlin)	ZAG-ḪI-LI-ŠAR	^{šam}saḫlê	
b	Ceratoria siliqua L.	ndm II.378.14	^{šam}ERI-TIL-LA	^{šam}ḫarubu (kasia)	
	Ficus carica L.	d3b V.417.11	^{iṣ}MA	tittu	Hebr. tĕēnāh
	Phoenix dactyli fera L.	bnr I.461.12	ZÚ-LUM-MA	suluppu	Hebr. dĕbaš
	Pyrus Malus	tph V.296.12 dpn V.568.10	^{giš}ḪAŠḪUR	ḫašḫûru	
ot	Prunus Armeniaca L.	—	^{giš}ḪAŠḪUR KUR-RA	armânu	
	Pirus communis L.	—	^{giš}ḪASḪUR-GIŠ-DA	kameššarû	
ry	Cerasus Mahaleb L.	—	—	karšu	
e	Cydonia Vulgaris Willd.	—	^{giš}ḪAŠḪUR ^{giš}PÈŠ	titânû	Hebr. tappûach
ar	Mespilus germanica L	—	ŠENNUR	šalluru	
h	Prunus Persica Tourn.	—	^{iṣ}DAR-RU-LG	darruqu	

cucumber, lettuce, endive and radishes as well as the fruit of the lotus tree join the more common vegetables already mentioned. Onions, garlic and leek were often added to these dishes. The fruit consisted mainly of dates, figs, nuts of the dûm palm, pomegranates and castor-oil berries. There was quite a variety of vegetable oils and animal fats to choose from [1]. Milk and cheese were produced and consumed and so was butter, at least in the form of a butter fat like the indian ghi.

Palestine, which was famous in Antiquity for its production of wine and oil ate very much the same food as Egypt, from which many foodstuffs were imported in exchange for wine and oil. Here too we find that bread and food are synonymous [2]. Like in the rest of the Ancient East grain was still consumed green or parched, concoctions of flour, honey and oil were very common and flans of dough were still baked on hot stones, embers or fires of dung. Olive oil was the principal vegetable oil used though nut-oil, fish-oil and coloquinth oil were known. Different nuts (walnuts) and mulberries were peculiar to this country. Just as in Egypt relishes and seasoning with salt were much appreciated and even indispensable in some cases. Sweets were made with honey and many other ingredients. Milk and butter were used and though camel and swine were known the only meat consumed was derived from cattle, goats and sheep. Pickled and salted fish formed a major constituent of the food of the poor, like in Egypt. The many types of geese and ducks eaten in Egypt did not appear so often on the tables of ancient Palestine.

In Mesopotamia fish was the general food in the extreme south, but further north fish is only exceptionally mentioned, possibly because the transport of fish caused grave difficulties as it did for many more centuries. Remains of meals found in the Uruk and Jemdet Nasr layers at Ur consist of fish, the meat of sheep and goats and vegetable matter. As stock breeding was one of the main bases of Mesopotamian economy, there is no doubt that meat of various animals was regulary consumed. Not only the wool of sheep and the hides of goats, oxen and cows were valuable but the meat must have been consumed too like in Persia. Pork must have been favoured as it is quite often mentioned in Babylonian texts, e.g. 92 pigs are allotted to a troup of soldiers (TCL X 54). The Amorite nomads must have consumed meat regularly and this custom must have persisted after their settlement in the Land of the Two Rivers. Tenants of the land belonging to naditu (priestesses) had often to add a piece of meat to the rent they paid. Milk and cheese were prepared and consumed from the earliest historical period onwards and Old-Babylonian texts mention butter (Sum. ì-nun; Akkad. ḫimetu) and cheese (Sum. ga-ḫar) but tell us little about their preparation (6).

Among the vegetable foods dates were of course most important and the texts from Mari give us a clear picture of the part they played in feeding the inhabitants of this town.

Though many vegetable oils were available sesame oil was the most common. The efforts to introduce olive oil production failed and this

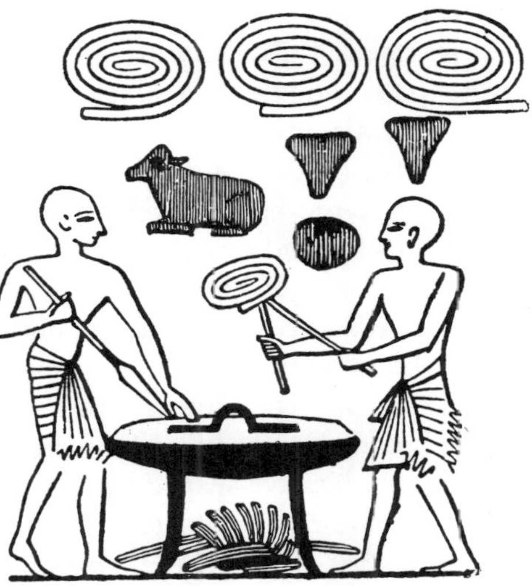

Fig. 11. Egyptian cooks frying cakes in fat

oil, though known, played a minor part only in consumption. In Mesopotamia there was a larger variety of fruit, most of the kinds we now eat were actually introduced from this very region through Greece to Europe (7). Grain in all forms remained the staple food. Here too it was eaten green, roasted, parched and bruished for porridges (thickened with milk, honey or oil) or baked into flans or loaves of many shapes.

The food mentioned above was prepared in many different ways. It shows that in early historic times many forms of cooking were already known and utensils had been developed to suit these techniques (Table VII). The oldest form, roasting, was applied to the preparation of beer [3] as well as to wild animals. In Egypt the pictures of the roasting of geese and ducks predominated in all periods. After being plucked they were stuck on a stick or spit (*without handle*) and roasted over a fire that was often fanned. After 1500 B.C. roasting beef was more commonly depicted though this may not mean a change in food habits. Meat was often beaten before cooking.

The development of the furnaces and the ovens can best be studied in the ancient bakeries. In Egypt, where no public bakeries throve, we find the simplest and earliest forms of heated stones laying flat on two or three vertical stones, between which the fire was lighted and regulated by raking by the attendant who was often depicted guarding his eyes from the glow of the fire with his left hand. Around 2000 B.C. a clay oven with a grate appeared on which a tray with the flans or loaves to be baked was placed. Brick furnaces come somewhat later as did special frying pans mounted on braziers or fires and other kitchen ranges, which did already form part of the kitchens of larger estates in the Pyramid Age (8).

In Mesopotamia where large bakeries formed part of the ancient Sumerian temple-economy we find furnaces built for mass production at a much earlier date. The temple kitchens of Ur had large beehive-shaped clay bread ovens and also clay cooking ranges with a flat top and circular flues. At the same time the more primitive braziers and stone hearths for cooking pots were in use. In Palestine the simple arrangement of heated stones, embers or dung fires served to bake the bread. At a later date the beehive-shaped furnaces were introduced, in which a fire was heated and raked out later, after which the flans are flung on the hot walls to bake. This way of baking flans descended from the simple device of a large pot preheated by the flames such as we find in Mesopotamia at an early date. It remained the common household bakery-oven in the Near East upto these days. The fire was kindled with the fire drill all throughout this period by the "bringer of the flame who rubs the drill" as the Egyptian texts have it.

These methods of baking bread in embers, ashes and furnaces were transferred to the making of pottery and later to metallurgy for they all date back to prehistoric times and it is difficult to establish their line of development in detail. We are not concerned here with the development of kitchen pots, cauldrons and the like but we should note here that in Mesopotamia the baker was not only the producer of bread but developed into a purveyor of food in general and a cook-shop keeper [4].

To the kitchen we also owe the development of grinding and crushing apparatus (Table IX). Mortar and pestle were the general tools for crushing and pounding flour, herbs, pigments and other materials in preclassical Antiquity. They differed little in form, higher forms were used in some cases but they mostly ressembled those still used in our days. In Mesopotamia they were probably preferred over the saddle quern for making flour in the earlier period for the miller took his name from the operation of "pounding" [5]. In Egypt pounding seems to have been limited to dehusking of grain, though herbs and the like were disintegrated in mortars. Nowhere do we encounter

TABLE IX

Evolution of the grinding of cereals

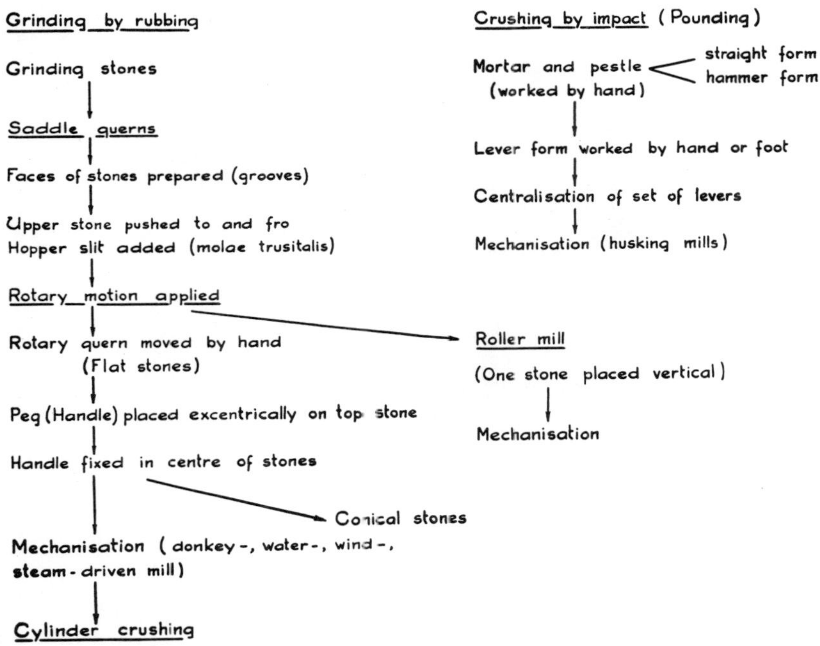

any sign of the mechanisation of the pestle in preclassical Antiquity, nor do we find the hammer-form pestle used in any of these countries.

The early story of grinding operations is still partly wrapped in mystery. Making flour, being a household operation in Egypt, was part of the task of the housewife, who ground the cereals on a saddle quern from the earliest historic times onwards. Only about 1500 B.C. do we hear of a "miller", grinding corn in larger quantities seems to have come fairly late here [6]. The miller had to kneel to grind his corn and soon a new form of saddle-quern was developed. Already in the

Pyramid Age we find the saddle-quern placed on a base, inclining slightly away from the miller, thus enabling him to grind more energetically. The mill-stone carried a cup on its further end in which the flour collected. There is no trace of the use of rotary querns in Egypt except in Hellenistic times, they seem to have been imported from Mesopotamia.

In the Land of the Two Rivers several forms of hand-mills were known besides the old saddle-quern, which always remained popular in the household [7], and which had three different forms each specially adapted to the corn, sesame or dates to be ground. We do not know whether the earlier handmills mentioned in the texts were

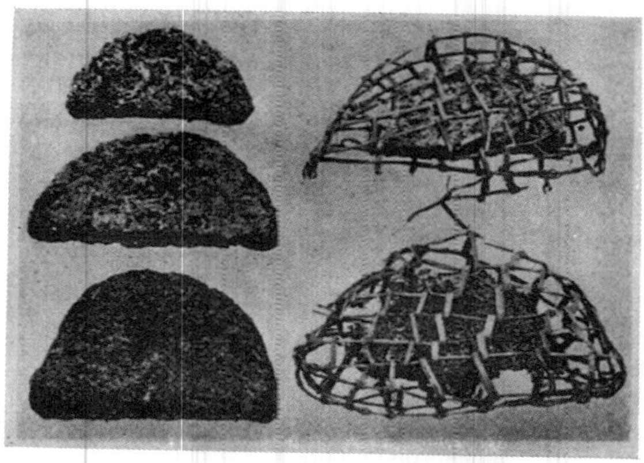

Fig. 12. Egyptian loaves

of the rotary type, which they certainly were in Assyrian times, that is after 1000 B.C. as we know from excavations. They were larger mills driven by donkeys, crushing mills, which were certainly of the roller mill type. The date when these rotary mills were introduced should be more closely studied with the help of excavated handmills.

In Palestine the rotary mill was introduced in Hellenistic times only, the saddle-quern being the common form (apart from mortar and pestle) which was used before that date. At Gezer a rotary mill was found (9) the upper stone of which had no peg or handle and which could therefore be moved to and fro only by the hands of the operator. It was probably used to grind small quantities of herbs or pigments. It may well have been then ancestor of the rotary mill, the only thing needed being the addition of a peg on the outer rim of the upper stone to make full revolution of this stone feasible and efficient.

A third important operation derived from the kitchen was sieving. Both in Egypt and in Mesopotamia sieves made of reeds, rushes or papyrus were in use, and different mesh sizes were made. That they were not very efficient is proved by the fact, that the ordinary bread was still full of grit. As a matter of fact winnowing the dehusked and crushed grain was usually considered sufficient and sieving was only resorted to for better qualities of flour and bread. The Old Testament term for sieve clearly shows that a grid of meshes was really aimed at [8]. The Mishnah speaks of a series of two or three sieves to be used in certain conditions.

The Egyptians had sieves in the form of very shallow baskets from the earliest historic times onwards and even developed metal sieves shortly before the Hellenistic times. Their two terms for sieving or grading corn perhaps denote winnowing and grading specifically. In Hellenistic times a new type of sieve, a deep basket the bottom of which held the sieve, was used. The Mesopotamian terms for sieves clearly show their manufacture from reeds and rushes and their use to sieve flour which was measured by the volume [9]. The term "sieved" is very aptly used by the Egyptians to denote the scintillating of little particles of dust in the sunlight.

The techniques of fermentation are closely connected with baking too. Fermentation is used when leaven is added to dough to bake loaves of bread, the gases evolved make the dough lighter and softer and contribute materially to the texture of the final bread. The application of this principle is clearly seen in the early history of baking, where at the beginning of historic times porridges are still very popular, which, however, gradually give way to flat and brittle biscuits and flans, which in their turn make place for the loaf of bread in the course of preclassical history though the three forms still continue in use side by side for many a century.

Fermentation and Alcoholic Beverages

Fermentation needs fire and pottery. Though simple forms of pottery were known by the end of the Upper Palaeolithic the plants collected in those days gave sweet infusions seldom suitable for fermentation, as in general they contain too little sugar. The techniques of fermenting came with organized agriculture, some traces of which go back the Upper Palaeolithic (Post Glacial period, Maz d'Azil, France). However, a more regular production of cereals suitable for fermentation came in Neolithic times only. Even the wild species of grapes, berries and other fruit collected and eaten in those days would hardly make a suitable base material for fermentation. The only material the fermentation of which may go back as far as early Neolithic times and even earlier is honey (10) (Table X).

TABLE X

Evolution of the infusions according to MAURIZIO (percentage of water indicated)

Stage of agriculture	Typical food	Sweet Infusion	Lactic acid Infusion	Alcoholic Infusion
Collection of wild grasses	Roasted wild grasses and malt (wild millet) (8 - 10%)	soup (also malt ?) (90-80%)	Acid Infusion	(mead) wild grasses (90 - 80%)
Hoe and stick agriculture	Cereals (roasted; dry porridge) (upto 5%)	Thick Porridges (70 -80%)	Sour cereal porridge (70 - 60%)	Cereal infusion (Thin beer, Ale, Chicha, Pombe) (upto 80%)
Plough and irrigation agriculture	Roasted flans Matzes (4 - 2%)	Thick dough Flans Bread (50 -40%)	Dies out in W. Europe	Food and luxury (Babylonian and Egyptian beer (95 - 92%)
Modern Times	Beer made from cereals and malt		Distilled Alcoholic Beverages	

The collection of wild honey in the forests along the clearings of the earliest prehistoric European farmers was soon followed by the domestication of bees, the straw hives of which were made from the straw harvested on the fields. Mead, the fermented drink made from honey (and grain) may even be older than agriculture, but this we will probably never know. It is quite certain that the alcoholic fermentation of sugary fruit-juices (such as dates) or honey was known to the ancient Egyptians when history began. The product was "self-generated" as the term reads literally [10]. Nectar and ambrosia were probably mead-like concoctions.

Food started with many forms of infusions and all primitive peoples knew that chewing the brew (that is mixing it with saliva) before cooking makes it "run to sugar". They were also aware that something similar happened in malting grain. They might not know "why" but they certainly knew "how" to make use of practical experience. They were also well aware of the fact that alcoholic fermentation (usually over in 3—4 days at the outdoor temperatures of the Near East) was later followed by a further fermentation forming acetic, formic and butyric acid. This was when the beer ran sour, and the Egyptians tried to prevent it by stoppering the beer jars [11] from the earliest period onwards.

Lactic acid fermentation was practised in Europe in early times but it died out quickly when alcoholic beverages were made from the modern grains. The Slavs still have their "kumyss" and similar drink based on this type of fermentation. A few traces of this type of fermentation in the Ancient Near East [12] point to the fact that it was known in the Pyramid Age in Egypt though not mentioned later.

Date wine was probably the most popular of fermented fruit juices. In Egypt the earliest method seems to have been pressing the liquid from soaked dates and leaving the juice to ferment by the wild yeasts introduced from the skin of the dates. About 2000 B.C. this manufacture was depicted on the wall paintings which show how the dates were soaked and left to ferment as such at that period. After fermentation the liquid was poured off, the dregs were pressed and the date wine filtered before filling it into jars, which were then carefully stoppered and placed on supports. Date juice itself had a high sugar content, it was used as a sweetening ingredient like honey and grape juice, but often honey was added before fermentation and the resulting alcohol content must have been high (Table XI).

This strongest drink of preclassical Antiquity was even more popu-

TABLE XI

Strong beverages and their ingredients

ENGLISH	EGYPTIAN	SUMERIAN	ACCADIAN
Honey	bj.t I.434.6	LÀL	dišpu
Sweet Sherbet	bnr I.462.9	KUKKU	matqu ṭâbâti
Mead	bj.t I.434.9 ḥḏ.t III.211.13	KÚRUN	kurunnu, šikâru
Date Wine	bnjw I.462.4 bnrṭ I.462.6		
Fig Wine (?)	dby (t) V.435.3		

lar in Mesopotamia, where between the Cassite period and the beginning of the Neo-Babylonian era it gradually succeeded in ousting beer from its leading position as a popular drink. Dates formed a major foodstuff in this country, the yield per palm being as high as 212 L. in some regions. The juice pressed from the dates was partly used to concoct sherbets (of which there were many kinds) partly to prepare the fermented "intoxicating drink" often mentioned in the texts and denoted with the same term as beer when it had outrun this drink in popularity. The dregs and kernels were used as fodder for the caddle, or the kernels were dried and used a fuel by the smiths.

The classical authors found this date-wine (or beer) "a pleasant drink causing headache" (XENOPHON, *Anabasis*, II.5.14). Special qualities of date-wine were made by adding herbs, cassia leaves and oils such as sesame oil to the brew. The secret of the manufacture of these special brands was well kept, for we have different names of date-wines concocted from exactly the same Dilmun dates, dried figs and raisins, which differed widely in taste [13]. We are informed that 1 Kur of dates (121 L) gives about one Ton of date-wine. The high alcohol content makes subsequent fermentation in storage impossible, and hence we hear of "one-year drink" and other terms which imply the holding and ageing of this drink over a longer period.

The "intoxicating drink" of ancient Palestine bears a name, that seems closely related to that of the Mesopotamian date wine [14]. It is often cited along with grape-wine and some have supposed that it was just old strong wine (11), but the storage of wine over a long period is most unlikely at this date. In Palestine these strong drinks were brewn not only from dates, but also from apples and even from barley. The mysterious Egyptian strong drink "brewn in the orchard", which was certainly not pomegranate-wine or date-wine, may be one of these fermented fruit juices, to which all kinds or herbs and honey were added, the secret of which has not been revealed to us.

A palm-wine is mentioned as early as the Pyramid texts and used in mummification (HERODOTUS, II.86; DIODOR, I.7). The sap is obtained by making an incision in the heart of the tree immediately below the base of the upper branches. By fermentation an intoxicating "wine" is then obtained, but it could never have become popular for the palm thus treated would die. PLINY (*Nat. Hist.* XIII.10) mentions a wine prepared from Cordia mixa, but this "myxa wine" must have been unknown in preclassical Egypt, for the "Egyptian plum" does not occur in our records before the Roman era.

Beer

The complexity of preclassical brewing is partly due to the facts, that so many terms for beer are given in the ancient texts. The old Sumerian texts mention no less than eight types of barley-beer, eight emmer-beers and three mixed beers. The Egyptian nomenclature is no less complicated [15]. This is probably due to the fact that we can no longer distinguish between real types of beer and proprietory brands, as details on many of these brews are sorely lacking. Hence there is much confusion in the older studies on this subject (12).

TABLE XII

Beer

ENGLISH	EGYPTIAN	SUMERIAN	ACCADIAN
Green malt		MUNU	buqlu
Malt	dḳw V.495.4	DUMGAL	sîrâšû
Beer-bread	bj.t (?) I.433.1	BAPIR	pappiru
Leaven	3ḥ I.12.14	BAPIR-KUR-GUB-A	šapulu
Barley beer	k3m.wt.t V.106 12 ḥḳt III.169.12	KAŠ, (TIN)(KÁŠ)	šikaru
Fine beer	ḥb3 III.62.5	KAŠ-SAG	šikaru rêštû
Types of beer		KAŠ-BIR (KAŠ-ZIZ-AN) ULUŠIN (KAŠ-Ú-SA-KA-DU) PIḪU	alappânu ulušinnu piḫu
Mixed beer		(KAŠ-Ú-SA) DIDA	billetu

The preparation of malt was the all-important process in preclassical brewing. When farinaceous grains germinate, an enzyme, diastase, converts part of the starch into maltose and dextrose. Malting is the reproduction of this natural process under controlled conditions. The maltose is an important factor in the final specific and sweet taste of the beer aimed at. Malting was not invented for brewing. This process is definitely older and belongs to the techniques of making food, cereals in particular, more palatable, when loaves of bread were not yet baked. Seeds and other hull protected (or bitter-tasting) fruits can be made palatable and easier to digest by simple, prolonged soaking in water (to which salt or lye might be added) without the application of fire. The nutritional value of farinaceous grains was thus greatly improved. The final product could be preserved after drying, it could be ground into groats or flour, but it could also be made into dough and baked into cakes. This germination could also be effected by sprinkling the grain with water and leaving it to germinate protected from the direct sunlight.

The cakes thus made form a king of "durable bread" [16] which in ancient times was used among other travel provisions such as groats and dried bread. Malted products such as green malt were often given as wages in kind to workmen and serfs of the temple administrations, but they disappeared as a food with the rise of the Third Dynasty of Ur. This shift of malted cereals from a food preserve to a basic substance for brewers may have been caused by the shift in food habits away from the preference of soupy cereal dishes, often seasoned by sour fermentation. The malted cereals now became "beer-bread" (see Table XII).

If not dried in the sun or roasted in kilns the malted product was dried, crushed in mortars and sieved to separate the hulls from the cereal. The malt thus treated was kept in earthen containers or sacks but was often baked into bread-shaped lumps, "beer-bread". It was aromatized by the addition of all kinds of herbs and spices, dates and other ingredients, each of these mixtures would give a special kind of beer.

In order to brew this beer-bread, green malt or hulled groats were mixed with cereals, soaked in water and subjected to fermentation, sometimes in the form of a solution extracted by filtration and pressing of the prepared mass. During this fermentation yeast was needed, the maltase of which converts the maltose into dextrose, which was then turned into alcohol and carbon dioxide by the zymase enzyme. During the earlier period the brewer could not yet control this fermentation by the addition of the yeast wanted. He was dependent on the microorganisms from the air of the skins and hulks of the fruits and cereals used, such as Saccharomyces Winlocki or Thermobacterium mobile.

These microorganisms were of course unknown to the ancients, no terms refer to them (13). They are often very strong and can stand the baking temperatures of the "beer-bread" (50—55° C) which would kill all yeast cells, of which hardly any were found in remains of ancient beer jars. In the case of wine the wild yeast Saccharomyces ellipsoideus which occurs on the skin of the grape would yield the proper fermentation. As far as Egypt is concerned there is evidence that a pure or almost pure yeast could be made by 1500 B.C. [17]. We have no direct evidence of this technique from Mesopotamia. Sour dough or leaven for the baking of bread was known about the same time all over the

Near East. The practical knowledge, that fermentation could be produced by human saliva, certain animal fluids and the like, was of course much older. Then the fact, that brewers in these ancient times carried their mashing containers along, might mean that the necessary microorganisms were carried from batch to batch by fungi in the cracks and recesses of these tuns. In a later stage some of the dregs or sediments of a previous fermentation were added to the "beer-bread" or mash.

The type of fermentation was of course directly linked to the length of time of storage of the beverage, the temperature of brewing and such factors. If the beer-bread after soaking was heated for a short time at some 50° C the quick conversion of the starch and hence later the rapid fermentation at low temperature would be ensured. In the case of a beer-bread with a high percentage of spices and dates, the ancient brewer may really have been a palm-wine brewer when he started out to make beer. The use of these mixes complicates our knowledge of the ancient fermentation techniques very much. The study of the selection and control of yeast cultures by the ancient brewers is still in its infancy. We may, however, soon be able to fix the decisive technological step which this control of fermentation meant in ancient brewing. In the past only too often the fact has been overlooked, that these processes did not take place in our climate, but at much higher temperatures such as were common in the Near East.

Both malting and practical fermentation were quite well understood early in the third millenium in Mesopotamia. In the fermentation or mash-tun the brew was stirred with a special stirrer and eventually transferred to a clarifying vat where the dregs and sediment were allowed to settle. The fermentation lasted some 3—4 days, and the vats were covered with mats during the night to keep the temperature as high as possible. From the clarifying vats the sieved liquid was transferred into pottery jars, 2—5 L if transported, larger ones if stored. Even at this early date we find a complex terminology varying according to period and region. We have many recipes mentioning the addition of certain odoriferous plants to give the beer a selected taste and also recipes varying the strength of the beer by mixing types of beer or adding water. Strong beers were obtained by adding honey to cereals or malt. The former mixture provided the strong beers of the prehistoric Germans and Celts, who apparently did not use beer-bread for brewing, though they aromatised their beers too by the addition of herbs to the brew.

The task of the maltster was, therefore, an important one particularly in Mesopotamia [18]. So was that of the brewer, who was always depicted with his mash-tun straining the mash through a sieve into the

TABLE XIII

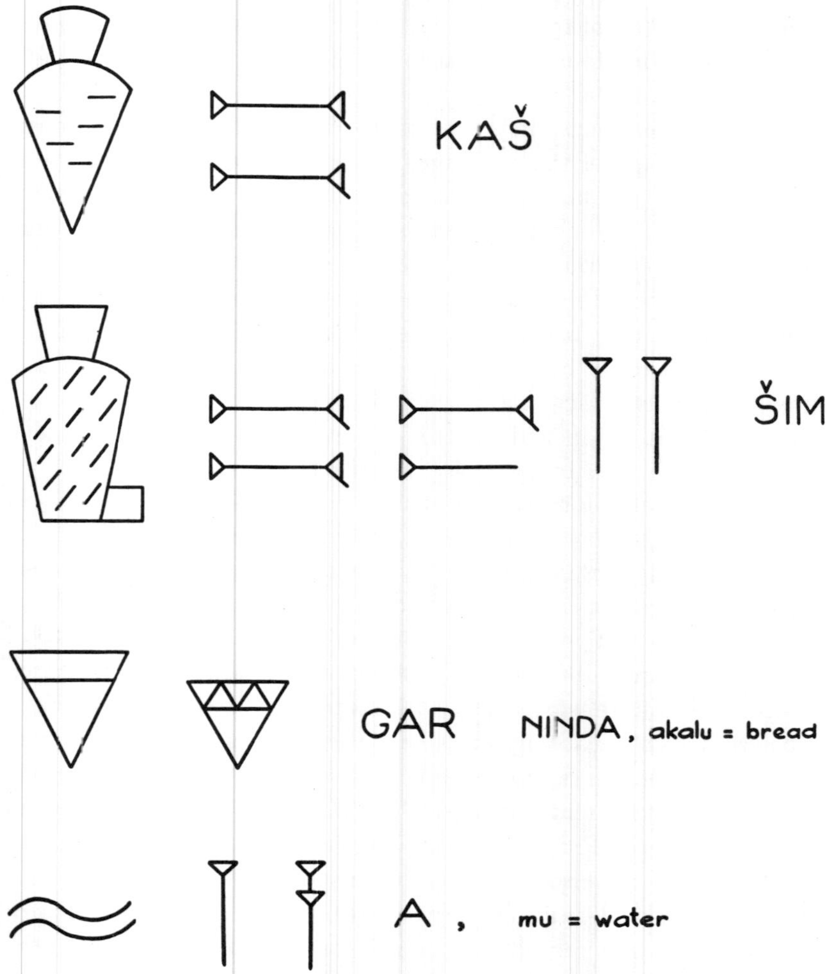

tun [19]. For in Mesopotamia about 40% of the production of cereals was used for brewing. Early in the third millenium 60% of barley and 40% of emmer made up the total, but in later periods less and less emmer or wheat were used for beer production. So-called emmer-beers always contained an appreciable percentage of barley (35—50%). In the Sumerian temple-economy a workman was assessed a ration of

1 L of beer a day, lower officials obtained 2 L, higher officials (including the ladies of the court) 3 L and the highest functionaries 5 L a day. Its production kept many hands occupied for the accounts show us that upto 60% of its cost went into wages.

The use of white, red and brown types of barley and emmer and their mixtures (husked or dehusked) allowed the brewer to prepare differently coloured and flavoured beers, as the extract in the mash tun would contain the dye and other components from the husk. He could, and certainly did, change his operating conditions during the preclassical period. Recent research has revealed several "revo-

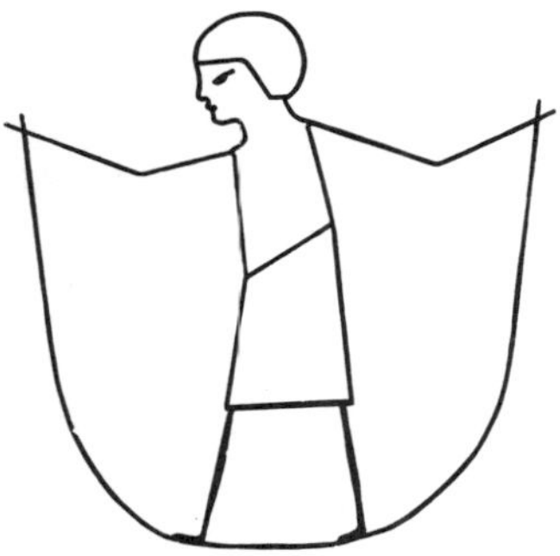

Fig. 13. Egyptian hieroglyph for "brewer"

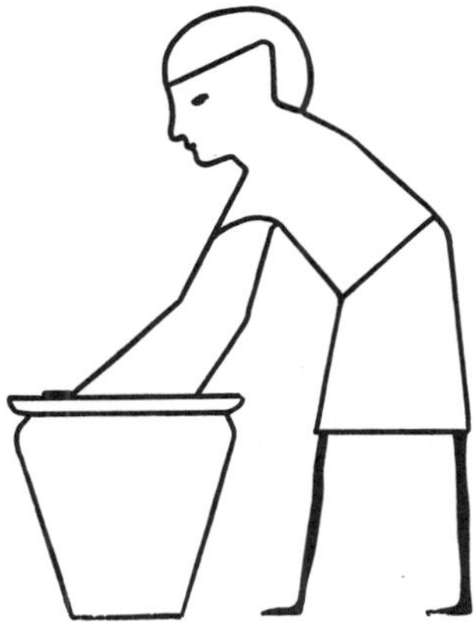

Fig. 14. Egyptian hieroglyph for "brewer"

lutions" in Sumerian and Assyrian brewing (14). "Beer" was originally written in cuneiform by inserting the sign for bread into the picture of the pointed brewer's vat (Table XIII). A change of the type of vat used in this sign [20] occurs between the reign of Urakagina and the kings of Agade. It probably meant that the druggist had taken over the preparation of alcoholic beverages of a novel taste or that the old ways of brewing had made place for one in which the addition of spiced ingredients and thermic processes played an important part.

Another change took place before 1000 B.C. [21]. The incorporation of aromatic ingredients by means of some thermic process took the place of the preparation of a beer-bread of different compositions before brewing, or it might refer to the use of a beer-bread now made up of malted substance plus dates and other ingredients baked into them.

The situation in the third millenium is further complicated by the brewing of beer from cereals which had not been dehusked. This type of beer is drunk by tubes or reeds. It seems at home in north-western Mesopotamia, Asia Minor and Syria and it is shown on Mesopotamian monuments upto the Agade period.

A fourth change in the brewing trade is a social and economic one, which happens at the end of the Old Babylonian period. The "female brewer" so important in older brewing texts disappeared from the scene. Not only did the brewing trade have two patron goddesses [22] but brewing seems to have been largely in female hands in these older times, who made and sold their home brew in their house. These small pubs had a bad reputation for "amusement", Hammurabi had to stipulate that they should not sell beer of too low a strength at too high a price (parag. 108 & 109 of his law) but his law (par. 111) also threatens them with death if political conspiracies were concocted at the bar. With the Semitization of the country, with the advent of mass production of beer too, the female brewer makes way for the male counterpart, as she did in practically all other countries, where "home-brewing" was the oldest form of beer-production.

Finally between the end of the Cassite period and the beginning of the Neo-Babylonian era beer (still denoted by the old term for this brew) came to be brewn of dates and other aromatic ingredients mainly, the use of cereals was more and more restricted to the baking of bread and other foodstuffs.

According to classical tradition Babylonian beer was slightly sour in taste but Egyptian beer was sweet and spicy. According to Jewish tradition the Egyptian beer was made of barley or wheat with saf-flower and salt. A similar type of beer was sometimes brewn in ancient Palestine, but it was never popular in a country that devoted much of its skill to vineyards. We have many pictures of the different phases of Egyptian brewing in the tombs of the Pyramid Age· During the Middle Kingdom many wooden models of breweries were buried with the dead in the rock tombs to show us even clearer what stages made up Egyptian brewing. We even have a fairly clear description of malting, still practised along the old traditional lines in Alexandria when Zosimos (fourth Century A.D.) wrote it down. Egyptian beer was much praised (and liked) by the classical authors "for smell and sweetness in taste make it not much inferior to wine" (Diodor, I.3). Many flavouring substances like lupin, skirret, rue, safflower, mandrake were used to prepare special brands of beers, which the Egyptian physicians used very frequently.

Brewing started in Egypt as a household operation and here too we see the female brewer disappear as beer comes to be made in larger quantities in breweries. It has been claimed that brewing came to Egypt from Mesopotamia in late prehistoric times with barley and other modern types of grains. However, Egyptian brewing does not show the great variety of techniques encountered in Mesopotamia. Though the recipes show that both barley and emmer (and their mixtures) were used and that white, red and darkbrown varieties of each grain give their colour to the beer brewn, husked grain was never used. Grain is always pounded and dehusked (often by hand), sieved and made up into a dough to which malt and other aromatizing substances were added. The dough was then lightly baked into a beer-bread.

This beer-bread was often crushed hot and straight from the baker's oven (or it was taken from storage and broken in four parts) and soaked, salt was added and the mash was mixed in the fermenting vat. This vat was a very large one in which the workmen tread the mash with their feet holding on to the rim. After fermentation the wort was kneaded through a sieve and the liquid was left to ferment again in a second vat. The mass on the sieve was sometimes washed and kneaded again with hot water, the liquid expressed being held apart as a second quality beer in the Mesopotamian manner. The dregs remained on the sieve was eaten or used as fodder.

After sieving the liquid was filled into pottery jars, which seemed to have been prepared in advance. Workmen were depicted with their arm in the jar and seem to have cleaned it or, as some supposed, to have applied a layer of resin to the interior as Egyptian pottery was usually rather porous. Pitch was certainly not used for this purpose. In some cases fuller's earth seems to have been used to clear the beer. The beer jars were then closed with clay stoppers, sealed and counted by the inevitable Egyptian official or clerk, as they were standing on racks or rows.

This method of brewing is still practised by the Egyptian fellahin making their "bouzâ" which is prepared from wheat part of which is malted, and part of which is baked into "beer-bread" flans about 10—12 cm high and 40 cm in diameter. This beer is fairly strong and contains 6—8% of alcohol (Lucas). With the ancient brewing methods the manufacture of stronger beers was certainly possible. We must realize that the digestion process at 40—56° C with wild yeasts from the husks of the grain (much less susceptible to the alcohol content than our cultivated yeast) allowed the ancient brewer to attain an alcohol content of some 12%, especially if he added substances rich in sugar to his brew. As early as the Pyramid Age he had five types of beer, several of which were said to be "strong", that is to contain more alcohol than the ordinary "bouzâ" type of beer.

Wine

Wine-like drinks may have been made from the species of prunes, cherries and grapes common all over Asia and Europe from Palaeoli-

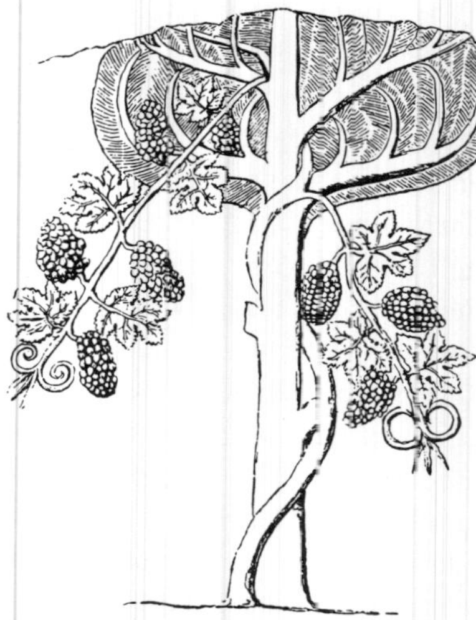

Fig. 15. Climbing vine on a bas-relief of the palace of Sennacherib (After Lenormant)

thic times onwards but we have no data on such fermented drinks until much later. Apples and pears were introduced from the Near East much later and hence they served as base materials in prehistoric Europe only at a relatively late date. In fact we have no information that cider was known in Europe prior to the fifth century A.D.

The species Vitis silvestris Gmel. grew all over Europe formerly, but it had to give way to the cultivated Vitis vinifera L., which was probably cultivated from the older species in the Caucasian region. For it is certain that viticulture was known (and wine was drunk) as early as the prehistoric Djemdet-Nasr period in Mesopotamia and brought to Egypt in proto-dynastic times, that is before 3000 B.C.

Greek tradition has it that the god Dionysos fled Mesopotamia in disgust because its inhabitants were addicted to beer. This is in a way true, beer always remained the popular drink there, but wine, an expensive commodity, was always highly appreciated by the rich. This is indicated by the very name of the vine and the grape [23]. Though Urukagina knew the vine and drank wine, we have the first definite data on viticulture from the reign of Gudea, which "lord of the city" built irrigated terraces protected by trees to grow grapes. Nabonid had from 50 to 100 bunches on his vines. Later we hear reports of vineyards in Singara with 2400 vines and in the neighbourhood of Harrân others with 15.000 and even 29.000 vines are mentioned. The Assyrian kings in particular were most interested in the "wine from the mountains", which could not be grown in the plains. Assurnasirpal (883—859) had vineyards near his residence, Kalah and Sanherib (705—681) tried to acclimatize exotic kinds of vines. Many good wines were imported by Nebuchadnezzar and Sargon II, who had large wine-cellars in his palaces, preferred the wine from the region of Lake Van. They even resorted to cutting off the enemies' wine supplies during their campaigns. Recent excavations in this region at Karmir-Blur (Teishebaini) have yielded remains of very large storage-rooms, where no less than 150,000 litres of wine was kept (15).

A wine-list in the library of Assurbanipal (668—626) lists the ten best brands of wine. This list is topped by the "pure wine from Izalla", followed by the wine from Helbon (near Damascus) which was well-known to the prophet Ezekiel (27.18), and finally by the wine of the Royal Vineyard. In Mesopotamia as in other countries spices and aromatic ingredients were often added to wine, the inhabitants of ancient Palestine knew such spiced wines, they had a "honeywine" prepared from wine, honey and pepper and a "vermouth" made of wine spiced with the herb Arthemisia Absynthium. Many names of ancient wines may be proprietary brands, others are poetical descriptions of its excellent qualities [24]. The officials declare in their reports that certain wines were "cellared in their presence". Wine is also used in Mesopotamia as an offering to the gods and libations of wine form part of the laying of the foundation stone of important new buildings.

There was no difference in the way in which wine was made in Mesopotamia and in Egypt. In both countries wild moulds (Saccharomyces ellipsoideus and apiculatus) which occurs on the skin of grapes converted the grape sugar into alcohol. The operations were pressing, fermenting, filtration, filling, and finally storage or transport. These operations are best illustrated from Egyptian texts which give much fuller information on viticulture in general. For Egypt (from which country Dionysios came to Greece according to tradition) loved wine better than Mesopotamia and consumed it in much larger quantities and among many more classes in that country.

As early as the First Dynasty seals and clay stoppers testify of royal vineyards. In a first dynasty tomb the body was buried with a layer of grapes to accompany him on his journey to the "western country". Originally the vineyards occur mostly in the Delta and in the surroundings of the capital Memphis, but gradually they spread south-

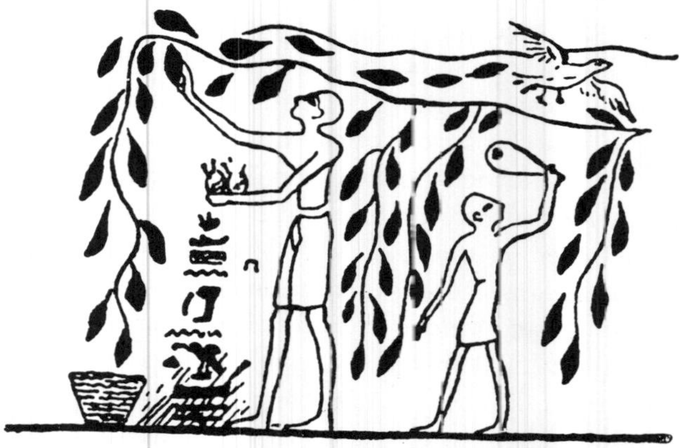

Fig. 16. Harvesting the grapes and chasing birds with a sling

wards to the First Cataract and even the Western Oases and the Fayyum, which still produces wine. The acreage devoted to viticulture was necessarily restricted in a country so densely populated. Vineyards were mostly situated in the higher parts of the Nile Valley, which had to be irrigated artificially, the so-called "sharaki land". Nor were they vineyards in our sense. Vines formed part of gardens or orchards where other useful plants were cultivated by careful irrigation and manuring [25]. Vegetables and fruits, oil and date palms, figs, melons and cucumbers were raised in these gardens, usually adorned with a pond with lotus flowers in the middle.

The nobleman Methen made such an orchard under king Sneferu and later built a vineyard of 2000 square ells. King Peribsen (Second Dynasty) had his vineyard "Prince of the boats" laid out in the form of a ship. King Zoser founded the famous vineyards "Praise of Horus the First in Heaven" and "Soul of Egypt" (in the Delta) both of which survived many generations. The kings of the New Kingdom (after 1580 B.C.) took particular pride in the vineyards they laid out for themselves and the temples of the great gods. Amenhotep III gave one to the temple of Luxor and its production of wine "was more plentiful than the water of the Nile at its highest mark, born from the Lord of Eternity". Private vineyards in Egypt date of Hellenistic times only. For wine was first used in the temple ritual only and later the rich began to drink it. The Greeks introduced wine drinking to all

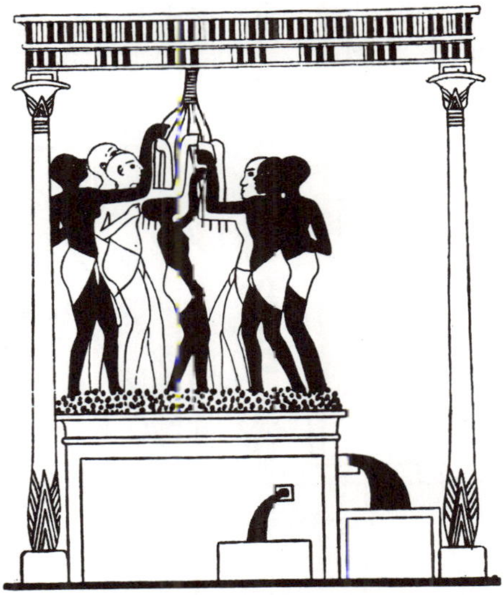

Fig. 17. Treading the grapes

classes and vineyards of 5500—13750 m^2 (though sometimes as large as 550.000 m^2) were now exploited by private wine-growers.

The ponds in the vineyards came in handy to irrigate the vines. These are illustrated in many tombs and thus we know that the Egyptians had, white, green, pink, red, deep blue and violet grapes.

In Palestine and Mesopotamia the vines would wind their way up trees or sticks with their tendrils. In Egypt, however, pergolas were constructed of sticks and the bunches of grapes could ripen in the shadow, whilst boys chased the birds away with slings and boomerangs.

The bunches of grapes are harvested with a sickle-form knife by men, women and children accompanied by singing and music. They are carried away in baskets covered with vine-leaves. Then came the "treading" or "scattering" of the wine-harvest as the pressing is called. The grapes are thrown into a wooden or stone vat, sometimes mounted on legs. Boys and men stand in it, music again helps them tread the grapes. They support themselves by hanging on to a bar or a set of ropes hanging down from such a bar. "Treading the grapes" even became a children's game in Egypt. From the lower part of this vat the juice flows into the fermenting vat.

The simple treading of the grapes is the beginning of the evolution of another important technological operation. It is the first stage of the press. Indeed right at the beginning of Egyptian history a start had already been made to mechanize this operation. It was the simple

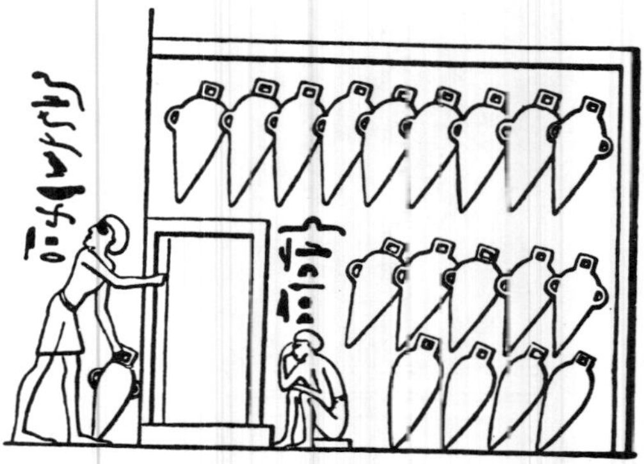

Fig. 18. Wine-cellar

"wringing of the cloth". The grapes were folded in a cloth, to the opposite ends of which two sticks were attached, which were turned in opposite directions by two men each, a fifth keeps the two sticks apart. As early as the Third Dynasty a hieroglyph shows this simple press in a better and more efficient form. The bag is supported on the two ends by two uprights. A further step was hanging the bag in a frame with one end attached to one of the uprights. The loop at the other end allows a stick to be passed through it to press the contents of the bag by twisting it. This was the ultimate stage of the press in preclassical Antiquity, spring presses used by present-day primitive peoples, were never found in excavations. The wedge-press, the beam-press and the screw-press are classical inventions of great importance in the story of the press.

It should be realised, that grapes were treaded all through Antiquity, for only thus the first quality wine was produced. The liquid pressed from the lees was kept apart to produce second-quality wine only.

Treading the grapes can still be seen everywhere in wine-producing countries.

We are not informed on the conditions in which the fermentation took place. We only know that the fermenting vats were placed in cool cellars and dark buildings, and sometimes we are shown the workmen creep out overcome by the carbon dioxide evolved. It is certain that a distinction was made between the fermenting vat and the storage vat. When the fermentation was completed the wine was carefully filtered through linen cloth on which the lees and marc were retained to be eaten or used as fodder. The wine was filled into jars,

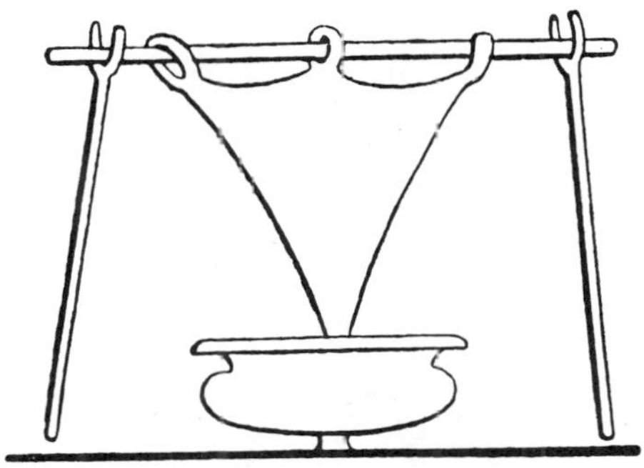

Fig. 19. Filtering the wine through cloth

most of which were sold directly. In some cases we still have traces of an ancient custom of drinking the fermented juice with tubes without filtering the liquid.

Part of the vintage was stored in jars in a cool place after being sealed with clay stoppers to prevent further fermentation. The jars were coated with resin, for they were fairly porous. The pitch so popular with classical vintners was unknown in Egypt and it was introduced in Hellenistic times only. The seals on the stoppers or inscriptions on the jars gave details of the vintage such as "In the year one. Good wine of the great irrigated vineyard of the temple of Ramses (II) at Per-Ammon. The chief of the wine-bottlers, Tothmes". Tax inspectors ("inspectors of the winetasting") assessed its quality and many wine-bottlers adopted more poetic titles such as "Weramon, prophet of the wine-cellar of the House of Amon". The pointed jars stood in sand or straw rings in the wine-cellar, "the place where the production of wine is (stored). One is glad there and the heart of those who leave it is in rapture".

A kind of "rouge pâle" was made by cooking the dregs with water. When taken out of the cellar to be drunk at dinnerparties the wine jars were put on stands and decorated with flowers and garlands kept wet to keep the wine cool by evaporation. At dinner wines were tapped from the jars with siphons and mixed according to tase. The grapes themselves were eaten, the juice was often used for sherbets and dried in the sun. The raisins thus obtained were kept in baskets in a cool, dark place.

The different qualities and brands of wines often carry fancy-names, in which the name of the god Horus is prominent [26]. The classical authors did not consider the Egyptian wines worth mentioning. MARTIAL declares that vinegar tasted better. STRABO says that Libyan wine tastes well when mixed with sea-water, it will not cause headache but helps digestion. Apart from these doubtful compliments we hear that a few wines are considered passable. As early as the Pyramid Age the Egyptians knew at least six different wines and they were less exacting than the Greeks. On the other hand we know that they imported wines from Palestine and Syria and even tried to obtain the vines to cultivate them in their own country.

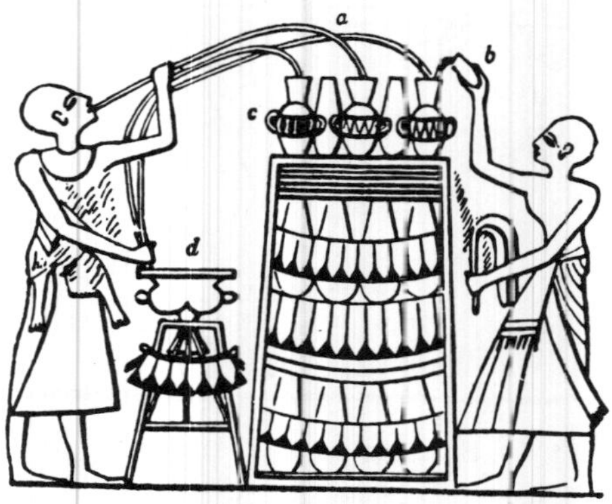

Fig. 20. Mixing wines with syphons

We have strong evidence that the original centre of viticulture lay in Syria. The documents recovered at Mari show that during the Old Babylonian period wine was already exported in large quantities from Carcemish, Aleppo and other cities in this region down the Euphrates to Mari and other towns in Babylonia.

In Palestine viticulture, known of old, was second only to the cultivation of the olive and the fig. Excavations at Gibeon showed that this region was a centre for the production of quality wines by the seventh century. B.C. and there is no doubt that there was even viticulture in the Negev (16).

When "spying out the land" the scouts of Num. XIII.23 arrive at "the time of the first ripe grapes". According to Jewish tradition the Tree of Life (planted in Paradise by the evil spirit Sammael) was the vine, which was saved from the Flood by Noah. Vines play a part in Jewish history and the Old Testament. Must, "blood of the grapes"

TABLE XIV

Wines and vinegar

ENGLISH	EGYPTIAN	SUMERIAN	ACCADIAN	HEBREW
Vine	i͗3rrt I.32.12 (b'ḥ I.450.4 š3 IV.400.13)	gišGEŠTIN	karanu	géphen
Grape	{i͗3rrt I.32.13 wnš I.325.7	GEŠTIN	karanu	eškōlōt
Grape-juice	wnš (wnš.t) I.325.8	gišGEŠTIN-ŠUR(-RA)	ṣaḫtu	májim
Must	mrśw II.112.15		mêrisu	tīrōš
Wine	ʾirp I.115.5	GEŠTIN (MU-TIN)	karanu (inu)	
Wine of second pressing	{ipw I.67.5 ipwr I.69.9	—	—	
Wine-water	mw irpw I.115.11	—	—	
Pharm wine	ʿwǝj.t I.172.8	—	—	jájim, mebussām
Date wine (palm wine?)	šdḫ IV.568.13 (?)	GEŠTIN-KALAG-GA	—	šekhār
Sweet wine	—	GEŠTIN-DÙG-GA	—	
White wine	šśp IV.284.12	gišGEŠTIN-HÁD-A	munzîku	
Rosé	inm.t I.97.1	—	—	
Dregs, Lees	{s'rmt III.463.7 g3š V.156.13	—	—	
Raisins	wnš I.325.7	gišGEŠTIN(-NA)-PAR-A	mu(n)ziqu	zebīb, ʿanābīm jebēšīm
Sour wine	—	gišGEŠTIN-BIL-LÁ	karanu enṣu	
Vinegar (from wine)	ḥmḏ III.99.13	{BÍL-LÁ A-GEŠTIN-NA	tâbâtu (ḫallu)	ḥômeṣ
Strong Vinegar	—	A-GEŠTIN-NA-KALAG-GA	—	
Mouthwash of diluted vinegar	—	A-UŠ-SA A-GEŠTIN-NA	—	

is produced by treading, and raisins were produced by drying the grapes. Jewish law tells us that the wine cellar contained two vats, the "upper" fermenting vat and the "lower" storage vat. These vats made of stone, wood or pottery were coated with resin. Sometimes special vats in which the wine was left to drop its sediment were used too. Many of these wine-vats were found by the excavators. Here too a second quality wine was made by pressing the dregs. From the texts we learn that wine could be stored upto three years, though many jars were found burst by the pressure of the gases developed by fermentation in the jar. It was well-known that the taste of wine improved on storage but reached a maximum after a certain period, after which it deteriorated. Wine was always drunk mixed with water as was the custom throughout Antiquity. Only "boozers" drank pure wine.

Vinegar

Though vinegar was important as the only strong acid known in Antiquity we hear little about its manufacture. It was known that fermentation if not stopped at the proper moment ended up in Mycoderma aceti converting the alcohol into acetic acid. Vinegar was therefore mostly prepared from date- or grape-wine leaving it to "turn sour". In ancient Mesopotamia "medical vinegar" was produced by fermenting an infusion of the root of Cyperus papyrus L., which vinegar was used "to remove poison from the body". The texts also mention the "inspissated acid vinegar" prepared from the juice of Acorus calamus. Vinegar was often used as a solvent for drugs and herbs.

In ancient Palestine and Egypt vinegar prepared from dates and grapes too. Likewise lees of wine were left to ferment. Vinegar, which was taboo to the Nazarites, was used as a dressing for salads, cabbage and turnips. It was rarely drunk in diluted state, though sometimes bread was dipped, in diluted vinegar (Ruth 2.14). Undiluted vinegar was applied to the "sponge of Good Friday (Matth. XXXVII.48)". Medically it was applied in certain cases, and it was generally used in the ancient East to preserve vegetables and meat.

Stronger vinegar was produced from the fermented liquid by inspissation, herbs being sometimes added. Distilling sour wine was not introduced until well in the Christian era. In ancient Egypt vinegar played a less important part, but it was known from a very early date onwards.

Notes

[1] See table IV in Chapter on "Cosmetics and Perfumes", p. 12
[2] Hebr. "lechem" is "food" and "bread", compare the Accadian "akalu" (NINDA, bread) and "ukullû" (ŠÀ - GAL, food)
[3] Compare the Sumerian KA - IZI (šumê, roast beef)

[4] The baker is the ^{lú}SUN - NINDA, nâdin akali or mušâkilu, a term also used for the proprietor of a restaurant.

[5] The Sumerian for pounding is ÀR, GAZ (-GAZ) (ḫašalu), hence the mortar ^{zá}GAZ (erettu), teh pestle ^{giš}GAZ - ZI - GAZ (kak madâkti ḫašlu) and the miller ^{lú}GAZ - ZI - DA (ḫâšil qêmi), which craftsman is, however, also supposed to grind, compare MA$_5$ (qamû, to grind). Mortars are used for grain, pigments and herbs.

[6] The female miller "ndw.t" (II.370.14) grinds her corn on the (lower) millstone "bnwt" (I.458.13) with the rubbing stone "s3ś" (III.42.26), which the Egyptian texts call the "son of the millstone".

[7] The millers often work in a E-ARÀ (bît erî, mill). There are basalt mills (^{a}ḪAR. AD. BAR, êru adbari), hand mills (^{a}ḪAR - ŠU, erî kalî) (erû habisi, baker's mill) as well as different mills for various type of flour. There was a larger mill ^{a}ḪAR zibu-um (erû zibi) and a ^{a}ḪAR.DUK.KA.BUR (erû paḫari, potter's mill) which was no doubt a roller mill moved by a donkey, as used in potteries. The ordinary saddle quern consisted of the lower ("female") stone (erittu) and the upper rubbing stone (narkabu). Three types are mentioned (for corn, sesame & dates).

[8] Hebrew "kebārā" (sieve) derived from "mikhbār" (window lattice, grid)

[9] The most ancient Egyptian word for sieving is "nḳr" (II.344.7) which also denotes sieving through a linen cloth, hence "nḳr" (I.344.11), sieve and the late expression "nḳr" for the dispersion of the Sun's rays by dust particles. Sieving corn is always expressed by "mnṭ" (II.91.17) (which should probably be more correctly rendered by "winnowing"), and "mfḫ" (II.55.13), actually sieving. The metal sieve is called "śḫnk.t" (IV.270.6) and the late basked-sieve ḫnmṭ (III.382.7). There is no specification of the late term for sieve "mrh" (II.112.12), but the contemporary term "d'r" (V.541.1) may be connected with the verb "d'r" meaning to search, to separate. The Sumerian for sieve GI - ŠÀ - SUR (nappû) is clearly connected with GI (qanû, reed), the Accadian equivalent napû, to sieve is probably connected with "nisip" (TA - LAM), a volume of 7.5 L.

[10] The fermentation product of dates and honey is called "ḫpr - ḏś.f" (III.261.10) that is "self-generated", "formed by itself".

[11] The souring of beer is expressed by "'m3 ('w3)" (I.185.1) connected with stoppering the beer jar "'mj" (I.185.7). The verb "'w3" (I.172. 3—5) is generally applied to express that bread, wood or beer have "gone bad" or "rotted". The term "'w3j.t" denoted a fermented liquid gone sour. Compare also the Accadian halla, vinegar, from the root hill "to go sour".

[12] The Egyptian alcoholic beverage "ḏśr.t" (V.616.7) is mentioned together with beer and wine as intoxicating. The drink that was "sweeter than honey", called "ḫwwij" (III.247.12) was probably a beverage, the percentage of alcohol of which had been raised by the addition of honey to the brew. See also K. Bühler-Oppenheim, *Die Rolle der Milch im Volksmedizin* (*Ciba Revue* No. 75, 1950, pags. 2628—2632).

[13] These drinks are called "sirdê" and "nâsu", date wine in general adopts the name of beer (KAŠ, šikaru) slightly before the beginning of the Neo-Babylonian era, that is about 700 B.C.

[14] This "šekhār" (compare the Accadian šikaru) gave its name to drunkenness (šākhar). It may be related to the Egyptian šdḥ (IV.568.12), but this may have been palm wine.

[15] Egyptians often refer to their beers by such poetical or fancy-names (or are they brands?) as "the beautiful, good" (nfr, II.261.7), "the heavenly" (ntrj, II.365.9), "the joy-bringer" (nḏm, II.381.12), "the addition to the meal" (III.18.7), "the plentiful" (h3m.t, III.362.11), "the fermented" (III.463.7).

They also knew beers for medical uses such as the aromatic "Ḫk.t - ḫ3" (III.332.1), the beer for liver-diseases (hk.t nḏ3ḏ3j, III.377.6), the beer that follows other medicines (ḫmt, III.285.1), the beer made with different herbs (tnm, V.312.12). Then there is the beer used for offerings which has a special name (hnms, III.295.10).

Terms applied both to wine and beer are "ḏsr" (V.616.14), "3h" (spirit?) (I.17.10) and "ḥnḳ" (sap, liquid) (III.117.4), all of which are late.

The beer called "hmt" involves something during its preparation which is done thrice or for three days.

[16] This "durable bread" is called NINDA-DURÚ-DURÚ-NA or NINDA-ḪAD (-DA), the "travelling bread" being NINDA-KAS-KAL. Malted cereals still appear as a seasonal delicacy for the fifth month in the calendar of the town of Lagash. Brewing was sometimes seasonal too, compare "sibûtum", the "mouth of brewing the sibû beer".

[17] Yeast (śrm.t, III.463.7) is mentioned from about 2000 B.C. onwards. It is semi-solid, stored in vats and sometimes eaten. The word is often incorrectly translated by "lees, dregs".

Leaven or sour-dough was known in Egypt at least from 1500 B.C. onwards (3ḥ, I.12.14) and made into oblong loaves or lumps.

In ancient Palestine leaven (seôr) is well-known.

[18] He is called MUNU$_4$ - MA$_4$, bâqilu.

[19] Compare the ideogram for brewer "'ftj" (I.183.9). He is sometimes called the "siever" ('tḫ, I.236.13/14) of beer & wine mashes.

[20] This corresponds with a shift from the sign KAŠ (the pointed brewer's jar) to ŠIM (the pointed jar on a low heating stove used to prepare decoctions from herbs).

[21] This corresponds with the change of the inscribed sign in that of the brewer's vat. This changes from GAR (bread) to A (water). Thus the old type of brewer BAPPIR (ŠIM + GAR), bappiru ("he of the beer-bread") becomes the LU-UM-GI (ŠIM + A), sirašu - ú ("he of the sira drink").

[22] ^{d}NIN - KA - SI and ^{d}Siris, patron goddesses of the female brewer" (SAL-KAŠ-TIN-NA, sabîtum) and her husband (sabûm).

[23] The vine and the grape were both called GEŠTIN (GEŠ + TIN = tree (wood) of life, a name which evokes memories of such Biblical

passages as Deut. 3, 24 & Rev. 2.7). Both in Egypt and in Mesopotamia man recognized a goddess protecting the vine: 'irp.t (I.115.12) and the "mistress of the heavenly tree of Life", the goddess Siris, living in the Hamrin mountains of north-western Assyria.

There is a second Accadian term for wine "inu" which may mean "the lordly" (compare enu, lord).

[24] Egyptians enjoyed wines and hence gave them such poetical names (or are they brands?) as "the blood-red (of the eye of Horus)" (wtr, 381.4), "the beautiful" (nfr, II.261.8), "the divine liquid" (rḏw - nṯr, II.469.8), "that which goes with the meal" (ḥ3w - iḫt, III.18.9), "the prominent" (ḥ3t, III.24.17), "that of the drinking-cup" (š3, IV.401.3) or "unguent of the heart" (irj - ib, I.106.2).

Other terms refer to the country of origin such as wine from Buto (im.tj, I.78.14), from Hām (ḥ3mj, III.32.8), from Pelusium (śnw, IV.155.8), Khor (Syria), the Oases, Busiris, Cynopolis or Imr in the same way as the Sumerians and Assyrians refer to the wine from Izalla, Tu'immu, Simminu, Hilbûmi (near Damascus), Arnâbanu or other mountain districts.

[25] The term for vineyard (k3m, V.106.6) is that for garden or orchard. There is no special term for vine-dresser for "K3mj" (V.106.10) means gardener in general. Viticulture was protected by the goddess Renenoetet (Greek Thermuthis), the "mistress of the barn"

[26] Such as "drink of the body of Horus", "gold of the body of Horus", "green eye of Horus".

Bibliography

(1) Remington, R. E., *The Social Origins of Dietary Habits* (*Scient. Monthly*, vol. 2, 1936, 193—204)

(2) See the chapter on "Cosmetics and Perfumes", p. 1.

(3) Stefansson, V., *Food of the Ancient & Modern Stone Age Man* (*J. Am. Dietetic Assoc.*, vol. 13, 1937, 102—119)

Helbaek, Hans, *Studying the diet of ancient man* (Archaeology 14, 1961, 95—101)

Cornwall, I. W., *The world of ancient Man* (London, 1964)

Andrews, A. C., *Acclimatization of citrus fruits in the Mediterranean region* (*Agr. History* XXXV, 1961, 35—46)

Braidwood, R. J., *The Near East and the foundations of civilisation* (1952)

Jensen, L. B., *Man's foods* (*Champaign*, Ill., 1953)

Braidwood, R. J., and Willey, G. R. edit., *Courses toward Urban Life* (Edinburgh, 1962)

(4) Maurizio, A., *Histoire de l'alimentation végétale* (Paris 1932)

(5) Casotti, L., *L'alimentazione nell'antico Egitto.* — Castalia, Rivista di Storia della Medicina, Milano, 35, 1951.

Keimer, L., *La nourriture des anciens Egyptiens.* — *Egypt Travel Magazine* no. 22, Mei 1956, 6—10.

Netolitzky, F., *Nachweise von Nahrungs- und Heilmitteln in den Trockenleichen von Naga-ed-dêr* (*Aegypten*). — *MDIÄA Kairo*, erstes Erg. Heft Berlin, 1943, p. 10/11.

Faucher, D., *La domestication des animaux* (Rev. Méd. vét. France 114, 1963, 8/9, 612—618)

Bühler-Oppenheim, K., *Die Rolle der Milch im Volksmedizin* (*Ciba Revue* no. 75, 1950, 2628—2632)

Leclant, J., *Le role de l'allaitement et du lait d'après les textes des Pyramides* (JNES 10, 1951, 123—127)

Elmer Marth, H., *The early history of cheese-making* (*Butter, Cheese and Milk Products Journal* 44, 1953, 10, 30—31, 46—49)

Ahmad Iskander Zaki, *Ancient Egyptian cheese* (ASAE 41, 1942, 195—313)

(6) Koschaker, P., ZA 47, 1942, 135

Ur Excav. IV,82

Bottéro, J., *Arch. R. de Mari* Vol. VII, 256—273

Figulla, H., *Iraq* XV, 1953, 91—122; 171—192

Landsberger, B., *MSL* I,200ff (JNES VIII, 284ff)

Levey, M., *Technology of Oils, Fats and Waxes in Ancient Mesopotamia.* — *Centaurus* vol. V, 1957, pags. 151—163

Levey, M., *Food and its Technology in Ancient Mesopotamia; the earliest Chemical Processes and Chemicals.* — *Centaurus* vol. 6, 1959, no. 1, 36-51

(7) CARNOY, A., *Origine thraco-phrygienne du vocabulaire de la vigne.* — *Muséon* LXXI, 1958, 161—171

CARNOY, A., *Substrat et adstrat en Grece, Noms grecs d'aliments végétaux d'origine orientale.* — *Orbis* VIII, 1959, 425—435

(8) HROZNY, B., *Das Getreide im Alten Babylonien* (*Sitzber. K. Akad. Wiss. Wien*, phil. hist. Kl., Bd. 173, 1914, No. 1)

WRESZINSKY, W., *Bäckerei* (*Z. Aegypt. Sprache*, Vol. 61, 1926, 1—5)

WÄHREN, M., *Die Backvorrichtungen des Altertums im Orient* (*Brot und Gebäck* 1960,5)

WÄHREN, M., *Typologie der altägyptischen Bröte und Gebäcke* (*Brot und Gebäck*, 1961, 1 & 2)

WÄHREN, M., *Brot und Gebäck im Leben der alten Aegypter* (*Brot und Gebäck* XVI, 1962, 1 & 2, 12—20, 30—38)

(9) MACALISTER, S., *Excavation of Gezer* (London 1912) vol. I, 96, 369, 392; vol. II, 36 & Fig. 228

SELLIN, E. & WATZINGER, C., *Jericho, Ergebnisse der Ausgrabungen* (Leipzig 1913, page 153 & fig. 41)

SCHUMACHER, G., *Tell el-Mutesselim* I (Leipzig 1908) page 62 & fig. 82

(10) MAURIZIO, A., *Geschichte der gegorenen Getränke* (Berlin 1933)

GARDINER, A., *Ancient Egyptian Onomastica* (Oxford 1947), vol. II, 233—237

HUANG TZU CH'ING and CHAO YÜN-TS'UNG, *The preparation of ferments and wines by Chia Ssu-Hsieh of the later Wei dynasty.* — HJAS vol. 9, 1945, 24—44

(11) DALMAN, G., *Arbeit und Sitte in Palästina* (Gütersloh 1936) Vol. IV, 291—437

(12) HUBER, E. & PHILIPPE, M., *Bier und Bierbereitung bei den Völkern der Urzeit* (Berlin 1926)

LUTZ, H. F., *Viticulture and Brewing in the Ancient Orient* (Leipzig 1922)

(13) GRÜSS, J., *Starkbier in vorgeschichtlicher Zeit* (*Forschungen & Fortschritte*, vol. XII, 1935/36, 110—112)

LINDNER, P., *Sawiq, das feste Bier der alten Babylonier* (*Deutsche Essigindustrie*, vol. 38, 1934, 413—414)

(14) HARTMAN, L. F. & OPPENHEIM, A. L., *On beer and brewing techniques in ancient Mesopotamia* (*Suppl. J. Amer. Orient. Soc.*, No. 10, Dec. 1950)

(15) PIOTROVSKY, B. B., *Fortschritte der Forschung des Urartu-Reiches* (*Vortrag* XXIV Int. Orient. congress 1957)

BARNETT, R. D., *Iraq* XXI, 1959, 1 ff.

(16) JOSHUA FINKEL, *An interpretation of an Ugaritic viticultural poem* (*Jewish Social Studies*, Publ. No. 5, 29—58)

PICCALUGA, G., *Numa e il vino* (Stud. Mat. Stor. Relig. XXXIII, 1962, 99—103)

SELTMAN, Ch., *Wine in the Ancient World* (London, 1957)

MAYERSON, Ph., BASOR 153, 1959, 27 ff

CHAPTER THREE

FOOD IN CLASSICAL ANTIQUITY

Roughly speaking classical diet consisted mainly of bread and porridge made from wheat or barley supplemented by vegetables, fish and spices and not much else as compared with our modern diet of white bread supplemented by a great variety of non-grain foods. Indeed most of the cereals we now produce are consumed as feed grain and only the smaller part is made up of wheat for human consumption. Before studying classical diet in details we must speak of the spread of the cereals in Antiquity and some of the factors that dominated classical agricultural trends so important in diet.

THE CEREALS OF PREHISTORIC EUROPE

The oldest form of wheat grown in prehistoric Europe was einkorn, which probably originated in Asia Minor and surrounding countries and thence invaded Europe ahead of emmer. It was cultivated in Central and Western Europe north of the Alps as well as in the Mediterranean basin, with the exception of Egypt. In the south it continued as a minor crop even in classical times and it still survived in Spain and Morocco when it disappeared from the rest of this region by the end of the classical period.

However, in prehistoric Europe emmer clearly dominated (1). In Neolithic Denmark and Britain most of the grain impressions on pottery proved to be emmer. Bread wheat and dwarf wheat were of minor importance. Wheat was certainly the most important crop in Neolithic times. The counts on neolithic pottery in Denmark gave: einkorn 5%, emmer 81%, bread wheat 11%, barley 13%. In England emmer with some naked barley was cultivated (2).

During the Bronze Age barley rose to pre-eminence. The percentages on Late Bronze Age pots (800—400 B.C.) in Denmark show 6% emmer, 3% bread wheat, 87% barley, 2% millet, 2% oats and also 10% of Polygonum seeds (cattle fodder) on the total of cereals. In England husked barley now dominated. In the Iron Age emmer and bread wheat regained some of their old importance on barley as far as England is concerned, but they remained quite secondary to barley in Denmark, probably due to the change in climate on the continent. In Roman times 81% of barley was grown in Denmark was compared with 2% of bread wheat, 5½% of rye and 9½% of oats, and barley continued to dominate in post-Roman times.

Club millet came to Europe from the East and penetrated the Danube basin to be cultivated in a few Neolithic sites north of that river. It was commonly used by the Lausitz people of central Europe as a minor crop and its cultivation then spread to Denmark as a subsidiary crop only in the Late Bronze Age, dying out completely during the Early Iron Age probably because of the onset of the Sub-Atlantic climate.

The cultivation of spelt in the Late Bronze Age was confined to Switzerland and southern Germany, it did not reach Denmark, but penetrated to England in the Early Iron Age.

Two important cereals seem to have originated in Europe, oats (from emmer) and rye (from barley) were originally mimics in the parent crops, spreading with them into Europe. With the worsening of the climate during the Sub-Atlantic period their greater resistance of cold enabled them to strangle their parent crops and emerge in their own right as cultivated cereals. Rye was first domesticated in northern Germany during the Hallstatt phase of the Iron Age, but not until the Roman Iron Age did it become common in southern Germany, Switzerland and Hungary spreading both north to Denmark and south to the Roman world.

Oats were first cultivated in Switzerland during the Late Bronze Age and to a slight extent in Denmark, but became important only during the Roman Iron Age (0—500 A.D.). Neither oats nor rye reached pre-historic England.

The cereals of the Ancient Near East

Einkorn, the one-kernelled wheat, was no doubt the oldest cereal in the Near East, where it was cultivated on a gradually decreasing scale until it disappeared at the end of the classical period. Together with barley, the husked two-kernelled emmer dominated agriculture in these parts from pre-historic times onwards. It probably came from the Zagros region and spread very early to the valleys of the Nile, the Euphrates and the Tigris. The prehistoric Fayyum people of Egypt cultivated 20% emmer, 23% two-rowed barley and 57% six-rowed barley, both cereals are found in prehistoric Mesopotamian sites too.

In historic times both were used for brewing beer and making all kinds of bread and cereal foods. Emmer, often misnamed spelt, slowly made place for more efficient naked wheats and disappeared by the end of the classical period. Spelt itself was known in Europe in prehistoric times and probably reached the Mediterranean area from the North very slowly, its penetration beginning just before the classical period, at the end of which it penetrated to Spain, but it did not reach Egypt much before Roman domination.

The naked wheats, which gradually came to dominate over spelt and emmer, are probably crosses of the wild species with wild einkorn or rather with grasses of the Aegilops family. The typical naked wheat of ancient Egypt seems to have been durum, though the excavations point to the possibility that some poulard was also grown. Durum was also grown to a certain extent in ancient Palestine and Mesopotamia but it had to yield to the naked spelts at the end of the classical period. Poulard wheat, probably split from durum in the process of transition to the moist conditions of the Western Mediterranean, together with durum represents the spring-sown wheat of the Greeks and Romans.

The wheats of the spelt group were found at Anau and the Indus valley at an early date, they seem to have penetrated Mesopotamia in the prehistoric Jemdet Nasr period and to have dominated there over the naked wheats of the emmer group. They do not seem to have been known in ancient Egypt nor in some other countries of the southern Mediterranean. Therefore it is very likely that they came from the North and they were slow to win out because of the great adaptability of the wheats of the emmer group to Mediterranean conditions. The latter were probably not grown north of the Alps in prehistoric times. The wheats of the spelt group provided classical civilisation with its fall sown wheat.

Both the two-rowed and six-rowed barley always occupied a prominent position in the Near East and even in the eastern Mediterranean countries by the end of the Roman Empire. Millet did penetrate slowly to the west and the north but it was only at home in a hot climate without winter cold. Rye and oats were unknown in pre-classical antiquity. Emmer, barley, durum and millet were the chief cereals of the ancient Near East.

Unfortunately, ancient nomenclature is not always applied very strictly and therefore Tables VIII and XV have a tentative character. The compounds with Sumerian še are more numerous than listed, še-bar was probably a special type of barley as the sign še (Akkad. še'û) often stands for barley too.

The cereals of classical Antiquity

Wheat and barley, the ancient staple crops of the farmers of the Near East, ultimately spread over the farming territory of western Europe mainly through the Mediterranean basin. The dry summer and the difficulty of raising any other than winter wheat had given rise to the Mediterranean two-fold regime in which crops alternated with fallow imposed by these conditions. The three-fold regime that gradually became characteristic of western European farming in the temperate zone depended on summer rains and the possibility of growing both spring- and autumn-sown crops. Like strip-cultivation and the four-sided plough also dependent on the conditions reigning in temperate western Europe the origin of the three-fold regime is still wrapped in mystery.

The use of bread made of wheat, the principal and superior food of Western Europe, was a cultural achievement of a high order, both from the consumption and from the production point of view (3). It meant making large stretches of poor, very acid, formerly forested soils (naturally adapted to rye, oats and buckwheat only) suitable for the cultivation of naked wheat.

The large gains of naked wheats on emmer and barley both in consumption and production in the classical world were less significant than those described above. These gains were primarily at the expense of emmer, but the shift was almost exclusively to a subspecies of naked wheat (durum). That is it was not a shift of one kind of grain to another but rather from a less efficient form of some kind of grain to a more efficient one. The type of food was little affected by this shift.

Besides emmer the only serious adversary of naked wheat in the Mediterranean region was barley. In so far as a shift from barley to naked wheat occurred it caused as significant a change in the type of food consumed as those brought about by a changeover from corn (maize) to wheat or even from rye to wheat. But a much smaller percentage of barley was involved in this shift which in this case was not mainly caused by a preference of wheat over barley as part of the diet. It was mostly brought about by the development of an international grain trade in the classical world in which the bulkiness of barley deprived it of a large proportion of its advantages over wheat in cost to the consumer at the place of destination. We will presently return to this transportation problem.

This rise of wheat in the ancient world is certainly also due to the fact that in ancient times wheat did not encounter here the competition of its present strong rivals in western Europe, rye and corn. Rye, the bread grain of the Germanic and Slavonic nations, began to penetrate as far as Campania towards the end of the Roman Empire. It then contributed heavily towards a considerable decline in the output of wheat and in the Middle Ages more rye was produced than all hulled and naked wheat put together. However rye is unadapted to Mediterranean conditions. Rice was still unknown in the classical world and so was maize. Both were excellent food grains for the underprivileged but both demanded artificial irrigation.

Now water conservation was the principle at work in the classical techniques of cultivation; irrigation, on which agriculture in the ancient Near East mostly depended, was only applied reluctantly if the climate proved all too arid or the type of plant grown demanded more water than usual. Classical agriculture was largely conservation of the winter and spring rains during a dry summer, which does not favour the cultivation of maize, sorghum or rice. Irrigation was not the strong point of the Greek or Roman farmer and though their engineers were quite capable of building the necessary dams, canals and aquaducts irrigation was applied only now and then to supplement "dry farming". Millet which does not survive the winter cold had to be sown in spring and hence remained a secondary crop, also due to its small return. Hence wheat competed only seriously with barley for acreage and consumption and its victory was attained "not so much by its own strength as by the weakness of its rivals" (3).

The Greek and Roman agronomists were not very precise in their terminology and this confusion becomes even greater when translation of classical works are consulted. Only gradually we are finding our way in this maze of terms denoting species and special types of cereals (4). However, it is quite clear that by 500 B.C. naked wheat was probably second only to barley both in production and consumption in Italy; millet, significant in the Po valley does not climatically belong to the Mediterranean region. In Spain whence Scipio got 270.000 modii of barley and only 40.000 of wheat barley remained the principal grain crop during the whole of the classical period.

A thousand years later (500 A.D.) naked wheat ranks first but its superiority is not very great. It is only positively first in Italy and

TABLE XV

The cereals of Antiquity

X = Known
— = Not known or proved

[Eng]lish Name	Botanical Name	Egyptian	Sumerian	Akkadian	Hebrew	Greek	Latin	Remarks
(in general)	—	npr II. 249.4 šś(r) IV.541.12	ŠE-PAD, ŠE	še'u	zê'raîm	sitos	frumentum semen	Naked wheat = Gr. pyros, L. triticum Hulled wheat = L. spica Hulled grain = L. spelta Winter wheat = Gr. cheimosporos Spring wheat = Gr. trimenos
WHEATS : EINKORN GROUP					(14 Chromosomes)			
[Eink]orn (hulled) [one-]seeded wheat"	Triticum monococcum	ihj I.118.10	X	X		tiphe	tiphe	"zeia aplè" (Dioscorides) often misnamed spelt Naked emmer does not exist
WHEATS : EMMER GROUP					(28 Chromosomes)			
[Em]mer (hulled), [two-]kernelled wheat"	Triticum dicoccum	bd.t I.486.14	ZÍZ-A-ÀN (NA)	alcpânnu kunašu buṭuṭṭu	kussèmeth	olyra (Aeolian) zeia (Ionian)	far	"zeia dikokkos" (Dioscorides) "far subtile = hulless emmer "alica" = groats, porridge
(Rivet, Poulard) [wh]eat (naked)	Triticum turgidum	X	X	X	—	semithalites (kritanias)	triticum (ramosum)	Also Gr. kagkrythias, drakontias Naked wheat = L. frumentum The spring-sown wheat (from III A.D.)
[Mac]aroni wheat (naked)	Triticum durum Desf.	sw.t III.426	X	X	(šehamtit) (lebânâ) ḥiṭṭa	semithalites	triticum	The spring-sown classical wheat
[Poli]sh wheat [(n]aked)	Triticum polonicum	—	—	—	—	—	—	Unknown in Antiquity
WHEATS : SPELT GROUP					(42 Chromosomes)			
[Sp]elt (hulled)	Triticum spelta	hrnt II.501.9 bd.t I.486.14	ŠE-IR-ZI	qutru	X	zeopyron (?)	brace, spica	Also Gr. sandala, scandala, scandula
[Com]mon (bread) [wh]eat (naked)	Triticum vulgare	?	ŠE-GIG (DUGUB-BA)	kibtu	X	sitanias	siligo	The fall-sown classical wheat Its flour = Gr. semithalites, L. semilago
[Clu]b wheat (naked)	Triticum compactum	—	—	—	—	sitanias	siligo (trimestre)	The fall-sown classical wheat
[Indi]an dwarf wheat (naked)	Triticum sphaerococcum	—	—	—	—	—	—	Cultivation in Mediterranean in Antiquity or later very doubtful
Barley	Hordeum vulgare	it I.142.11 'nḫt I.205.10	ŠE-BAR (-SE)	uṭṭatu	śe'ôra	krite	hordeum	Arab. shaeir
[Six-]rowed barley	Hordeum hexastichon L.	šm'j IV.476.8 śr.t IV.524.2	ŠE-IN-NU-HA	innunu	śe'ôra	krite	hordeum (grandias)	
Millet	Paniceum miliaceum L.		ŠE	duḫnu (arzik)	dâhan dôhân	kegchros	milium	Setaria italica = Italian millet, Arab. dúra, duḫn L. panicum, Gr. elymos, melime
Rye	Secale cereale	—	—	—	—	briza		Imported from Europe in Roman times only
Oats	Avena sativa	—	—	—	šiphôn	bromos	avena	Not cultivated in Mediterranean in Antiquity
[Fl]our (in general)		·nḏ	ZID-QU (ŠE)	qêmu			farina, ador pollen, flos	Dehusked wheat = Gr. tragos Pounded wheat = Gr. pistikion
[G]roats (general)		X	BULUG (pearl-barley)	buqlu (pearl-barley)	hâriphot (barley) sôlet (barley)	chonthros alphita	alica	

Egypt, probably in Sicily and North Africa too. In Greece, the Aegean, Crete, Syria, Palestine and Spain barley was very much first, wheat then follows up as a poor second. The production of wheat then begins to decline due to the invasion of rye.

We must, however, remember that a considerable part of the barley grown, but little of the wheat, was used as a feed grain, thence the ratio of wheat to total grain used for food was much greater than the ratio of production. This made the wheat trade even more important to the social structure of the ancient world, given the great part the annona played in Roman politics and the imports of grain in ancient Athens.

Unfortunately, we can not yet assess precisely the part transportation played in this corn trade. We know, for instance, much about the vehicles and techniques of road building in ancient Rome but little about the cost of transportation of different goods except that it was costly and difficult, and that it stood in direct relation to the production and consumption of food in ancient Italy. The few data we possess all point to the fact that the price of a heavy commodity was doubled or more after being hauled over a distance of 100 miles. The high price of Italian wheat was the result of constant scarcity due to the persistent demand of Rome and the armies and of the low yield per acre. This price was of course only relatively high (6—10% of the modern one) and had nothing to do with the fantastic prices paid by a small minority for exotic luxury goods.

Large scale production of Italian wheat for Rome and the army was made impossible by the high cost of transportation on pack animals or by oxen-teams. The rates of transport finally fixed by Diocletian could have applied to very short distances only, no large scale transport of low-cost bulky materials was possible under these economic conditions.

This must have had a revolutionary effect on Italian farming. The farmer was diverted from producing wheat for sale to the big cities and induced to produce grain for feeding livestock, since it was easier to drive cattle and hogs to the market over the roads of Italy than to transport grain in large quantities. It is a reasonable guess that the abnormally high production of barley (and later oats) in northern Italy was used for the feeding of livestock mainly. Thus we also understand why no protests were raised against imports of grain from Sicily as grazing and breeding must have begun to flourish even before the large-scale import of foreign grain. Oxen were anyway needed in the farm for draft purposes and the steadily rising demand for milk, cheese, beef and poultry in the cities made breeding a valuable adjunct to the growing and more profitable wine and olive farming. Manure was in heavy demand for viticulture also, and barley was grown to feed both the stock and the slaves on the new farms (5). The "frumentum Siculum" of Latium was giving way to that of Sicily and Egypt.

The competition of more cheaply produced and more easily transported grains of Egypt and Africa evidently brought about a similar transformation of agriculture in Sicily later on. These imports did not only consist of the Egyptian emmer called olyra (tragos) and the African emmer (zeia, semen) but mainly of naked wheats of the durum type. It is true that the speed of ancient ships was no more than an average 3—4 knots, but then this remained so until well in the eighteenth century. Also ocean freights were very high in Antiquity, but we have to take into account the difference between private shipping and the fiscal cargoes of the ships commandeered for the annona.

This trade also makes us understand the use of an artificial port with a stormy entrance like Ostia. The ever-present threat of famine in Rome discouraged the use of the much better harbour of Puteoli for the annona, for though a deep-sea harbour the choice of Puteoli would have meant 150 miles of landhaulage. Seen in this light Nero's plan to connect Ostia and Puteoli by a canal was economically sound. It would have made possible direct grain-transport to Rome in barges without transfer at Ostia.

The cheap Egyptian and African grain led to the quantitative decline of wheat-growing in Italy except in the interior, where cities and towns could be profitably supplied and slaves and livestock were to be fed. Vineyards, olive plantations, orchards and stock farms became the dominant part where slave labour proved profitable only because it could be employed the year round, whereas cereals demand intensive activity only at planting and harvest time. Hence the use of the dwindling and expensive slave force for the production of wine, oil and perfumes rather than for the production of cheap grain which could be produced more economically in Egypt and Africa and landed at a cheap rate in Italian ports. However, this policy spelt the same trouble for Italy as it had caused in ancient Greece.

The policy of "bread and games" imposed a constantly increasing burden on the Roman politicians which was not easy to solve. Its story, which is in reality a socio-economical problem rather than a matter of cattle-breeding and agriculture, has not yet been fully studied.

Many false ideas are still rampant. Only recently did White demonstrate that there was no decline of cereal-cultivation in Italy during the first century, but rather a widespread practice of intercultivation and changes because of demographic shifts and the decline of formerly important centres rather than exhaustion of the soil. The yields mentioned by Varro and Cicero agree with those in parts of the present Italy and Sicily where tools and methods have hardly changed (5).

The production of flour and bread

We can interpret our data on flour prices as corresponding to 8 sesterces per modius of the cheaper kind of Roman wheat and almost 10 sesterces per modius for the more expensive one. Sicilian and Egyptian wheats belonged to the cheaper kind. The high cost of transportation and storage and the heavy risks involved in the grain trade may well have brought the price of Sicilian and Egyptian wheats in Rome close to the one mentioned above and the free market price in that city was certainly considerably higher than the 3—4 sesterces per modius mentioned by the historians (6).

Apart from the farming policy, social and economic changes in classical farming and transportation problems we also have to consider milling technique if we want to have a clear picture of the food of the classical world. Flour in those days was very much poorer than commonly assumed for the wheat was not thoroughly cleaned before the rather coarse grinding and sifting. Our modern white flour means a 70—75% extraction of the wheat. Most of the ancient flour was simply whole-grain meal, among the sifted flours an 80% extraction was most common. Grinding wheat to three grades of flour as described by Pliny (7) was probably only found to a moderate extent in the larger cities, nor did this mean an extraction percentage below 80%.

The cereals to be ground were emmer, triticum in the narrow sense (durum and poulard wheat) grown mostly as fall-sown wheat in the area around Rome, Sicily, Egypt and Africa and siligo, raised as a spring- of wintercrop in Central Italy, the Po valley and some parts of Sicily, Greece and Asia Minor. As siligo was softer, it gave a whiter flour which was preferred.

In our days wheat is thoroughly cleaned and even part of the outer skin is removed with the dirt adhering closely to the kernels. It is then washed, cleansened and tempered, that is moistened, conditioning it in such a way that the skin strongly resists pulverisation but not the interior which are then easily separated by grinding. In classical times cleaning before grinding is mentioned in Egypt for flour made for the kings and nobles. The Mishna instructs millers to pick stones from the grains used for sacrifice. GALEN describes details of washing grain in baskets before grinding but this pertains only to certain cities in Asia and Egypt, which used more refined milling techniques than Greece and Rome. In fact flour in classical times was inferior in colour and above all it contained all or most of the impurities of the wheat, some poisonous, some harmful to the teeth.

Tempering wheat before grinding was common practice in Babylonia, Palestine and Egypt in PLINY's time but not in Rome. Moreover the ancient miller did not possess the steel rollers and modern machinery but only a stone mill, very primitive hand-sieves, vessels for measuring the grain, a ruler used with these vessels, baskets and the like. Most of these were thousands of years old and only the hand-mill had been improved. The rise of the professional miller did not mean a better grinding job, for animal mills required more power and did a poorer job than hand-mills for several centuries to come. The inefficient use of animal power in Roman mills partly accounts for the fact that human labour was so largely used for grinding. The reasons why grinding (though relatively considerably more expensive than nowadays) meant no more than a relatively small percentage of the free-market price of wheat were the high wheat price, the cheapness of

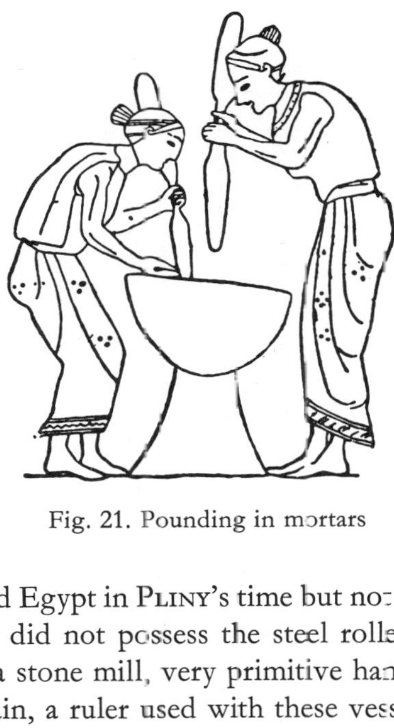

Fig. 21. Pounding in mortars

slave labour and especially the small amount of power utilized per bushel of the coarsely ground wheat.

Jasny (6) has calculated that a two-donkey mill in Rome used no more than 0.4—0.5 HP as compared with the 1.5—2.0 HP per bushel of wheat consumed in a modern factory 60% of which are used for cleaning and 40% in grinding operations. The animal in the ancient rotary mills exerted its force by means of a sweep with a small circle and could not give more than 1¼ HP/hour a day that is sufficient to

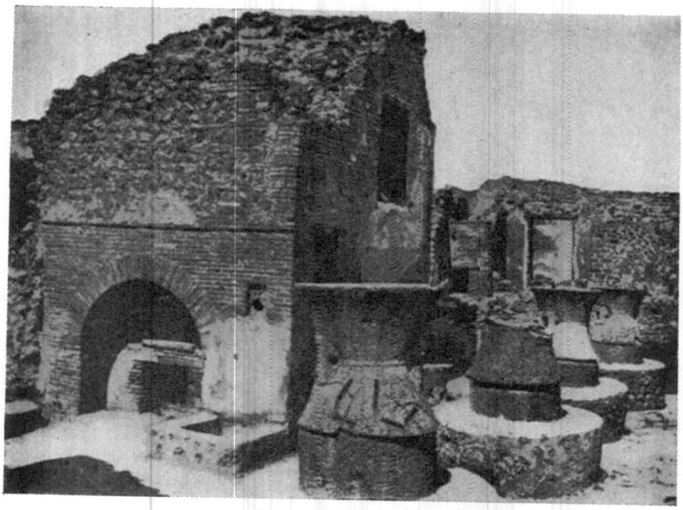

Fig. 22. Hourglass-mills in a Pompeian bakery

grind 3½ bushels. About ten pounds of wheat per working day went to take care of the cost of food, housing, interest and depreciation of the donkey per day. As the maximum daily wage of the pistor in Diocletian's Edict was fixed at 20 pounds wheat's worth it meant that he could hold about two donkeys on the average. A horse would be able to grind about 5 to 6 times the amount of wheat but consumed much more than a donkey. Grinding costs then could have amounted to 10% of the cost of wheat maximum.

Sieves had not improved very much since pre-classical days. "The Gallic provinces invented the kind of bolter made of horse-hair, while Spain made sieves and meal-sifters of flax and Egypt of papyrus and rush" says Pliny (8). These sieves were very coarse. The "farinarium" used to separate bran from flour was also used for "alica" a kind of semolina, with very large bits. Cato used the farinarium to force cottage cheese through it in the way in which certain ingredients were pressed through a coarse cloth ("colare"). The "pollinarium", a linen sieve used for separating first grade flour, pollen or flos, from second-grade one was not a fine one according to our standards for it was used to separate chalk from "alica" (9).

Again ground wheat was generally sifted only once. Repeated grinding and sieving is mentioned only for very special occasions in classical texts as well as in the Mishna, where the most refined flour of Antiquity, "sôlet", is said to be ground but once and sifted 11 to 13 times. The yields of the different types of flour according to the classical authors can be judged from the table given by JASNY (6) (Table XVI), the terms used for the different grades of flour are:

Type of wheat	*Triticum*	*Siligo*
First flour grade	pollen	flos
Second ———	similago	siligo
Third ———	secundarium, cibarium	
Bran	furfur	

Moritz has both modified and amplified this valuable pioneer work of Jasny, their works (6) contain various details on the types of flour produced, the yield, etc., partly obtained by working with actual querns of the Roman period.

Bread always remained the staple food of classical Antiquity. The Greek "artos" means both "bread" and "food in general". In Bronze Age Greece a coarse unleavened bread was eaten in the form of flat cakes or flans like in the rest of prehistoric Europe (10). The lighter leavened bread, the manufacture of which was introduced from the East, was still a luxury in the days of SOLON. PLINY (11) devotes an entire paragraph to the manufacture of leaven.

"Millet is especially used for making leaven; if dipped in unfermented wine and kneaded it will keep a whole year. A similar leaven is obtained by kneading and drying in the sun the best fine bran of the wheat itself, after it has been steeped for three days in unfermented white wine. In making bread cakes made of this are soaked in water and boiled with prime flour of emmer and then mixed with the flour, the process being thought to produce the best bread. Moreover though these kinds of leaven can only be made in the vintage season, it is possible at any time one chooses to make leaven from water and barley, making two-pound cakes and baking them in ashes and

TABLE XVI

Extractions in the Three-Grade Grindings of Unmoistened Wheat in Rome

acc. to Jasny (Pliny 10.39 and 9.86-87)

From triticum			From Pisan siligo		
Ground produkt	Sextarii per modius of wheat	% in terms of weight of wheat	Ground produkt	Sextarii per modius of wheat	% in terms of weight of wheat
pollen	5	27	flos	8	44
similago	8	44	siligo	5	27
secundarium	4	15	secundarium	4	15
Bran	4	11	Bran	4	11
Waste	—	3	Waste	—	3
Total	21	100	Total	21	100

charcoal on a hot hearth or an earthenware dish till they turn brown, and afterwards keeping them shut up in vessels till they go sour; then soaked in water they produce leaven. But when barley bread used to be made, the actual barley was leavened with flour of bitter vetch or chickeling; the proper amount was two pounds of leaven to every two and a half pecks of barley. At the present time leaven is made out of the flour itself, which is kneaded before salt is added to it and is then boiled down to a kind of porridge and left till it begins to go sour. Generally, however, they do not heat it up at all, but only use the dough kept over from the day before; manifestly it is natural for sourness to make the dough ferment, and likewise that people who, live on fermented bread have weaker bodies, inasmuch as in old days outstanding wholesomeness was ascribed to wheat the heavier it was."

Yeast was known in later days, Pliny (12) tells us that the Gauls and the Iberians when making beer from corn used "the foam that forms on the surface in the process for leaven, in consequence of which those races have a lighter kind of bread than others".

The diet of ancient Greece

There is no doubt that even the prehistoric Greeks were familiar with the general methods of boiling, baking and frying food. Even when more modern baking ovens spread after 600 B.C. primitive methods like baking in hot ashes remained in use locally until the

Roman period (13). As baking became a profession larger baking ovens were built, large forms of which were discovered in Roman excavations. A rich Roman "director of bakeries" even left us a monument in the form of a large baker's oven. As private baking by the house slaves or by the women became less common other phases of bread making such as kneading were also mechanised. Several Pompeiian bakeries had such kneading machines built on the principle of our mixers (14).

Apart from bread groats were very popular, both in Greece and Rome. Its manufacture is described in detail by PLINY (15): "Alica (groats) is made from emmer. Its grain is pounded in a wooden mortar so as to avoid the hardness of stone grating it up, the motive power for the pestle, as is well known, being supplied by the labour of convicts in chains; on the end of the pestle there is a cap of iron. After the grain has been stripped of its coats (deshusked), the bared kernel is again broken up with the same implements. The process produces three grades of alica — very small, seconds and the largest kind which is called in Greek "select grade". Still these products have not yet got the whiteness for which they are distinguished, though even at this stage they are preferable to the Alexandrian alica. In a subsequent process, marvellous to relate, an admixture of chalk is added, which passes into the substance of the grain and contributes colour and fineness. (The chalk came from a hill between Puzzuoli and Napels.)

A spurious alica is manufactured chiefly from an inferior kind of emmer growing in Africa. The ears are mixed with sand and pounded and even so there is a difficulty in rubbing off the husks, and only half the quantity of naked grain is produced; and afterwards a quarter the amount of white lime is sprinkled into the grain, and when this had stuck together with it they bolt it though a floursieve. The grain that stays behind in the sieve is called residuary and is the largest in size. That which goes through is sifted again in a finer sieve, and is called seconds, and likewise the name of the sieveflour is given to that which in similar manner stays behind in a third extremely fine sieve which lets only grains like sand through. There is another method to adulteration which is everywhere used; they pick out from wheat the whitest and largest grains, half boil them in pots and afterwards sprinkle them with water and crush them in a mill. A more attractive kind of groats called tragum is made from emmer, although it is in fact merely a spurious alica; but it is given whiteness by an admixture of milk boiled in it instead of chalk."

In ancient Greece as in the East similar methods, though on a smaller scale and with more primitive household instruments, were used to produce groats. Those from Thessaly and Megara were highly in favour in ancient Greece. Groats were certainly not produced in the same type of mill as ordinary flour, for special terms are known both in Greek and Latin for groat-mills, though none have survived (16).

A large proportion of the farinaceous food was, however, still consumed as porridge, such as the "maza" compounded of flour, honey, salt, oil and water and the "turon" made of flour, cheese-gratings, eggs and honey. Indeed a greater variety of porridges appeared when the quality of flour was improved by better production methods. Both porridges and broths continued in favour until the end of the Roman period. In early Greece many dishes were sprinkled with barley flour before being cooked. Even in the Bronze Age the inhabitants of Greece had a considerable variety of vegetables at their disposal, which they seasoned with different spices. Mutton and beef were added but beef was costly and rare. The upper classes were able to afford fowl and game. Dishes made with milk and cheese were generally appreciated and fish and other sea-food quite common. Apples, pears, plums, pomegranates and almonds were eaten as the excavations prove (10).

The Homeric poems give the impression that meat (lamb, pork and beef) were devoured in quantities by all and that fish was consumed by the poor only, a fish diet being synonymous to poverty. However, the main food was farinaceous, barley porridge, bread and groats. HOMER specially mentions barley-groats as the typical food for men and warriors. These porridges and broths were eaten with meat, fish, cheese and vegetables, all embraced in the Greek term "opson" which originally meant "boiled meat", then "fish" and finally any seasoning agent like salt. Meat was certainly less common than HOMER's lines would suggest. The Greek have no word for "animal killed for food" but the word "hiereion", which actually means "victim for sacrifice". Meat was therefore mostly eaten at occasional sacrifices but as religious festivals abounded it figured quite frequently on the menu.

Still the diet was mainly vegetarian in early Greece, the porridges of corn-flour and broths of beans and pulses figuring very largely (17). They were seasoned with dried fish, fresh fish, oysters and other shellfish, vegetables, fish and honey. Game was rather a luxury and appeared mainly on the tables of the rich who preferred the hare and the thrush. Very few other wild birds were eaten, and that only in times of distress. The rich also indulged in the meat of ewes and kids and the better types of fish such as eels from Lake Copais. Nuts, acorns, chestnuts, almonds and other fruit were very popular, onions were often eaten raw even with wine. Salads were known in many varieties.

The Greeks had a curious abhorrence of cow's milk which was considered unwholesome. The consumption of neat milk (akreton) was considered intemperate since the days of HOMER and both milk and cheese were mainly produced from ewes and goats (17a). Wine, however, was the main beverage, it was also never drunk as such but diluted with 1—3 times its volume of water. Barley-water was sometimes drunk.

With the expansion of Greek civilisation, its contacts with the Mediterranean world and its dependence on grain imports diet changes in the course of the sixth and fifth centuries B.C. Wheat bread and porridge came to dominate. Bakeries become more common in the rich ports, fish is eaten more frequently. Spices such as cummin, coriander, sesame and silphion (from Cyrene) were grown or imported. In the fifth century barley-bread was generally considered fit for the poor or the barbarians of the North only. White wheat-bread and all kinds of cake compounded with oil, cheese, milk, wine, pepper, anise were now considered normal. Pulses were no longer regularly eaten by the well-to-do. Salted fish such as tunny, herring and sardines now appeared more frequently as well as all kinds of sauces of which the most famous was "garon", prepared by leaving fish immersed in a salt brine to ferment for some two to three months. A much greater variety of vegetables now appeared on the menu such as cabbage, aspergus, gurkins, artichokes, spinach, celery and spices like fenchel, mangold, mint, and others imported from distant countries. As a reaction local herbs such as thyme, garlic, cress and others were favoured in certain circles (17).

This rapid extension of the diet, is accompanied by the publication of cookery-books, by the appearance of special famous cooks working either as private artisans or attached to a great household and by the organisation of dinners and symposia. We also find the first inklings of the science of dietetics in the writings by HIPPOCRATES (460—377 B.C.) (18), whose name is attached to such treatises as *On Nutriment* and *On Regimen in Acute Diseases*, which lightly touch the value of diet for the sick. However, to the ancients "diet" meant something quite different. If DIOCLES of Carystos speaks of the diet of the healthy, this "diaité" means a description of the spread of the meals over the daytime or in general the way of life and later the rule of life, which includes the proper way of using air, exercise, sleep, rest and food in daily life. Only very gradually its original meaning 'when to eat' changes into "what to eat", a change which was not even complete some 150 years ago. The Greek doctors touch only lightly on fasting and special food for certain diseases and here and there we find some indications of the proper diet for specialists such as professional sportsmen.

The diet of ancient Rome

A similar evolution can be observed in ancient Rome. The stock dish of the ancient Roman farmers was a thick porridge called "puls" and made of flour prepared from emmer or beans, eaten with salt. Later wheat-flour was used for this "puls" which was eaten with green vegetables but seldom with meat. It still figured on the tables of the poor in the Imperial period and it survived very long as it plays a part in the Roman religious rites.

The Roman "puls", the equivalent of the Greek "maza", was supplemented by dishes made from groats like the "puls punica". The ancient Roman bread was a flat, hard cake called "libum" which was baked in hot embers and ashes and which continued in favour even when wheat-bread and leaven was introduced. The professional baker (at the same time a miller) appears around 174 B.C. Barley-bread was then only eaten by slaves and gladiators, the coarse flans were sopped in milk before eating. Beans (which also played a large part in Roman religion) peas, turnips and onions completed the mainly vegetarian diet. The leaves of beets were at first the only part eaten. Fruit such as apples, plums, pears, pomegranates and figs were well known, spices such as garlic, salt and garden herbs completed the menu. Milk, cheese, honey and olive oil were generally used. The most ancient drink was milk diluted with water, wine came later. Fish was little valued by the ancient Romans, game was seldom eaten and most of the meat consisted of goat, lamb or pork.

The change in diet occurs about 300 B.C. when the Roman state had come to power and Greek civilisation spread from the south. Wheat now generally began to displace the older emmer and einkorn. The taste for white bread and pastries increased with the absorption of Greek civilisation. The imports of Egyptian corn began during the second Punic war (209 B.C.).

These imports of the competitive Sicilian, Egyptian and North African wheat and rye from Gaul not only spell the death of Italian corn-farming but the production of pulses, beans and vegetables also suffer from the change in taste, which becomes more and more sumptuous and refined. Though cabbage, leek, pulses and peas are still eaten by the poor in large quantities, fruit-culture is now intensified. Almonds, chestnuts, hazelnuts and walnuts are now produced in much larger quantities. During the first century B.C. new fruit such as cherries, peaches and apricots are introduced in the orchards of Italy. Citriculture did not succeed until the fourth century A.D.

Bigger supplies of meat were now needed for game and meat began to figure largely on the tables of the rich. Italian farmers began to specialize in fattening-techniques for geese and fowl. Fish-dishes and sauces were now introduced from Greece and they gave rise to the introduction of fish-ponds and all the techniques associated with fish-farming. With the fall of the Roman Republic and the beginning of the Empire extravagant tastes of the new rich stimulated the imports of luxury food such as oysters from Britain and the building of cellars in which snow and ice served to preserve such delicacies. Cookery-books like that of Apicius are now published and famous symposia are mentioned in literature, culminating in the satyre on such upstarts as Trimalchio (A.D. 65) (19). The first cooks were imported from the East about 190 B.C.

Not until the Imperial period did Roman doctors bother about diet for the sick. The first realistic though empirical rules were given by CELSUS (53 B.C.—7 A.D. in his *De Re Medica* (20)) which supplemented by GALEN's (A.D. 130—200) three books on *the Faculties or Power of Aliments* became the basis of medieval dietetics. The often over-refined taste of the Romans in the Imperial period led to the improved grinding and sifting of flour which, however, meant the discarding of the nourishing bran. The common people still ate the old-fashioned food and this is particularly true of the army. The soldier's diet was still based on a daily ration of two pounds of barley and wheat, the soldiers carried their own rotary querns and prepared their own flour, which they baked. Beans, pork-fat, beer, wine and oil supplemented this diet. Meat was considered an extra and Scipio still grumbles about the spits, which the soldiers would have to carry in order to roast their own meat. Even during the late Roman Empire a tactician like VEGETIUS still considers meat an "adminiculum", that is an "addition" to the vegetarian diet of the soldier.

The production of olive oil

The ancient world disposed of certain limited amounts of animal fats such as lard but it depended mainly on olive oil for its supply of fats. Butter, though known, was used in certain religious rites and medical recipes only but not consumed on any large scale. The modern species of olives, which western civilisation has spread far beyond the Mediterranean basin even into the Western Hemisphere all seem descended from the wild Oleaster or Olea. Palestine and Syria seem the homeland of the spineless types of Olea Europeana L. Another type

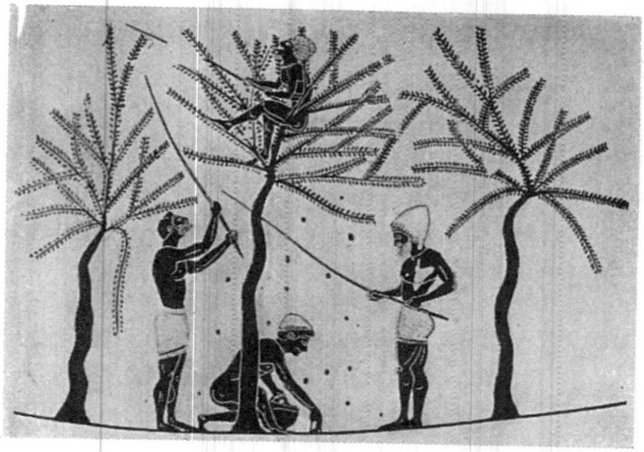

Fig. 23. Olive-gathering

with spines seems to originate in Crete, where the olive was cultivated as early as 2500 B.C. and where enormous pithoi used for the storage of olive-oil and other archaeological evidence point to the fact that the wealth of the kings of the famous Cretan palaces was certainly partly based on the export of olive-oil to Egypt and other Mediterranean countries (21). Certainly its name even in Turkish goes back to a West-Semitic original "zajit", and in ancient Egyptian a related term "ḏt" is used since about 1500 B.C., when olive-oil comes into more common use in that country. The Greek for olive oil "elaia" and the Latin "oleum" (whence all the terms in Western languages) seem to go back to a Semitic term for oil "ulu".

From the Eastern Mediterranean the use of olive-oil in cooking slowly spread westwards and the cultivation of the olive went with it and reached Rome later than 580 B.C. when the vine came to that city though some hold that the olive was introduced in Etruria and

Latium during the seventh century B.C. (21a). By the classical period it was common in all coastal regions of the Mediterranean and its cultivation and use spread into northern Europe stimulated by its ritual use in the Christian Church. Its cultivation was even attempted in southern Britain but olive-oil never dominated the fat supply of western Europe, as the olive was not suited for these northern latitudes and imports came too expensive. During the Middle Ages rapeseed-oil and mawseed-oil came to be cultivated and started to compete with animal fats during the thirteenth century to hold their ground since.

The use of olive-oil is therefore typical of the Mediterranean countries. Though in the Homeric world olive-oil was still a luxury of the wealthy and not yet cultivated in Greece, by the days of SOLON its cultivation in Attica was so intense that laws regulating its production had to be enacted. To Italy the olive-culture came with the Greek colonists in southern Italy and thence to Rome, where exports begin by the first century B.C. Spain and Africa probably received the olive from Phoenician traders and settlers.

Syria must have been a centre of olive-growing for centuries as the Mari texts and other local archives show and probably the techniques went back to the second millenium, though we do not have material proofs yet.

However in Greek and Roman days the production of olive oil slowly grew into the industry which it certainly was during the Roman Empíre, when the centre of production shifted back to the East again and Syria became an important centre of this monoculture again (23).

There is no essential differences in the techniques of production of olive-oil in the Near East (22) or the classical world (23). The first stage was the picking of the olives which was preferably done by hand, shaking the branches when the olives were too far off for picking or striking the branches with pliant twigs in order not to spoil the olives. Figures on pottery vases show us how the olives were tested by squeezing the juice out of a few specimen through a funnel into a little flask and by inspecting the taste and smell of the separated oil. Such tests were also to find out whether the olives were sufficiently ripe for picking.

The problem after the picking consists of separating the oil from the flesh, separating it from the bitter watery liquid which the ancients called "amurca" and avoiding to crush the kernel. As the skin is fairly tough, this is achieved by first partly crushing the olive, extracting the kernel and the liquid and then expressing the oil. These processes are described in great detail by such Roman agronomists as Cato, Columella and Pliny.

The freshly picked olives were sometimes stored on the floor (tabulatum) of the press-house, but it was recommended to crush them immediately. This was achieved in different types or rollermills, in fact the production of olive-oil was the main incentive for the evolution of this type of mill. The original type in which a vertical mill-stone was made to turn and roll in a stone basin containing the olives was not

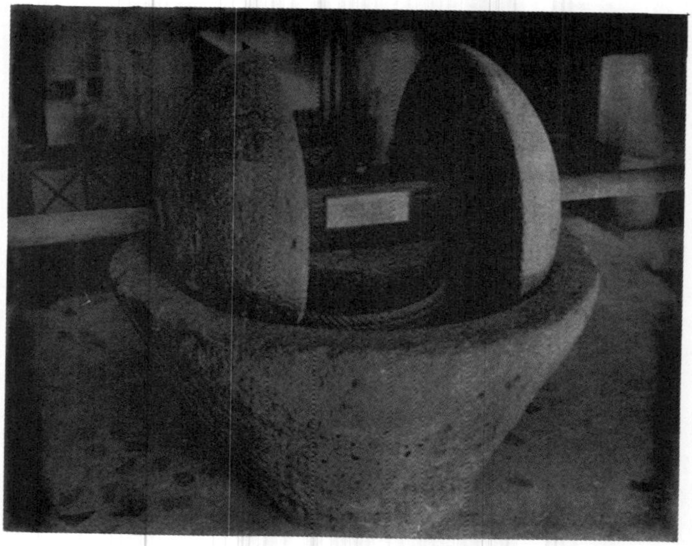

Fig. 24. The trapetum

satisfactory when the production of olive oil became more refined. As the distance between stone and basin could not be regulated too many kernels were crushed and the quality of the oil spoiled. Hence the classical world and probably Roman inventors developed the "trapetum" in which a pair of stone turning round a solid column in the middle of the basin could be adjusted to a given distance from the walls of the basin thus achieving the correct degree of crushing the olive without spoiling the juice.

Then the kernels were separated from the pulp and the first oil recovered. The pulp was then often soaked in hot water and subjected to a second pressing in the type of press (beam-press or screw-press) that was commonly used in the production of wine. Here again olive-oil production was a strong force behind the gradual perfection of the press. The oil and juice separated from the pulp ("sampsa") like that of the first treatment was stored in settling vats. As early as the Bronze Age the Cretans had already used settling vats in which the water could be drawn off through a spout in the bottom and the pure oil collected after it. Between these two pressings the crushed pulp was usually spread on mats raised slightly above the floor in order to get rid of the larger part of the bitter "amurca" contained in the olive, the taste of which might spoil that of the olive-oil.

The second pressing could be carried out in different stages by raising the pressure. In each case more oil but of lower quality was obtained. Usually three qualities of olive-oil were produced, the first quality being that which was drawn from the pulp directly after the crushing in the trapetum, the other two qualities being expressed in the beam-press after soaking the pulp with water. The many qualities distinguished by ancient authors are related to the fact that olive-oil was not only used for cooking, but also in the many unguents, cosmetics and toilet preparations in which they indulged and which demanded a high purity of the oil, which served as a carrier or body of the perfumes and essential oils only.

Bibliography

(1) Cecil Curwen, E., *Plough and Pasture* (London 1946)
Slicher van Bath, B. H., *The Agrarian History of Western Europe, 500—1850* (London, 1963)
(2) Clark, J. G. D., *Prehistoric Europe, the economic basis* (London 1952)
(3) Jasny, N., *Competition among grains in classical Antiquity* (*Amer. Hist. Rev.* 1942, 747)
(4) Jasny, N., *The Wheats of Classical Antiquity* (Baltimore 1944)
Helbaek, H., *Ancient Egyptian Wheats* (*Proc. Preh. Soc.* N.S. Vol. XXI, 1955, 93—95
Helbaek, H., *Domestication of Food Plants in the Old World* (*Science*, Washington, vol. 130, no. 3372, 365—372)
Helbaek, H., *Early crops in Southern England* (*Proc. Preh. Soc.* XVIII, 1953, 194—233)
Helbaek, H., *Queen Ichetis' Wheat, a contribution to the study of Early Dynastic Emmer of Egypt* (Copenhagen, 1953)
Ehrenberg, P., *Neues zum Vorkommen und Bedeutung des Spelzes* (*Dinkel, Triticum Spelta*) *im Altertum so wie jetzt* (*Z.*f. *Acker- und Pflanzenbau*, Berlin, Bd. 98, 279—288)
Helbaek, Hans, *Studying the diet of ancient man* (*Archaeology* 14, 1961, 95—101)
Montet, P., *Landwirtschaft und Viehzucht im alten Aegypten* (*Die BSAF*, vol. XI, 1961, 1, 13—17)
Mohamed Riad, *Native plough in Egypt* (*Bull. Soc. Géogr. Egypte* 33, 1960, 241—277)
Furio Jesi, *I primi silos dell'umanità* (*Sapere Italia* vol. LII, 1961, no. 621, 471—473)
(5) Yeo, C. A., *Land and Sea transportation in Imperial Italy* (*Trans. Amer. Phil. Soc.* vol. LXXVII, 1946, 221—244)
Gagé, J., *Frumentum Siculum* (*Ac. Inscr. Belles Lettres, Bull. Fac. Lettres* 1950, 347—359)
Chastagnol, A., *Le ravitaillement de Rome en viande au Ve siecle* (*Rev. Hist.* CCX, 1953, 13—22)
Nebbia, G., *Aspetti storici del problema del controllo della qualità delle merci nel mondo antico e nel medioevo* (*Quaderni di Merceologia* I, 1962, (1), 327—380)
Yeo, G. A., *The development of the Roman plantation and marketing of farm products* (*Finanzarchiv*, Tübingen, NF XIII, 1952, 321—342)
Raffo, G., *Sulle distribuzione di viveri a Roma nell III secolo d C* (*Gior. Ital. Filol.* IV, 1951, 250—255)
Smith, E. M., *Some Roman dinner tables* (*Class. Journal* L, 1955, 255—260)
White, K. D., *Wheatfarming in Roman Times* (*Antiquity* XXXVII, 1963, 207—212)
(6) Jasny, N., *Wheat prices and milling costs in Classical Rome* (*Wheat Studies*, vol. XX, 1944, No. 4)

MORITZ, L. A., and JONES, C. R., *Experiments in grinding wheat in a Romano-British quern* (*Milling* 114, 1950, 594)
MORITZ, L. A., *Grain-mills and Flour in Classical Antiquity* (*Clarendon Press*, London, 1958)
(7) PLINY, *Nat. History* IX, 86—87; X, 89
(8) PLINY, *Nat. History* XVIII, 108
(9) PLINY, *Nat. History* XI, 108 & 115
(10) VICKERY, K. F., *Food in Early Greece* (Urbana 1936)
HANNESTAD, K., *Evolution des resources agricoles de l'Italie du IVe au VIe siècle de notre ère* (*Hist.-filos. Med. Danske Vid. Selsk.* Copenhagen, 1962, XL, 1)
ADRIAN, W., *So wurde Brot aus Halm und Glut* (Bielefeld 1951)
MCCANCE, R. A. and WIDDOWSON, E. M., *Breads, white and brown* (London, 1956)
JACOB, H., 6000 *Jahre Brot* (Hamburg, 1954)
JACOB, H. E., *Six thousand years of Bread* (New York, 1944)
JASNY, N., *The daily bread of the ancient Greeks and Romans* (*Osiris* IX, 1950, 227—253)
LURASHI, A., *Il pane e la sua storia, l'arte bianca* (Torino, 1953)
STOKAR, W. VON, *Die Urgeschichte des Hausbrotes* (Leipzig, 1951)
WÄHREN, M., *Römisches Brot* (*Suisse Primitive* XX, 1956, 19—22)
(11) PLINY, *Nat. History* XVIII, 102—104
(12) PLINY, *Nat. History* XVIII, 68
(13) OVID, *Fastes*, V. 315
(14) MAU, *Pompeii* (2e edit.), page 410, Fig. 425
(15) PLINY, *Nat. Hist.* XVIII, 112—116
(16) "chondria" (POLLUX, III. 78; VII. 19);
"alicaria" (PLAUTUS, *Poen.* 266)
(17) BONNER, S. & L., *Die Ernährung der Griechen und Römer* (Planegg 1943)
GLOVER, R. T., *Feeding the Athenians* (In: *The Challenge of the Greek*, Cambridge, 1943)
GLOVER, R. T., *Diet in History* (In: *Greek Byways*, Cambridge, 1932)
SPARKES, B. A., *The Greek kitchen* (JHS LXXXII, 1962, 121—137)
GRIMAL, P. et MONOD Th. *Sur la véritable nature du garum* (*Revue Etud. Lat.*, vol. 54, 1952, pages. 27—38)
ANDRÉ, J., *L'alimentation et la cuisine à Rome* (Paris, 1961)
ANDREWS, A. C., *The carrot as a food in the classical period* (*Class. Phil.* 1949, 182—196)
ANDREWS, A. C., *Celery and parsley as foods in the Greco-Roman period* (*Class. Phil.* 1949, 91—99)
ANDREWS, H. N., *Ancient plants and the world they lived in* (*Ithaca*, 1947)
ANDREWS, A. C., *Hyssop in the classical era* (*Class. Philol.* LVI, 1961, 230-248)
ANDREWS, A. C., *Majoram as a spice in the classical era* (*Class. Philol.* LVI, 1961, 73—82)
ANDREWS, A. C., *Thyme as a condiment in the Greco-Roman era* (*Osiris* XIII, 1958, 150—156)
ANDREWS, A. C., *The mints of the Greeks and the Romans and their condimentary use* (*Osiris* XIII, 1958, 127—149)

ANDREWS, A. C., *The parsnip as food in the classical era* (*Class. Phil.* LIII, 1958, 145—152)

ANDREWS, A. C., *Acclimation of citrus fruits in the Mediterranean region* (Agric. History XXXV, 1961, 35—46)

BAAS, J., *On kinds of fruit eaten by the Romans* (*Saalburg Jahrbuch* X, 1951)

LAUR-BELART, R., *Gallische Schinken und Würste* (*Suisse Primitive* XVII, 1953, 33—40)

MILHAM, M. E., *A glossarial index to De Re Coquinaria of Apicius* (Madison, 1952)

MINGAZZINI, P., *Gli antichi conoscevano i maccheroni?* (*Arch. Class.*, Roma, VI, 1954, 292—294)

PARRY, JOHN W., *The Story of Spices* (New York, 1953)

BEATTIE, A. J., *The spice tablets of Cnossos, Pylos and Mycenae* (Minoica, *Festschrift Sundwall*, 1959, 6—34)

TELLEZ, R. & CIFERRI, F., *Trigos arqueologicos de Espana* (Madrid, 1954)

JOHNSTON, L. D., *Glandium, what piece of pork?* (*Class. Philol.*, vol. XLIX, 1954, pags. 244—250)

MYRES, J. L., *Ancient Groceries* (*Greece and Rome* vol. XXII, 1953, pags. 1—10)

BALIL ILLANA, A., *Un estudio sobre el garum* (*Arch. Espan. Arqueología*, vol. XXVI, 1953, pags. 183—185)

(17a) USSHER, R. G., *A comment on unmixed milk* (*Hermathena* LXXXIX, 1957, 59—64)

BEHRENS, G., *Römische Milchkocher* (*Germania* XXX, 1952, 110—111)

(18) HUTCHINSON, R., *The History of Dietetics* (*The Practitioner*, Jan. 1934)

(19) PETRONIUS, *Satyricon* (edit. HESELTINE, *Loeb Classical Library*, 1919)

(20) RIDDELL, W. R., *The Dietetics of Celsus* (*Med. J. and Record* CXXXIV, 1931, 247)

GALENOS, *Die animalischen Nahrungsmittel und Getränke: Werke* vols. III & IV (Stuttgart, 1952)

(21) HOOPS, W., *Der Oelbaum* (In: *Forschungen und Fortschritte* 1947, p. 35 and *Heidelb. Akad. Wiss.* 1942/43, p. 3)

(21a) VALLET, G., *L'introduction de l'olivier en Italie centrale d'après les données de la céramique* (*Mélanges Grenier*, Bruxelles 1962, 1554—1563)

(22) DALMANN, G., *Arbeit und Sitte in Palästina* (Gütersloh, Part IV, 206, 221)

(23) BLÜMNER, H., *Technologie und Terminologie der Gewerbe und Künste bei Griechen und Römern*, Vol. I (2nd Edit.) (Leipzig, 191, 332)

CAMPS-FABRER, H., *Une nouvelle huilerie romaine dans la région de Périgotville* (*Libyca* V, 1957, 43—47)

CAMPS-FABRER, H., *L'Olivier et l'Huile dans l'Afrique Romaine* (Alger, 1953)

BOTTERO, J., *Archives R. de Mari* vol. VII, 266

TCHALENKO, G., *Villages antiques de la Syrie du nord. Le Massif du Bélus a l'époque romaine* (2 vols.)

BENNETT, E. L., *The olive oil tablets of Pylos* (*Suppl. to Minos* II, 1958)

SARAH, B. PORGES, *A Lease of an Olive Grove* (*Trans. Amer. Phil. Soc.* 92, 1961, 469—480)

VALLET, G., *Introduction de l'olivier en Italie centrale* (Mélanges Grenier, Bruxelles 1962, 1554—1563)

CHAPTER FOUR

FERMENTED BEVERAGES 500 B.C.—1500 A.D.

Wine

There is considerable truth in the Greek tradition that Dionysos the god of wine, fled from the homecountry of "froth-blowers", Mesopotamia, to Thrace. This god of classical tradition was the results of the merger of two slightly differing older gods of Thracian and of Lydian-Phrygian origin. This god who brings orgiagism, the godly frenzy, whom the Silenes and the Satyrs accompany, brought the beauty of spring flowers and was a fertility god of trees. Only later did he become a god of the vine, and characteristically he is not connected with the great Greek wine-festivals.

Philology tells us that the Latin, Greek and West Semitic words for wine are independent borrowings from Asia Minor. The technique of viticulture too reached Rome and Greece by different ways, as is proved by small differences, Rome probably inherited viticulture from the Etruscans who may have come from the eastern Mediterranean. In Greece wine belonged to the ancient Aegean culture with its strong Anatolian bonds, it played a large part in chtonic worships and Greek colonists brought the vine to southern Italy and Sicily.

Archaeology suggests that the vine was cultivated in the Aegean in the Early Bronze Age. It may have come from Syria and Egypt by the way of Crete, where wine seems to have been used for libations to the gods (1). However, it is more probable that wine came to Greece by the way of Asia Minor. The oldest grape-seeds found on such Mycenean (pre-Greek) sites as Orchomenos, Tiryns and Mycenae belong to the Middle Helladic period or Late Bronze Age. In the Mycenaean town on the Menelaion-hill near Sparta clay stoppers were found which bore the imprints of vine-leaves (2). Greek viticulture was centered on the western and eastern shores of the Aegean thus confirming the tradition of the Anatolian origin of the vine.

There is no doubt that *the Greeks* were great wine-lovers even in the days of Homer. The Eupatrids, the leading hierarchy in the state of Attica owned vineyards. However, the Greeks paid dearly for their wine. When the reforms of Solon the law-giver of Athens broke the power of the Eupatrids it became clear how deeply viticulture was influencing their economy. A densely populated country like Attica with an average farm-size of 10 acres only could ill afford producing wine when it was short of corn to feed its population. Hence the economy of classical Greece depended on the import of cereals which were paid for by exports of wine, olive-oil, figs and pottery. Greece was therefore in great danger of specializing in products for export only and losing control of the production of food necessary for its own population.

However, only in Attica did the vineyards encroach seriously on the corn-fields. In most other Greek states the area planted with corn remained practically constant and the vineyards increased their area at the expense of forests or shrub-covered hill-sides. Nevertheless Greek colonisation and the introduction of Greek wine are practically identical. Thus soon after the foundation of Massalia (Marseilles) about 600 B.C. the Greek colonists started to export wine to the Celtic tribes of Gaul. The typical wine-vessels called "amphorae" and bronze flaggons with beaked spouts are found in excavations in prehistoric Europe. They prove how wine penetrated into central France by way of the rivers Rhône and Saone and by crossing the Belfort gap in the mountains reached the upper Rhine region. Along with the wine went the drinking ritual and all the vessels connected with carrying, storing, mixing and drinking it. These beautiful pottery or bronze vessels had a profound influence on the art of the European barbarians and a famous archaeologist (3) has truly said that "la Tène (Celtic) art may have largely owed its existence to Celtic thirst".

By the fifth century B.C. Greek wine from the islands and coasts of the Aegean went to Sicily, south and central Italy, Gaul, the Iberians of Spain, the Illyrians and Thracians on the Adriatic coast, the Danube and the Balkans, the Scythians of southern Russia, Asia Minor, Cyprus, the Syrian coast and Egypt. The reckless civil wars in Greece ruined private farming to a large extent. By the end of the century viticulture was more or less industrialised. Professional wine-merchants buy the produce and sell it overseas. The wine trade is regulated and most islands sell their wine only in sealed and stamped jars (Thasos, Cnidos, Rhodes, Sinope, etc.). We possess the full trade regulations for the isle of Thasos. Sale of the crop before its reaping in May and June is forbidden. Wine may be purchazed in sealed jars only and Thasian ships shall ply no foreign wine between certain points of the Greek mainland. Greek wine was extremely popular in Egypt where local viticulture was not so successful. These imports arrived at the Greek colony and port of Naucratis in the Delta. The island of Naxos rich in vineyards became the centre of the cult of Dionysos.

By the fourth century B.C. the defects of Greek economy begin to show up. In the course of this century many wineloving districts start to produce their own wines. Thus the emancipation of the Pontic (Black Sea) markets becomes apparent though they still remained an important factor in the exports of better Greek wines. The Bosporean Kingdom starts its own viticulture. The profitable markets on the Adriatic were cut off by Dionysos of Sicily who started to flood them with his native products. Large quantities were still shipped to the

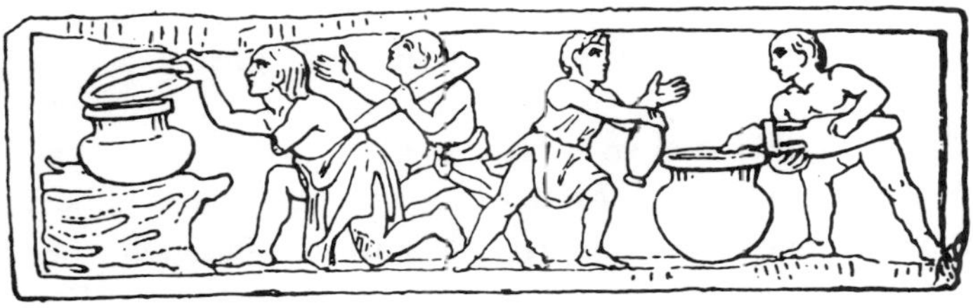

Fig. 25. Wine being decocted

East and to Italy, but it became evident that only quality wines could help to maintain the Greek markets.

The Greek viniculturists, stimulated by the natural "curiosity" of the Greeks, studied and perfected their art driven by these economical changes.

Unfortunately we have no early documents on the art of viticulture and we can therefore only guess that this was a development based both on the practical experience of the wine-growers and the theoretical interests of the botanists. This assumption seems well-founded if we turn to the first essays on this art. They were written by THEOPHRASTUS of Eresos (370—385 B.C.), ARISTOTLE's most famous pupil. Many remarks on the vine and viticulture in his *Enquiry into Plants* (4) show the blend of practical experience and theory, but it is proved even more fully in his *On the life of plants* (III.11—16) which contains very detailed observations on viticulture (5). These observations were only partly culled from the writings of earlier wine-growers, most of them, however, were derived from his own experiments on his Stagira farm.

His theories are profoundly affected by PHILISTON of Locri (S. Italy)'s views on respiration and diseases of the respiratory organs, written about 388 B.C. He believes that plants derive their "vital spirit" (pneuma) from the soil and draw it up through the pithy parts of the stalk together with water. Hence the quality of grapes is largely determined by the ratio of wooden and pithy parts of the stalk. The more pith the stalk has the juicer the grape, though at the same time this engenders the danger of evaporation and loss of juice during summer.

From this theory THEOPHRASTUS then deduces the correct way of striking cuttings from good vines, the conditions under which they should be planted, the porosity and moisture of the soil and the care to be spent on the cuttings during the first few years. THEOPHRASTUS rejects grafting which will never give good vines. Though he does not yet recognize the part leaves play in plant growth his advice is generally admirable and often very modern.

He also discusses in great detail the art of pruning, which should not only be confined to the barren wild tendrils. It should be attuned to the type of grape and soil. In dry, hot soils the vine should be pruned in autumn, in wet, cold soils in spring according to his "pneuma" theory. Finally he discusses the value of sprinkling the bunches of grapes with pulverized earth to protect them from the heat of the sun, a common practice in classical viticulture. On the whole his essays show how little practical experience of wine-growers has changed during the last 2200 years. They also demonstrate how Greek genius was able to raise viticulture from a craft to a science. All throughout classical Antiquity Greek wines managed to hold their enviable reputation.

Greek wine-growers avoided propping, trellising or festooning their vines, a practice typical for Roman vineyards where the "pergola" originated. They favoured layering their vines along the soil except where summer moisture made propping necessary. Hence mice and foxes were great enemies of the wine-growers who invoked the help of Apollo Smintheus the "mouse killer". Low-growing vines saved money and escaped the summer winds, but they demanded very careful hoeing to keep the soil free of weeds and to pulverize it sufficiently to retain water. This hoeing was repeated twice or trice a year. In summer all unnecessary leaves were primed to avoid evaporation. Sometimes green manure was used or greens planted between the rows of vines were broken up instead. Women often worked in the vineyards of Greece. September was the vintagemonth, the grapes were collected early that month in the plains and towards the end in the hills. It started with an important festival during which a boy sang the song of Linus, god of the wine-press to the tune of a lyre surrounded by a circle of boys and girls stamping the earth with their feet and ending by dancing and shouting. The bunches of grapes were collected

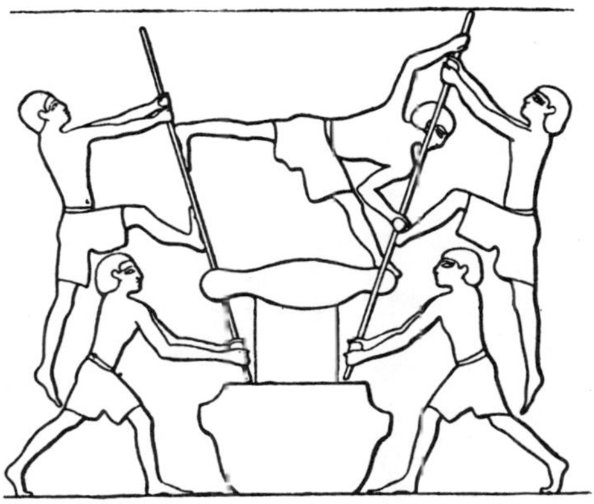

Fig. 26. Egyptians "wringing the cloth"

in baskets and brought to the "wine-press", that is to low cement vats slightly inclined towards one corner. Thence the grape-juice flowed when the grapes were tred with the feet of the workers. Sometimes

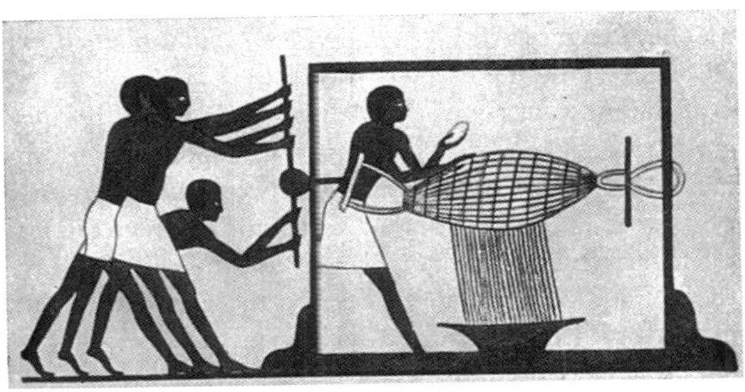

Fig. 27. Last stage of the bag-press

these vats were made of accaciawood. This first must, more particularly the juice extruded from the grapes by their own weight (the "prodomos" or "protopos") was especially valued as it could be kept fairly long.

The rest of juice was extracted in the same primitive press which the Ancient East had used. It was wrung from the treaded grapes in a bag-press made of cloth or in a plaited mat. However, the Greeks soon invented a new type of press, the beam-press, in which a long beam having its turning-point at one end and loaded by heavy stones on the other compresses the layers of grapes separated by mats piled up about half-way its length. It is claimed that it goes back to the Mycenean period but real proof of its existence is obtained only from pictures on early Greek vases. A third-grade wine was prepared by mixing or even cooking the lees with some water and expressing this

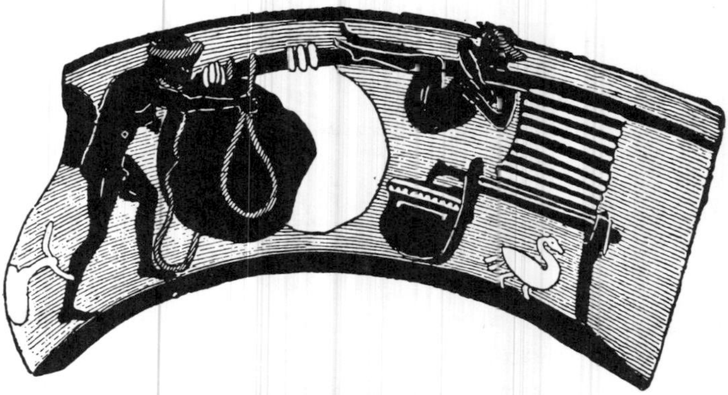

Fig. 28. The Greek beam-press

mixture. The "deuterias" or "stemphylites" thus obtained was only drunk by the very poor.

Some of the must was consumed after treating it with vinegar but the larger part was then stored in cellars in huge pottery fermenting vats. These "pithoi" of considerable size were the common storage vats for oil, wine and the like in the Greek world, which did not know the wooden barrel, and later only seldom used this northern invention. Often these "pithoi" were buried deep in the ground after they had been smeared with pitch or resin inside and outside. This was not only done to correct the porosity of this type of pottery but also because the ancients appreciated the peculiar taste thus imparted to the wine, a flavour still characteristic of the Greek "retzinato".

These "pithoi" were often upto 10' high with a mouth of 3' diameter. After the civil wars when there was a severe housing shortage in Athens many citizens slept in such vats. The Greek poet ARISTOPHANES (6) mentions "the vat-sleepers" (pithaknai) living on the suitable spots in town", and the philosopher DIOGENES probably never slept in a barrel but in one of these pithoi.

During the six-month fermenting period the liquid was constantly skimmed. Then the fermenting vats were opened during the spring festival of the "pithoigia" or "opening of the vats" on the eleventh day of the month Anthesterion and corresponding with the Roman "Vinalia" celebrations. The wine was then transferred to skins (askoi) or pointed pottery jars (amphorae) for transport and sale. The handles

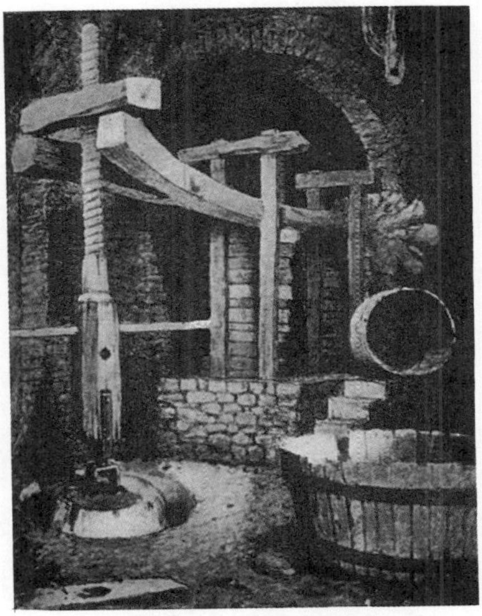

Fig. 29. The beam-press of Boscoreale

and stoppers were stamped to indicate the brand, the origin and the vintage. During this transfer the wine was filtered through perforated metal sieves or cloth as the fermented juice contained much dregs and other contaminations.

The main difficulty of the Greek vintners was the instability of their wines. As cork stoppers were still unknown, it was practically impossible to stop fermentation during storage. Hence wines had to be consumed within three, at most four years. Nestor may have drunk a ten-year old vintage and ATHENAEUS, the wine-expert, may mention a 16-year old wine, these are exceptions to the rule given by the poet THEOCRITOS. The second problem that puzzled even such expert vintners as SERAMBOS, whom PLATO mentions (7) was the acidity of their wines. They tried to correct it by treating the wine with sea-water, turpentine, pitch, resin, chalk, gypsum, lime prepared from marble or shells and aromatic herbs. Usually resin gave the Greek wine its peculiar "bouquet". In certain cases wines were specially prepared as ingredients for unguents and cosmetics.

The Greek poets give us much information on the different types of wines produced. They are distinguished by their colour (black, red, white or yellow) or by their taste (dry, harsh, light or sweet). The

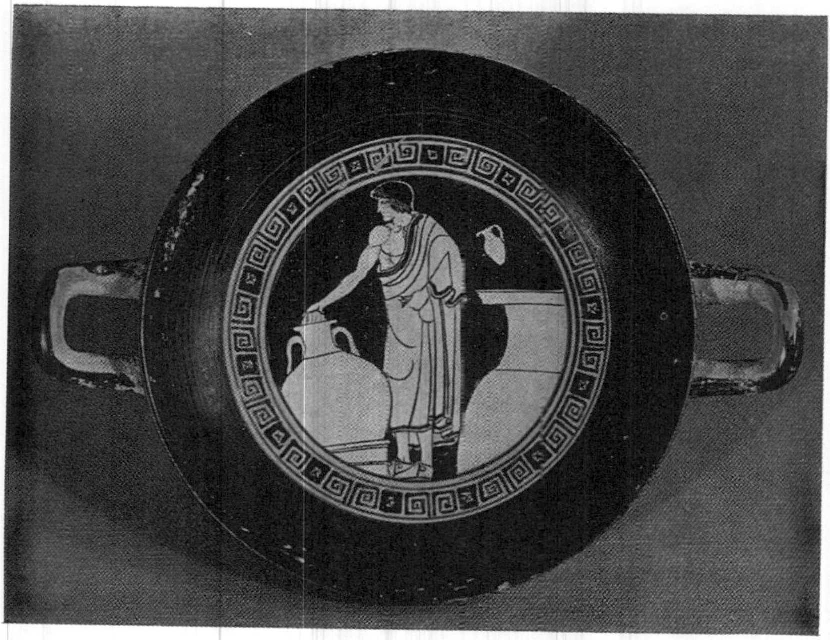

Fig. 30. Testing wine

different brands are discussed by many authors, above all by ATHENAEUS who mentions no less than 85 different wines (9); drugs preventing alcoholism such as owl's eggs are mentioned.

The producers and wine-merchants bought their wine after testing a sample (deigma), and even clients tested their wine occasionally. It was done by dipping a sponge into the large pithoi and then testing taste and bouquet of the wine. Often the "taste-vin" would spill a few drops on the back of his hand to test it, as he did with olive-oil (9). It was then sold over the counter in the wine-shop (kapeleion) mostly in units called a "kotyle" (475 cc), thence the verb "kotylizein" came to mean "selling wine". Wine was never drunk as such but always mixed with water. At dinner-parties the toast-master indicated the dilution-ratio. We are told that certain wines were so strong that they had to be diluted to a twenty-fold volume!

It has been claimed that the expansion of Greek civilisation in the wake of Alexander the Great's conquest, which we call Hellenism, was determined by the natural limits of viticulture.

The Chinese general Chan K'ien on his mission to the West spent a year in Bactria in 128 B.C. and reported that grape-wine was made and drunk in Ferghana and Parthia. Seeds were sent home and planted by the Emperor (10). Though this was the beginning of the cultivation of the grape in China and Japan, and various wild grapes had been known for centuries, the art of making or drinking wine was adopted much later during the reign of T'ai Tsung (A.D. 640) who himself became a great connoiseur.

As Alexander and his successors dumped the wine of their domains on their natural markets, the new Hellenistic cities sprinkled throughout the Near East they were slowly undermining Greek viticulture. At first their policy brought wealth to Greece and the islands Chios, Samos, Lesbos and Thasos throve. When the Ptolemaic kings of Egypt temporarily dominated some of these islands they were constantly in desparate need of silver to pay for their wine-imports. However, here again, the development in the Black Sea area and other regions repeated itself. The Greeks in the Near East began to grow their own wines and imported top-qualities only from the home-land.

In Hellenistic Egypt, for instance, there was an extensive planting of vines on the recently reclaimed lands in the Delta, especially in the Mareotic and Arsinoite nomes (provinces). The Zenon papyri show that Zenon the landowner bought wine from Thasos, Cnidos, Chios, Leucas & Lesbos. But a large land-owner like Apollonius sent messengers to obtain cuttings in Cilicia, Chalcidice, Thrace, Phoenicia and Alexandria, in total eleven varieties. One letter mentions 10.000 vine plants and 1700 shoots, another 20.000 vine-cuttings. He was finally able to export wine to Palestine and Suria.

The Ptolemies took great care to promote this trend. The usual wine-tax (apomoira) was $^1/_6$ of the produce of the vineyards to be paid in kind. The Greek settlers concentrating on wine-growing had to pay only $^1/_{10}$ and heavy import duties helped to protect them against the competition of imported wines.

Wine remained a necessity in Greek diet together with fish, bread and oil. But in the course of the second century B.C. conditions deteriorated in the homeland. The price of grain rose, that of oil and wine fell to unknown depth as did wages and finally the rents of vineyards had to follow. The wine-merchants of Cos, Delos and other islands in despair continued to dump their wine at any price. Finally through fallen wages and landrevenues the Greek wine-growers managed to survive. Exports to the Balkan countries, the Danube and Celtic lands in the West continued on a smaller scale and exports to Italy began to dwindle away. Indeed from 150—80 B.C. Roman wine-merchants and agents living in Delos played an important part in this centre of the wine-trade but bought only small quantities of first quality wines for their home-country.

The fame of these wines continued but Greek viticulture itself was more and more thrown back on its home-consumption and the "vin ordinaire" for the ordinary citizen became its main product. The "kapelos" was no longer a merchant of wine, oil and corn but he had to become dealer in general foodstuffs, a tavern-keeper and caterer in order to survive.

With Roman domination of Greece in 148 B.C. the end came and the importance of the Greek wine-trade and its centres passed away slowly. The Romans rewarded Rhodes by making it the centre of the wine trade in the Aegean and by-passing Delos. Exports continued to come from several islands but wine-growing for export seems to disappear from the mainland of Greece. However it never fell so low as to import Italian wines.

In the Hellenistic period the experience of wine-growers all over the civilised world was pooled. Chaereas the Athenian was well-acquainted with Babylonian practice and Bolos of Mendes (200 B.C.) reported on Egyptian viticulture. However, the practical and theoretical system devised by the Greek wine-growers and so admirably expressed by THEOPHRASTUS continued to dominate the art. It was adopted with minor modifications in Egypt and in the Western Mediterranean in Hellenistic and Roman Times.

The Romans inherited viticulture from the Etruscans. Tradition has it that Mezentius, king of Etruria, helped the Rutuli to throw the Latin tribes back on the south bank of the river Tiber (11). He was rewarded by a yearly tribute of wine at the feast of Vinalia, besides receiving all the wine then found in the conquered Latin territory. The Romans too were great wine-lovers, but like the Greeks they turned their wine to many uses. Undiluted wine "per se" was used as a medicine (12), as a sweetening ingredient when honey was too expensive and for the manufacture of vinegar. Wine was also an important ingredient in the composite fish-sauce "oenogarum" so dear to the Romans and used as frequently as we use ketchup, Worcester sauce and such concoctions.

Though the soil in many districts of Italy is eminently suited for viticulture and though we hear of wine-growers in early Roman history the rise of this art dates of the second Punic war only (242 B.C.). Hannibal and his African troops had washed their horses with wine at Picenum and they cut down the vineyards of Campania like they destroyed the farms of southern Italy. The fact that Sicily took over the corn-supply of Rome at the end of the war is in itself an indication of the shift of Roman agricultural policy. Vine- and olive-raising increased and the value of land quadrupled because of these profitable occupations. The replanting of Luciana and Apulia with vineyards counterbalanced Hannibal's wanton destruction of these areas.

The Roman playwright PLAUTUS (254—184 B.C.) mentions but Greek wines but this soon changes. Greek and Carthaginian treatises on viticulture are now translated and applied. After the fall of Carthage (146 B.C.) MAGO's work on farming and viticulture is translated into Latin by order of the Senate, though it was mainly important for information on dry-farming as applied in the recently conquered Africa. The Greek books such as those of THEOPHRASTUS, however, were of vital importance. Cuttings were imported from foreign countries and the vineyards began to grace the hill-sides. The grades and vintages of Italian wines also begin to be differentiated during the second century B.C. The vintage of 121 B.C. "the year in which Opimius was consul" was the most famous one and a few samples seem to have survived(?) in the Imperial Age when they were tasted and admired by connoisseurs. Italian names appear on wine labels. However, the rich still preferred Greek wines. The censors of 89 B.C. had to curtail the import of luxury wines by fixing a maximum price and even LUCULLUS or Caesar still resorted to Greek wines if they wanted to cajole the plebs of Rome. During the first century B.C. Italian wines can be said to have come in their own, (13) though sometimes subject to economic crises.

Roman agronomists now begin to write their own handbooks. CATO's book gives many details on wine growing in the second century B.C. (14). He tells us about the labour, traction-animals and equipment needed and gives a good budget and schedule for a 66 acre vineyard. VARRO (37 B.C.) adds but few details. More instruction can be obtained from Columella (A.D. 65) (15) and Pliny devotes the entire fourteenth book of *Natural History* to this art. Other data are scattered throughout Strabo's *Geography* and the verses of such poets as Martial (40—104 A.D.) and Virgil (70—19 B.C.). All these texts demonstrate that Greek viticulture was taken over but supplemented with minor improvements.

In contrast to Greek practice the Romans propped or trellised their vines. Very often the elm, ash or poplar appears as a support of vines in the "arbustum". In close-set vineyards chestnut or willow poles with cross-pieces or cane reeds were commonly used. The leaves of the trees were used for feeding cattle during the dry seasons. Sometimes corn is sown between the rows of vines as a secondary crop. Later generations often overlooked the detailed prescriptions of the classical wine-growers but they proved very practical hints. The maturity of the grape was judged by the colour of the stones and great care was taken in harvesting. The Romans maintained that the first grapes harvested gave the largest percentage of juice, the second lot was the best and the last harvest gave the sweetest wine. In some cases the grapes were harvested one by one, and anyhow all the branches and stalks had to be carefully removed. In Italy too harvesting began early September but might last until the first frost period like in the region of the Thurii.

The first juice obtained by treading or extruded by the grape's own weight in the press-room (vinum primarium, lixivum) was immediately bottled in amphorae and very carefully handled. Then the grapes were usually pressed in beam-presses; after adding some water to the lees a second pressing could be obtained. The press-room was a separate part of the "wine-factory", the juice obtained was sieved and then collected in a large vat or container (lacus) whence it flowed by gravity through channels or pipes into the fermenting vats. Sometimes force-pumps were used to displace these liquids. The Greek beam-press was considerably improved by the Roman engineers. In order to get a constant pressure during the entire pressing period they not only loaded the beam-end but often pulled it down with pulleys or screws so that constant adjustment was possible (16). The screw invented by Greek mathematicians about the lifetime of Archimedes (300 B.C.), was first used to press down the boards of a press and the mass of grapes or olives between them at then end of the first century B.C. Wedges were sometimes driven between the boards of the presses to exert extra pressure on the compacted bags of grapes.

Roman fermenting cellars ("cellae vinariae") were seldom as deep as the modern ones, though they were built away from trees and dung-heaps which might influence the taste of the wine. Later large amphorae were placed on a rack in the storage-room or attic ("apotheca") or even in a room that could be heated ("fumarium"). For the Romans carefully adjusted the conditions of fermentation ("efferviscatio") to the nature of each type of grape. In Campania this took place in the sun in the open air. The grapes of the Po valley would soon turn sour by this treatment so they were fermented indoors. The Falernian wine with a high initial sugar content fermented very quickly and completely in the open air. Pliny claims that no further fermentation was possible and that it could burn because of the high alcohol content. On the other hand rapid fermentation may affect the bouquet and this the ancients knew quite well. They also observed very strict hygienic rules in the fermentation room, some of which were of a religious nature. During fermentation the wine was mixed and the froth was removed. If the fermentation did not take place properly fresh must was added.

Careful precautions were taken to prevent after-fermentation. The fermenting vats were drawn in May-July when northern winds prevailed and the weather was dry. The amphorae were filled and marked, but often decanted later on. During the tapping the liquid was filtered ("liquare") and all yeast cells removed ("defaecato"). Too much handling was avoided in order to retain the bouquet. White of egg was sometimes used to obtain a clear wine.

In order to obtain a fully ripened wine there was usually a final heat-treatment in the "fumarium". The idea was to hasten the ripening, to kill all bacteria and to make the wine keep its qualities longer. In fact it was one of the first steps on the way to pasteurization. Not all wine was treated "in a bottle in the smoke" (Ps. 119.83), some wines were simply exposed to the sun in jars, again must might be inspissated in jars immersed in hot water. Unfortunately this process was also used to speed up ripening of second-class wines, changing their flavour to obtain a higher price if necessary by adding other wines or sherds of old fermenting vats during the process.

In fact Roman wine-merchants knew many tricks to change the flavour of their wines. A test involving a 40-day immersion of a strip of copper, tin or lead was used to detect tartar. Wines were often mixed with inspissated must ("defrutum") to obtain a higher alcohol content. Resin was often added to wines, notably to those of Gaul, which were liable to suffer from after-fermentation by insufficient treatment. Wood-tar pitch was used for the same purpose and the word "crapula" (hang-over) was often used for pitch. Adding lime (Chaptalize) was common in some areas, gypsum improved the lustre of the wine (vin plâtré). Sea-water was added to improve its clarity. Herbs and flowers imparted an artificial "bouquet" to the wine. Essences were concocted from "defrutum", herbs and berries. Vermouth was imported from the Pontic or Alpine region. This addition of herbs and sweetening ingredients was called "condire". Diluting wines and adding "defrutum" or honey (the modern "gallisation") was also practised. Hence most of the modern tricks of the trade were well-known to the Roman vintners.

Some wines took 10—15 years to ripen and the risks were so great that these tricks were often resorted to. Certainly the more scientific handling allowed the Romans to keep their wines longer than the Greek, but the labels and inscriptions of wine-jars show us that 3—4 years was the rule. These trade-marks were usually written on the body of the jar in ink, red lead or white paint, though wooden labels were sometimes attached to the neck of the jar. They inform us on the vintage, the origin, the date of tapping and who tapped them, the purity, the name of the vintner, the colour, the type of grapes, the number of the jar and the name of the cellarer.

Trade used pottery amphorae, the metal flaggons were for domestic use only like the glass amphorae which were occasionally used for high quality wines. The amphorae contained 26 L of wine, the larger unit being a leather bag or skin, the culleus (of 20 amphorae). The tonnage of wine-ships was measured in thousands of amphorae (16a). Mass transport was usually done in leather skins or in wooden barrels. The barrel or cask was a gift of the Northern peoples to the Roman world. STRABO is the first to mention these "wooden pithoi" and he adds that the Celts are excellent coopers and use their wood-tar pitch. "For their casks are larger than houses and the excellent supply of pitch helps them to smear (the cracks of) these pithoi". (17).

Making wooden barrels and casks dates back to the Late Bronze Age inhabitants of Switzerland and it gained very much by the advent of iron tools by the La Tène Age. Now good barrels built up from dowelled staves and strengthened with hoops and metal bands penetrated southwards about the beginning of our era though they remained expensive. The cask is called "cupa" (18) and they become so common soon that the emperor Maximus could bridge a river near

Aquilea with old wine-casks (19). The word "tun" is derived from a late-Latin "tunna" which is not used before the ninth century A.D. The Late-Latin "butis" (wooden cask) is the ancestor of the English "butt" and the French "bouteille" (bottle) but it dates of the same period. Wooden barrels were now used for storage and transport more particularly in northern Italy and we have indeed a Roman relief showing a rowing vessel transporting wine-casks.

Some amphorae were protected by plaited straw. We have here the origin of the Italian "fiasco". Some amphorae contained a thin layer of oil to shut out the air. In most cases, however, clay or cork stoppers were used supplemented with pitch, resin, cement or gypsum. In his 4,000 *years under the Sea* Ph. Diolé mentions that many amphorae have been recovered from wrecks near the Riviera coast which were either stoppered with cork and covered by a disk of pozzolana on which the trademark was stamped or with stoppers of terra-cotta covered with vine leaves, daubed with clay and kept in position with twine. Cork stoppers seem to have come into use in the first century B.C. This more efficient stoppering of the amphorae was of considerable assistance to the Roman vintners in storing their wines without trouble. Hence the Romans use oblinere (to daub) or gypsare (to plaster) for "corking", and deradere (to scrape) or relinere (to break) for "uncorking". The Roman soldier may have had his pottery hip-flask, the wine-grower wanted large capacity vessels. A Roman villa at Boscoreale had 84 dolia of 315 gallons each, 72 of which had contained wine. Usually wine-growers had 30—50 of these huge vats in their cellars. Most wine-growers sold their product to retail-dealers or directly to the public through a slave tavern-keeper in a pub adjoining their house. Some sold the crop on the vine.

Classical authors praise many brands. Pliny discusses 150 wines and varieties of grapes though some of his "foreign wines" were culled from obsolete Greek books. Athenaeus knows of 85 brands of wines, Galen enumerates 60, Strabo 30 varieties. Very few came from "slave-run factories", small wine-growers who produced one or two special brands abound. Wine-growing became so attractive because it paid well. Generally speaking 18% was obtained yearly on the capital invested. The yield per acre was some 4000 l for high-grade wines and double the amount of other wines. Only piracy was more profitable but far more risky. The vintners became mighty and wealthy men, many obtained a knighthood. They were a power in Roman politics, notably when they formed a trust in the third century A.D.

(20). The power of the "corpora vinariorium" was based on the fact that wine was Italy's most important export product, though over 30.000.000 hl were consumed yearly in the homeland.

Africa had a small production of no remarkable quality. It was Rome's granary rather than a wine-growing country. In the Imperial period the coastal strips were partly converted into vineyards. Africa produced excellent smoke-died grapes which the emperor Tiberius loved. In Syria and Palestine there was extensive local viticulture particularly on the large estates. Talmudic authorities forbade the export of local production. Mesopotamia, lost to the Romans after the Parthian wars, with Parthia played a large part in the transmission of Greek methods to the Far East. In Asia Minor and the countries on the Black Sea local production continued though sometimes threatened by Spanish exports. From Egypt we have many papyri informing us on details of local vineyards. However this country was mainly important as a trade-station between Rome, India and the East in which wine also played an important part. From Egyptian sources (20a) we know that wine formed part of the pay of farm-labourers and soldiers, who could exchange their wine "coupons" for money or other goods. Most of the Near Eastern countries lost their vineyards with the Arab conquest, viticulture barely survived the sword of the Prophet.

When Spain was conquered by the Romans (133 B.C.) the Iberians had some vineyards but their favourite drink was a kind of mead (21). During the Imperial period viticulture made such rapid strides that Spanish wines became severe competitors for Italian brands not only in Gaul, Britain and Germany but even in the East. Enormous quantities of these second quality wines were imported in Italy, sherds of the jars which contained them form the largest percentage of the 150 foot high Monte Testacio at Ostia, the main harbour of Rome. The vine was even carried to Britain where a quantity of vine-stems were found in the immediate neighbourhood of a Roman villa at Boxmoor (Herts.) on a sheltered slope facing west and south. However viticulture disappeared with the Roman conquerors.

When the Romans dethroned the Greek vintners in the world, they did not learn the lesson of history. In the face of competition from the provinces they tried political force and the law. The emperor Domitianus tried to forbid viticulture in the provinces during an Italian wine-crisis and even ordered vineyards in Gaul and Spain to be cut down (22) in 92 A.D. This was more or less a repetition of an older Republician edict forbidding the Gauls to cultivate the vine or the olive-tree (23). Neither could nor was properly enforced and the emperor Probus in 282 A.D. officially withdrew it. In the Imperial period free wine had become so important a part of the policy of "panem et circenses" that large imports in Italy had to be tolerated, lest the plebs might revolt (24). The results of this policy came in the third and fourth centuries A.D. when the value of money fell quickly and the political situation became unstable. The troubled times that followed led to neglect of the irrigation system and proper care for the vineyards. The times when Italy could exchange its wine for Danubian slaves, cattle and hides, Celtic honey and ailver and other goods had passed away.

Roman penetration of Gaul transformed this country of beer-drinkers into the traditional land of wine-lovers. It became the centre of the reconquest of *Europe as a wine-growing country*. The Romans had furthered the production of second-class wines in the province of Narbonensis (Gaul south of Lyon). In the trade-centre Lyon the powerful wine-merchants and their allies the skippers (nautae) handled the import- and export-trade to northern France and Germany. Lyon's decline dated from the years 197 A.D. when Septimus Severus took and sacked the town. Meanwhile local production of better wines by more scientific Roman methods had started all over Gaul. When we hear of the wines of Beaune (Burgundy) in the third century A.D. (25) the vines are "of a hoary age", and the wines of Bordeaux (26) and of the Mosel (27) are certainly several centuries older than the fourth century A.D. texts that first mention them. It is certain that not only were there brewers in Metz and Trier early, but that Caesar's legions brought the vineyards to the Rhine (28).

The fall of the Roman Empire, the incursions of Germanic and Asiatic tribes, of Moslem armies and Vikings meant a severe set-back for viticulture. The vine finally disappeared completely from regions like southern England, northern France, Swabia and eastern Bavaria which it had conquered in Roman or later times. Indeed medieval viticulture meant but a slow rediscovery of the excellent classical techniques. In many places Christianity assisted the survival of the vineyards as every parish tried to produce its own wine needed for the Catholic ritual. The recovery was greatly assisted by the fact that Spain, France and part of Germany had been definitely converted to wine-drinking. Wine also remained a major ingredient in pharmaceutical and medical recipes and therefore many treatises were devoted to its medical use (29).

The Barbarian invaders had never destroyed an appreciable percentage of the vineyards and they were soon keenly interested in the wine which many Imperial edicts had formerly withheld from them, as were Charles the Great and his successors. During the ninth century viticulture began to flourish again in the regions of Worms and Speyer, spread into the Rheingau and even reached Swabia, Franconia and Thuringia. By 1200 it had crossed the Elbe river into the middle Oder district. During the Middle-Ages wine-growing was still practised in England, Flanders and the Pyrenees, since lost to the vintner.

In France there was a considerable extension of vineyards especially in regions where the soil yielded less corn, particularly in the West. Religious houses held vineyards as distant as the Rhine, Moselle, Champagne and the region of Paris and met severe difficulties in managing estates so far apart. More important, however, was the fact that France and Germany were trying to improve the quality of their wines. True, the flavour, thinness and roughness of second-quality medieval wines was often concealed by special treatments or by the addition of herbs or spices such as honey, cinnamon, sage or coriander. Grapes that did not ripen and green grapes formed the base material ("verjuice") for vinegar production. Better types of grapes were grown and selected. Classical methods were adopted in these regions. We find a full programme of work based on classical experience in the eleventh-century charter of the abbey of Muri (Zürich) and similar foundations Willow plantations usually accompanied the vineyards in order to supply the withes and barrel-hoops. Italy where many municipalities frantically tried to revive classical viticulture during the fourteenth century fell behind.

The Middle Ages produced few books on viticulture and wine that could cap the classical essays. ARNALD DE VILLANOVA (1235—1311) when shipwrecked on the coast of Africa wrote a book *On Wine*, describing medical wines and their uses. In 1478 VON HIRNKOFEN added to this book another Latin manuscript on wine-growing, the production and preservation of wine and beer also ascribed to VILLANOVA, translated the whole into German and had it printed in Esslingen (Germany). It became a best-seller, no less than 21 editions were produced within a century (30).

His contemporary PIETRO DEI CRESCENZI (1233—1320) composed a *De vineis et vito*, an excellent book on vines, viticulture, wine-production, preservation and correction compiled from observations in Italy and Provence, more comprehensive than VILLANOVA's. Neither book contains any technological innovation in the production of wines One generation later the Muslim historian and physician IBN AL-KHAṬÎB (1313—1374) was the first in the eastern world not to decry wine officially but to justify the use of wine for Christians and Jews in his medical treatise of 1360.

The fermentation of grape-juice being so successful many peoples have tried making *wines from other fruit* like apples and pears. These attempts were not always successful as they depend on the sugar content of these fruit. Though wild pears and apples grew in prehistoric Europe we find that no such drinks were produced in appreciable quantities, until cultivated apples like the Pirus Malus L. pumila were introduced from the East by way of the Mediterranean world. The Romans knew many kinds of apples but the Gauls had no cider though they had imported new kinds of apples and pears.

More serious cultivation of apples and pears hardly started before the fifth century A.D. and a hundred years later we hear of the first cider in Europe. In regulations for his estates CHARLEMAGNE (800—812) speaks of brewers who prepare fermented drinks from grapes, apples, pears and other fruit. Old French documents more frequently mention "pomatium" and "piracium". However both cider and perry were poor man's drinks. When ST. GÚEGOLÉ of Brittany (464—532) wants to chastise herself she lives on water and perry. ST. RADEGONDE (513) and ST. SÉGOLÈNE (753) drink only perry. Then these drinks often seem to have been brewn from wild fruit. Another second-grade brew was called"dépense" and consisted of a decoction of sliced apples, grapes, etc.

Though some claim that better apples and pears came west with the Crusaders, it seems that several came from the Basque country where cider brewing was very old in the eleventh and twelfth centuries. Normandy became the home of the new types of cider and from there it came to England in the thirteenth century. However as late was 1486 the archbishop of Rouen still had 70 bushels of (wild) apples from his forest, though he improved his orchards by planting and grafting new kinds of apples. The new cider won much ground with the farming population whose corn was often too expensive and sometimes too short to be used for home-brew. Thus cider established itself firmly in the countryside.

We should also mention a side-line of viticulture. In the period we are discussing sugar was either unknown or an imported luxury. Hence honey was its substitute but as supplies were rather short, grape-juice was used as a substitute and often called so (mellis vice) (31). Must could be kept a year, the Romans filled it in jars, shut and sealed them tightly and immersed them in cold river or sea-water, thus stopping fermentation. It could be evaporated in leadlined vessels and used as a sweetening ingredient. Reduced to half its volume it was called "defrutum", to $^2/_3$ "sapa". Quite an appreciable percentage of the most of the vineyards was turned into "defrutum" and "sapa". We even know of factories of this substitute honey, some was imported from Syria. It was used to preserve olives and all kinds of food. The production of "save" continued well into the Middle Ages and it was still used in eighteenth century France.

Beer

Beer may have been consumed in ancient Crete. Pots with spouts very suitable for beer were found and some archaeologists deem that some kind of beer, may be imported from Egypt, preceded wine in the island (32). However, the Greeks knew beer (zythos) only as a barbarian product and very rarely drank it. Nor did the Romans like it. Tacitus (33) informs us that the Germans drank "a liquor drawn from barley or from wheat, and like the juice of the grape, fermented to a spirit". When the Roman Emperor Julian the Apostate drank "cervesia" for the first time in Gaul he wrote a satirical poem (34) on its tendency to cause flatulence. This deep rooted aversion of beer in the classical world survived until the nineteenth century in Italy and Greece.

In its homeland, the Near East, beer continued to be very popular. In the Hellenistic period brewing was a royal privilege in Egypt. It was brewed from barley and consumed in large quantities during the hot season. Professional brewers organised in local guilds were in the service of the state. In certain cases licenses seem to have been given for home-brewing. The brewers and their guilds were concessionaires of the government, receiving a certain quantity of barley and sold their beer to retail dealers and consumers. Contractors underwote the collection of the beer tax, for every Egyptian had to pay for the right to buy beer.

Hellenistic and Roman brewing methods did not differ much from more ancient ones, nor from those still in use. Zosimos, the famous chemist of Panopolis (Egypt) is reported to have written a book on brewing (300 A.D.) (35). The Romans continued the policy of their

Ptolemaic predecessors. Their capitation tax "zytera" was 4 drachmae per person, where the price of beer was 1 drachmae per 3 choes (10 l). The individual consumption varied from 1—3 choes per month. Topers paid on account. Then in the third century A.D. prices of beer rise with those of cereals. We also find that beer is frequently purchased privately and distributed to workmen engaged in the home and the fields.

We have little detailed information on brewing methods in Roman times. Some private brewers were attached to the larger estates. Sometimes the temples have breweries endowed to them by the king and not operated by them. The taxes paid by these temples may represent the capitation tax collected, the licence fee or both, as brewers seem to have been used as tax collectors by the state.

From the papyri we also know that the brewing trade flourished in Babylonia in Roman times. In Syria and Palestine fruit-wines and fruit-beers are mentioned in our sources and may even have been exported. Many Roman estates in these regions have their own brewery for home production.

Millet-beers were known in China several centuries B.C., but we do not know whether the cultural exchange between the Near and the Far East involved any exchange of brewer's techniques. The art of beer-making came to Tibet by the way of China about 650 A.D. and involved both barley- and millet-beers.

In the West the Celts had known the art of brewing before the Egyptian methods could have been transmitted by the Greeks and the Romans. The classical authors, who are not interested in beer, report little on their brewing methods but that they used barley or corn. "The nations of the West have their own intoxicant made from grain soaked in water; there are a number of ways of making it in the various provinces of Gaul and Spain and under different names though the principle is the same. The Spanish provinces have by this time even taught us that these liquors will bear being kept a long time" (36). The German tribes adopted brewing in the first century B.C.

The Celts had discovered the preparation of beer yeast for we are told (37): "When the corn of Gaul and Spain of the kind we discussed is steeped to make beer, the foam that forms on the surface in the process is used for leaven, in consequence of which those races have a lighter kind of bread than others."

We do not hear of great breweries in these parts. Probably most beer was produced as home-brew, though the cornmarkets of Cologne,

Metz and Trier showed inscriptions of brewers ("cervesarii"). The oldest sample of beer dating of 353 A.D. is shown in the museum of Alzey, though many dregs of evaporated beer were found in Celtic and German graves. In many cases honey was found to have been added to sweeten the beer, a custom still surviving in certain regions on the continent. Our word "beer" is derived from the Latin for drinking (bibere). The break in brewing tradition during the classical period is further demonstrated by the fact that our brewing terms have been created in the Middle Ages when the monasteries were great centres of beer production, where large scale production and cleanliness contributed greatly to modern brewing technique (38).

The most important medieval discovery in brewing was hopped beer. The addition of hops to beer means not only a change in taste but also the possibility of keeping the beer much longer. We know from PLINY's note on the beer of the Iberians that this was not an innovation. From times immemorial herbs had been added to alcoholic infusions to flavour and to preserve them. Some of these herbs contained narcotic substances or they were considered to be magically potent (39).

Hence hop, a creeper (Humulus, Lupulus L.) the top leaves of which contain an alkaloid called lupulin, had to fight its way to the top. It had to compete with ling or heather and with mixtures of herbs, such as the "gruit" of medieval Germany which contained sweetgale or bog myrthe, marsh or wild rosemary, milfoil or yarrow and other herbs. It was most important in German breweries. As late as 1380 the Archbishop Frederic of Cologne ordered all his subjects to buy their gruit from his episcopal "gruithouses" only and he forbade all imports of Westphalian hopped beer. Hopped beer came from Hamburg and Bremen to Holland to compete with the local gale-beer.

Hops were known to the classical world as a kind of vegetable, but mostly as a herb used in medicine (40). It definitely first belonged to the herb-garden. It is first mentioned in the charter of Pepin II of 768 in which hop-gardens (humlonaries) are given to the abbey of St. Denis near Paris (41). In 822 the abbot Adalhard of Corvey releases the millers of their duty to grind malt (malce) and hop (humlo), probably the first time hop and brewing are linked together. The number of hop-gardens seems to have increased quickly and early in the ninth century the abbey of St. Germain des Prés had sufficient supplies from its own garden. The abbey of St. Gallen grows its own hops about 1030.

Hopped beer is said to have been made in Bavaria between 859 and 895 but our earliest definite reference to hopped beer dates of the eleventh century botanist HILDEGARD of Bingen (42), who claims that hop preserves barley beer because of its bitter taste. About 1031 the monastery of St. Emmeram had its hop-gardens near Regensburg and Straubing in order to produce hopped beer. The codex of Niederalteich (1260) mentions hop and beer and the herb begins to appear in many judicial documents. It is now grown in many regions without vineyards such as Magdeburg (1070), Silesia (1224) and southern Sweden (end of the thirteenth century). Curiously enough some of the most famous medieval botanists such as Albertus Magnus (43) (1260) describe hops, but do not mention its use in brewing. This is, however, recognised by Conrad of Megenburg (44) in 1340.

The cultivation of hops extended to northern Germany, Bohemia and Flanders where it gained commercial importance in the fourteenth century some 400 years after its introduction, when hopped beer begins to appear frequently in documents and laws. A letter of the bishop of Liège and Utrecht of 1304 complains that hopped beers "are now competing on the market some 30 or 40 years". A century later French brewers at Dieppe import it from Holland and England. Therefore it must have been imported into England before or shortly after 1400, though the first king to prohibit the use of hops was Henry VIII (1530). The word "hoppe" in English documents dates of the fifteenth century only and occurs frequently in the regulations of the London Brewers of 1418, 1442 & 1483.

There is considerable confusion in the older documents on beer. Usually the word "ale" is applied to an unspiced malted beverage and "beer" to a spiced one, later hopped beer is called "beer" and "ale" denotes beer made without hops. Earlier documents mention "strong beer" (the first strainings from the mash-tun) and "small beer" (the later washings), qualities probably coinciding with the "bitter beer" and "penny ale" of fourteenth century documents, the price of which is 4 d. and 1 d. a gallon. Still beer is often called "porter" and strong-vatted ale is denoted as "beer". This confusion is gradually dispelled as the trade is regulated in the fifteenth century and the law controls brewing which is to become an excellent object of taxation under Charles II. We can therefore state that hopped beer had slowly won its way to the top of the ladder by 1500, when the cultivation of hops was mainly centered in western Germany.

It would seem from Dutch medieval texts that originally wort and malt were boiled together in the beer kettle. Much later malt was treated with hot water in a mash-tun, the wort being sieved and the liquid filled into the kettle, sometimes together with hops. In some cases the wort was boiled as such, "medulla brassii" seems to indicate wort, "soppa fermenti" the spent grains.

We have hardly any complete medieval description of brewing, the scraps of information we have show that no important change in technique occurred except the introduction of hops. A few incunabula deal with the medieval use of beer (45).

Bibliography

(1) Evans, A., *The Ring of Nestor* (*J. Hellenic Studies* 1925, p. 19)

(2) Fimmen, E., *Die Kretisch-mykenische Kultur* (Leipzig 1924, 118)
Leonardi, C., *Ampelos. Il simbolo della vite* (Roma 1947)

(3) Navarro, J. M. de, *Massila and Early Celtic Culture* (*Antiquity*, 1928, 423—440)

(4) edit. Sir Arthur Hort (*Loeb Classical Library* Nos. 70 & 79, 1916)

(5) Senn, G., *Der Rebbau im antiken Griechenland* (*Gesnerus*, Vol. I, 1944, 3, 77—91)
Dion, R., *La viticulture dans l'Antiquité Grecque* (*Revue des deux Mondes*, 1952, 465—486)
André, J., *Contribution au vocabulaire de la viticulture, les noms des cépages* (*Revue Etud. Lat.*, Vol. 30, 1952, pags. 126—156)
Piccaluga, G., *Numa e il vino* (*Stud. Mat. Stor. Relig.* XXXIII, 1962, 99—103)
Barzen, R. M., *Das Winzermesser und andere Schneidgeräte im römischen Weinbau* (*Trierisches Jahrbuch* 1957, 85—90)
Parruzot, P. et Leber, P., *Outils de vignerons gallo-romains* (*Revue Archéol. de l'Est* V, 1954, 147—152)

(6) Aristophanes, *The Knights*, line 795

(7) Gorgias, 518 B
Boyancé, P., *Platon et le vin* (*Bull. Assoc. G. Budé* 1951, 3—19)
Salvi, C., *Rosin in amphorae* (*Pitture e vernici*, 6, 1950, 104)

(8) *The Deipnosophists* (edit. C. B. Gulick) (*Loeb Classical Library*)
Steiner, G., *Owl's eggs and Dionysus* (*Classical Weekly* vol. 44, 1950/51, 117—118)

(9) Immerwahr, H. R., *An Athenian wine-shop* (*Trans. Amer. Phil. Assoc.*, Vol. 79, 1948, 184—190)
Brouette, E., *Vinum Falernum, contribution a l'étude de la sémantique latine au haut moyen âge* (*Classica et Mediaevalia* X, 1949, 267—273)
Durry, M., *Les femmes et le vin* (*Revue Etud. Latines* XXXIII, 1955, 108—113)
Schnur, H. C., *Vinum Opimianum* (*Class. Weekly* ,L 1957, 122—123)

(10) Laufer, B., *Sino-Iranica* (Chicago 1919, 220—245)
Huber, E., *Die Einführung des Weinbaus in Türkestan* (*Die Umschau* 31, 1927, 528—533)

(11) Pliny, *Natural History* XIV, 88

(12) Pique, R., *Le vin et la médicine dans* l'*antiquité* (*C.R. IV Congrès Chim. Ind.* 1925, 552—560)
Lantronici, N., *I vini medicinali nelle storia e nelle scienze* (Milan, 1947)

(13) Remark, P., *Der Weinbau im römischen Altertum* (München 1927)
Dalmasso, L., *La viticultura ai tempi dell' Impero romano* (Roma, 1941)

Aymard, A., *Les capitalistes Romains et la viticulture Italienne* (*Annales Economies, Sociétés, Civilisations* vol. II, 1947, 257—265)

Barzen, R. M., *Neue Arten der Rebenveredlung nach den antiken.... Columella* (Neustadt, 1958)

Bellini, L., *La viticoltura nella politica economica di Roma republicana* (*Mem. Accad. Lincei ser.* 8a *I*, 1948, 387—432)

Christoffel, K., *Durch die Zeiten strömt der Wein* (Hamburg, 1957)

Diolé, Ph., *4000 years under the sea* (New York, 1954, 46—48)

Seltman, Ch., *Wine in the ancient world* (London, 1957)

Galtier, G., *Le commerce des vins dans l'empire romain* (*Bull. anc. élev. École sup. Commerce de Montpellier* No. 207, 4e trim. 1951)

Heurgon, J., *Les lassii pompéiens et l'importation des vins italiens en Gaulle* (*La Parole del passato*, 1952)

Isnard, H., *La vigne en Algérie* (*Gap*, 1952)

Gerov, B., *Zur Frage des Weinbaus in Untermösien* (*Bull. Inst. Archéol. Bulgare*, Sofia XIX, 1955, 187—193)

(14) Cato the Censor, *On Farming* edit. E. Bréhaut (New York 1933)

(15) Columella, *De Re Rustica* (edit. H. B. Ash) (*Loeb Classical Library*) Books V & VI

(16) Drachmann, A. G., *Ancient Oil Mills and Presses* (Kopenhagen 1932)

Hörle, J., *Cato's Handbücher* (Paderborn 1929)

Juengst, E. und Thielscher, P., *Catos Keltern und Kollergänge, ein Beitrag zur Geschichte von Oel und Wein* (*Bonner Jahrb.* CLIV, 1954, 32—93)

(16a) Wallinga, H. T., *Nautika (I), The unit of capacity for ancient ships* (Mnemosyne, XVII, 1964, 1, 1—40)

(17) *Geography*, Book V, cap. 214 & 218

(18) Cicero, *In Pisonem*, 27

(19) Herodianus, 8.4.9; Capitolinus, *Maximus* 22

(20) Lampadius, *Alex. Sev.* 33,2

(20a) Eitrem, S. & Amundsen, L., *Sale of Wine on Delivery* (*Eos*, 48, 1956, fasc. 2, 77—81)

Erichsen, W., *Ein demotischer Brief über eine Weinlieferung MDAI(K)*, Bd. 15, Festschrift Junker Teil I, 1958)

Turner, E. G., *The Hibeh Papyri Part II* (*Graeco-Roman Memoirs* No 32, London, 1955)

(21) Columella, 5.5.15; Diodor, 5.34

(22) Suetonius, *Domit.* 7.2

(23) Cicero, *De republ.* III, 9, 16

(24) Ammianus Marcellinus, 19.10

Chastagnol, A., *Un scandale du vin à Rome sous le Bas-Empire* (*Annales, Sociétés, Economies, Civilisations*, Vol. V, 1950, 166—183)

(25) Panegyr, V.6.4

Dion, R., *Les origines du vignoble bourguignon* (*Annales, Economies, Sociétés, Civilisations* vol. V, 1950, 433—439)

Lantier, R., *Le vin et l'huile en Bourgogne au temps gallo-romains* (*Rev. Arch.*, Vol. 40, 1952, pags. 103—105)

Dion, R., *La vigne en Gaule à l'époque romaine* (*Rev. Deux Mondes*, 1954, pags. 106—116; 499—515)

DION, R. *Histoire de la vigne et du vin en France.*
DION, R., *Le commerce des vins de Beaune au moyen Age.* — *Rev. hist. Fr. oct.—dec.* 1955, 214, 209—21.
NIERHAUS, R. *Kaiserzeitlicher Südweinexport nach dem freien Germanien?* — *Acta Arch. XXV*, 1954, 252—260
ROBERT, J. B. *Une contribution à l'histoire et à la géographie du vignoble européen.* — *Revue de Géographie de Lyons XXVIII*, 1953, 349—352
RÖPER, J. *Bodenspuren alten Weinbaus am Nördlichen Mittelrhein.* — *Rhein. Vierteljahrsbld. vol. XVIII*, 1953, 3/4, 170—193.
THÉVENOT, E. *Les importations vinaires en pays bourguignon avant le développement de la viticulture.* — *Revue Archéol. de l'Est IV*, 1953, 234—239
THÉVENOT, E. *Deux figurations du Dieu au maillet accompagné de tonneau ou amphore.* — *Gallia XI*, 1953, 293—306

(26) AUSONIUS, *Epist.* 9.18; PLINY, *Nat. Hist.* XIV.27
(27) AUSONIUS, *Mosella* 21, 160
(28) VARRO, *De Re Rustica* 1.7.8
(29) KLEBS, A., *Incunabila scientifica et medica* (*Osiris* IV, 1938, 1—359)
(30) *The earliest Book on Wine* (edit. H. E. SIGERIST) (New York 1943)
(31) *Palladius*, XI.19.1
(32) EVANS, Sir A., *Palace of Minos* Vol. I, p. 415
(33) *Germania*, chap. XXIII
(34) *Anthol. Palat.*, IX.38
(35) *Chr. Gott. Gruner: Xosimi de zythorum confectione*, Sulzbach 1914
(36) PLINY, *Nat. History* XIV.149
DIODOR, V.26.2
STRABO, *Geography* 3.3.7. cap. 155
(37) PLINY, *Nat. History* XVIII.68
FORBES, C. A., *Beer, a sober account* (*Class. J.*, Vol. 46, 1951, pags. 281—285, 300)
(38) KING, FRANK A., *Beer has a History* (London 1950)
(39) MAURIZIO, A., *Geschichte der gegorenen Getränke* (Berlin 1933)
(40) The "lupus salictarius" of PLINY (XXI, 86) and the "lupus" of MARTIAL IX.296)
(41) KILLERMAN, S., *Zur Geschichte des Hopfens* (*Tageszig. f. Brauerei*, Vol. 31, 1933, pags. 320—321 & 403—404)
KING, FRANK A., *Beer has a History* (London, 1947)
KOCH, R., *Die Untersuchung der Britzer Grabfunde* (*Berl. Bl. Vor-Frühgesch.* No. 1, 1952, 16—20)
DORKA, G., *Britzer Bier aus der Völkerwanderungszeit* (*Berl. Bl. Vor-Frühgesch.* No. 1, 1952, 10—16)
DOORMAN, G., *De Middeleeuwse Brouwerij en De Gruit* (*with a preface in English and German*) (Nijhoff, The Hague, 1955)
(42) *Physica*, II.27
(43) *De vegetabilibus* (edit. JESSEN, Berlin 1867) Liber VI cap. IX
(44) *Buch der Natur* (edit. PFEIFFER, Stuttgart 1861) IV B, No. 43
(45) KLEBS, ARNOLD C., *Incunabula scientifica et medica* (*Osiris*, Vol. IV, 1938, 1—359)

CHAPTER FIVE

CRUSHING

Introduction

Crushing or disintegration can be achieved by exerting pressure, by grinding and by impact. The development of the different crushing operations is closely related to the evolution of agriculture and the kitchen.

Pressure was needed to collect the juice or oil from grapes and olives. It led to the invention of the bag-, the beam- and the screw-press.

Grinding is needed for the preparation of the daily bread. From the mortar and pounding stone the saddle-quern and the rotary mill sprang which later also ground ores and minerals.

Impact as used in the mortar and pestle was used for herbs and seeds too, and sometimes for ores. Its mechanised forms are at the bottom of our hammer- and stamp-mills. Treshing was another form of impact crushing used to dehusk corn first of all. In Antiquity development was not carried further than the flail, a late-comer in history.

Disintegration by fire-setting was confined to ancient mining but very widely used since mining began and still surviving in our days. Its method was so simple and effective that no further development took place on this line.

Pressing

The press was not invented for compaction but in order to perfect the expressing of juice or oil from fruit and seeds. Expressing [1] was originally achieved by treading, as is clearly proved by the expressions used by classical authors for the production of olive oil [2]. In ancient Palestine the prophet said: "Thou shalt tread the olives" (Micah 6.15) using the term "dārakh" which translators have often rendered as "expressing". However the modern Arab "daras" means both "crushing olives in a mill" and "threshing corn with oxen treading it". In the case of olive oil this is a less efficient way of expressing the oil, as the hard skin of the fruit has first to be crushed in order to get the full yield of oil later.

In the case of the soft-skinned grape, however, no pre-crushing was needed nor was the pulp ever expressed in a basket by the weight of a stone. Ancient Egyptian reliefs show us how the bunches of grapes were thrown into a wooden or stone vat sometimes mounted on legs for the "treading" or "scattering of the wine-harvest" as the texts call it. Boys and men stand in it and music assists them to tread the grapes. Often they support themselves by clinging on to a bar or a set of ropes hanging down from such a bar. From the lower part of this vat the juice flows into the fermenting vat.

a. *The bag-press.*

This simple treading of grapes, olives and the like was mechanised right at the beginning of Egyptian history (3000 B.C.). The Egyptians discovered that more pressure could be exerted by torsion than by weight. Their operation of "wringing the cloth" consisted of filling a cloth with grapes or other ingredients, and folding it in such a way that the two ends on each side enfolded a stick. The two sticks were then turned in opposite directions thus expressing the contents by torsion at much higher pressures than could be achieved by treading.

This scene is very often depicted, each stick being twisted by two men, the fifth trying to keep the sticks at their proper distance as the effect of torsion is to make them approach each other. As early as the Third Dynasty (2700 B.C.) a hieroglyph depicts a better and more efficient form of this bag-press, the two ends of which are now supported by uprights.

Very soon after a further step improved its efficiency again. The bag is still hung in the frame but one of the sticks is now replaced by a noose attached to one of the uprights. The other end of the bag still holds a stick that is twisted by workmen, whilst an inspector is usually depicted testing the bag for possible holes or cracks. This bag-press is used for grapes, olives, flowers and herbs and represents ultimate stage of the press in the pre-classical world.

The ancients never hit on the idea of the spring press now used by primitive peoples. Nor did they hit on the idea of the flexible bag-press used by the Arawaks of Guiana to express the poisonous juice from manioc-flour. The root of the manioc or cassave is ground and mixed with water. This pulp is then introduced into a long spirally woven cylinder, which is then hung by a loop from a branch of a tree. The loop of the lower end is then pulled down with force, sometimes by means of a long lever attached to the tree. The extension and constriction of the woven cylinder is able to exert considerable pressure on its contents and leaves dry, edible manioc behind free from its poisonous juice. This ingenious device seems an independent invention of these South American Indians (1).

b. *The beam-press.*

The Aegean world seems to have invented and developed the beam-press, but how far back this invention goes, we do not know for certain. However, the cultivation of the olive and the use of olive oil dates back to the early part of the Bronze Age, at least in the southern Aegean (2). It is not until much later that some evidence of the machinery for crushing the olives is found. The early pressing operations may have been quite primitive until Middle-Minoan times (2200—1600 B.C.), the probable date of the remains of an olive press and a through for crushing olives found at Palaikastro (Crete) (3). Unfortunately few of these archaeological reports are sufficiently clear to identify the detailed construction of these presses.

What actually must be a beam-press used for olives was found in the Aegean island of Thera, one of the Cyclades (5), its date is late-Helladic (1600—1100 B.C.). After that date they grow more frequent and their construction is revealed as soon as they are depicted on vases such as the black-figure ware of the Athenian (early sixth century B.C.) potters. This beam-press applies the principle of the lever. One end hinges in the recess in a wall or between two stone pillars, the other end is drawn down (sometimes with a rope) and it is often loaded with heavy stones. The middle of the 20′—30′ beam presses down a packet of bags of olives or layers of olives separated by planks or strips of wood (regulae), which may rest on an elevated bed or table. This is not only shown on these early vases but fairly well-kept remains of such a press dating from the second century B.C. were found at Praesos together with separating vats for the expressed water and oil and storage vats for the oil (6). These presses have survived in viticulture in many regions upto the present day (7).

Then data on the further evolution of the beam-press begin to flow from the pen of classical authors (8). These data have been fully discussed by modern authors (9). In fact Pliny gives a very valuable summary of this evolution which enables us to date several of these stages. This is what he has to say:

"Some press the grapes with a single press, but it pays better to use a pair, however large the single beams may be. It is length that matters in the case of beams, not thickness; but those of ample width press better. In old days people used to drag down the press-beams with ropes and leather straps, and by means of hand-spakes; but within the last hundred years the Greek pattern of press has been invented, spars with furrows running round them in a spiral, some people putting handles on the spar, others making the spar lift up chests of stones with it, an arrangement which is highly approved. Within the last twenty-two years a plan has been invented to press with small presses and smaller press-houses, with a shorter spar straight in the middle, bearing down with the full weight from above on the lid laid on the grapes and to build a superstructure above the press."

The difficulty in translating this passage into technical language is not only due to the fact that PLINY was not a technician but an encyclopaedist. The main trouble lays in the shift of meaning of certain technical terms. Thus the Greek "lenos", originally the treading-vat came to denote the entire press or the press-house. The Latin torcular (press-house) (compare the German "Torkel") is used for the press itself, and so is prelum (press-beam). Again pressorium is used for the twin-screw cloth-press from the sixth century A.D. onwards.

PLINY clearly describes four types of presses. The first one is the old beam-press slightly mechanised, the type usually called the Catonian press because CATO describes it so clearly. Two timber uprights (arbores) stand close together and carry a cross-piece in slots. In countries poor in timber slots in the wall or stone pillars are used. The end of the heavy press-beam (now often upto 50') is caught under the cross-piece. The other end is drawn down by means of a leather thong or rope (topeion, funis torculus) fastened to a horizontal 6″—9″ drum, carried by another pair of uprights (stipites) and turned by means of handspakes (vectes). The mass of crushed olives (sampsa) or grape pulp (pes) is placed on a $4^1/_4'$ stone press-bed (ara, forum vinarium) and a 4′ wooden lid (orbis) covers it and distributes the pressure exerted on it by the press-beam. After the pressing is over the beam can be raised by means of a tackle and rope. Two such presses were found in the neighbourhood of Salona (10).

The mass to be pressed was often enclosed in rings woven of espartograss, in baskets or kept together with ropes, sometimes a wooden framework (galeagra = "weasel-trap") is used (HERON, III. 16—17), even two or more on top of each other. This was a new invention to HERON and to PLINY who says (XV.2): "Olives are crushed in wicker baskets or by enclosing the mesh between thin bars, a method recently invented." Ropes wound around a mass of pulp under a press beam is shown on a Greek relief now in the British Museum. One or two gutters (lacus) cut into the press-bed collect the juice and conduct it to the storage-vat which usually had a capacity of 20 cullei (10 m³). This simple method of pulling down the press-beam which sometimes weighed over 525 kgr was used until the end of the Roman Empire. It is depicted in a wall-painting in the house of the Vettii at Pompeii. However the pressure thus exerted on the mass could not be kept very constant.

The second improvement is embodied in so called Heronian press, a lever and weight press. The stone weight, which is to give constant pressure on the press-bed, was raised by means of a rope running from a drum via a pulley on the prelum and another one fastened to the stone back to the prelum. Once the drum was wound sufficiently to free the stone from the ground, it could then act on the press-beam. A press of this type is shown on a relief in the Villa Albani near Rome. This mechanisation of the old stone-weighted press seems to have been invented in Greece, it is quite familiar to Heron in 50 A.D. but must be considerably older seeing the application of its principle to the screw-press about the beginning of our era.

c. *The screw-press.*

The application of the screw to haul down the free end of the lever press can of course not antedate the invention of the screw. This dates back to the generation of ARCHIMEDES (300 B.C.) and by the time of HERON screw-cutters to make inner screw-thread were known (11). This fits in excellently with the description of the screw-press by PLINY, who died during the catastrophe at Pompeii of 79 A.D. Their introduction in Rome therefore dates back to about the end of the first century B.C. and their probable invention in Greece to the second or first century B.C.

The simplest application was that of a single screw to supersede the drum and handspakes for drawing down the beam. The screw is fixed to the floor in such a way that it can turn without giving way upwards. The end of the beam is forked and the nut of the screw placed across the fork. The screw is then turned by means of handles on it below the beam and thus lowers the beam. We have a modern example of a similar press at Fenis near Aosta.

A further improvement of this type of press is the one in which the screw draws up a stone weight or chest of stones. It is described by HERON and still to be seen in use in Egypt, the Aegean, the Alps and Italy (Boscoreale). The weight is released from the floor by turning the screw and the beam is lifted by turning the screw backwards. It is sometimes called the "Greek press" (torculum graecanicum) but it was common enough in Rome in the days of VITRUV (25 B.C.). A press of this type of Roman date was found in Palestine (12) and they are mentioned in Jewish law. Less complete examples can be traced in Greece and North Africa (13) as well as in the Near East (14).

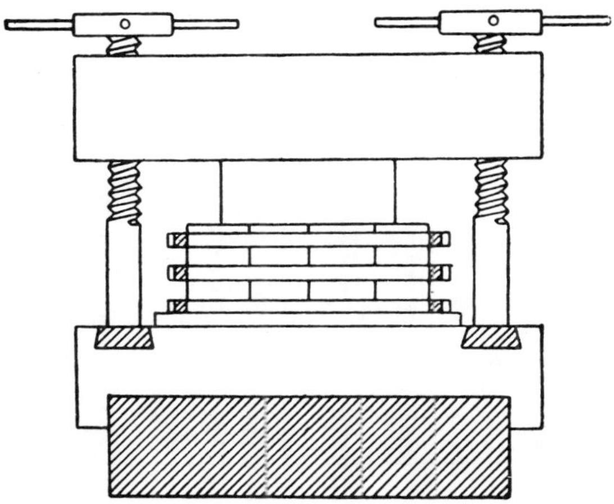

Fig. 31. Heron's screw-press

The Zenon papyri and similar documents (P.S.I. 624) show that the Egyptians of the turn of our era followed these developments and build, lease and reconstruct oil-presses.

The application of the screw as a source of direct pressure on the mass is a very important step taken at Rome about 50 A.D. according to PLINY, and possibly a Greek invention of the latter part of the first century B.C. or about the beginning of our era. HERON knows two forms. In the first (unknown to PLINY) two screws each at the end of a short beam press it down. The other press had only one screw, the nut of which is cut into a solid beam fixed to the press-bed by two stout uprights like the modern copying press. The press lid (called the tympanum) is pressed down by turning the screw (coclea, cochlea).

The superstructure (congeries) mentioned by PLINY was necessary only when a lever press had to be transformed into a direct screw press. The most practical way to counter the upthrust of the screw was to prolong the uprights and build above the beam a weight of stones and bricks. An actual well-preserved single screw press was found at Herculaneum and a double screw press as described by HERON (III.19) is in the Museum of Alexandria. A wall painting in a fuller's shop of Pompeii show a cloth-press of this type. The typical bed of such a press would measure 45 × 60 cm.

Apart from the beam-press and the screw-press classical Antiquity knew a third type, the wedge-press [3], not mentioned by the classical authors but depicted on ancient monuments (15) and described in later pharmaceutical literature. Two strong frame works of timber

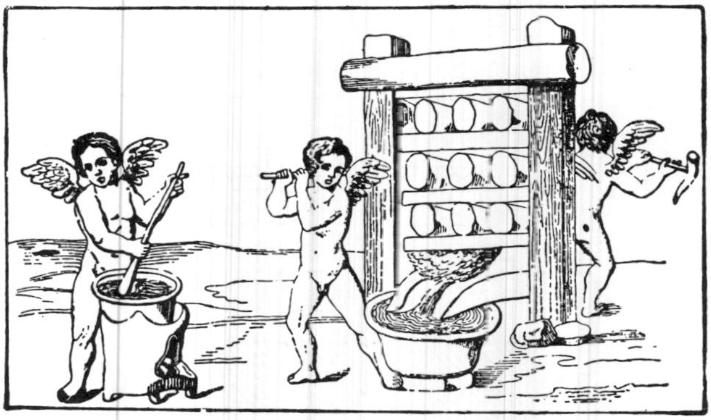

Fig. 32. Wedge-press on a mural at Pompeii

are built over a square foundation of stone which contains a depression to hold the pulp or herbs to be pressed; a spout conducting the juice to a receiver. On the pulp a plank is placed on which there are alternate tiers of wedges and planks, the upper plank being held by the upper cross pieces of the two frames. The wedges are driven in with hammers with long handles by men on each side of the press thus exerting pressure on the mass to be expressed.

The screw- and wedge-presses were used mainly for oil-seeds, sheets of papyrus, cloth, herbs and roots and the preparation of essential oils. The beam-press were particularly suited for large-scale pressing of olives or grapes. We are informed that a team of four men could finish every day 23 pressings of 100 bushels (VARRO says 120—160) of olives, each bushel yielding about six pounds of olive oil. In the case of grapes each pressing yielded 100 L of must from 300 bushels of grapes.

This most important unit operation like that of pounding is from the very start closely connected with the preparation of food. From Palaeolithic times onwards man has used stones to disintegrate foodstuffs like acorns, nuts and wild grasses by using a pear- or pestle-shaped stone to beat and rub the material laying on a flat stone sometimes showing a natural or an artificial depression. This original combination of grinding and crushing can still be found in the Latin word for baker "pistor", which actually means "one who pounds". Though both operations are thus intimately connected with the preparation of food and of corn in particular grinding by rubbing became the operation used in making flour for baking whilst crushing or pounding by impact was mainly used for dehusking cereals. They also came to be used for fine and coarse disintegration in pharmacy, mining and many other technologies.

This distinction of coarse grinding or pounding for the production of every-day qualities of flour and of finely ground flour for ritual or special purposes pervades the whole of pre-classical literature. In Mesopotamia pestle and mortar were sometimes preferred over the saddle-quern in the earlier period when the miller took his name from the term for "pounding" [4]. Evidently this was connected with the different types of cereals cultivated in Antiquity. The later types of naked wheat needed grinding and sieving or bolting only, the earlier husked cereals like emmer and spelt demanded a proper cleaning (winnowing) and conditioning (roasting), a pounding to separate the husk from the grain and a final grinding [5]. It seems that the finer flours were prepared from the naked wheat type of cereal (16).

The process of making flour was definitely a household operation for many centuries, a major task for the housewife. Only about 1500 B.C. do we begin to hear of professional millers in Egypt [6]. In Mesopotamia professional millers are older. As in other countries it originated in the household but became a woman's profession, the ṭeinatum, though some texts mention a ṭeinu. They used different kinds of flour and produced various types of bread and cakes [6a]. The "house of the mill" [7] that is a centralised place for grinding corn is even older and later even became a monopoly for the production of certain types of flour. This centralisation of grinding and building of mills annex to the temple belonged to the ancient Sumerian temple-economy and did not release the housewife of her heavy duties until much later (17).

This limitation of the quantities of corn, herbs, etc. to be ground or pounded necessarily slowed down the evolution of more intricate forms of mills and mortars. Pounding and grinding slowly dissociated, some peoples still produce their flour by pounding alone. The oldest grinding stones consisted of a flat or slightly concave lower stone and a concave runner with a flat top which both ground and crushed by a combined oscillatory and rotating movement (18). Such grain-rubbers have not only been found in pre-historic Europe or the Near East, but they are still used by primitive peoples.

a. *The grain-rubber and the saddle quern.*

Most peoples, however, use rubbing stones in which two flat surfaces grind because of the oscillatory movement of the runner. The earliest form was a flat lower stone on which the runner was moved

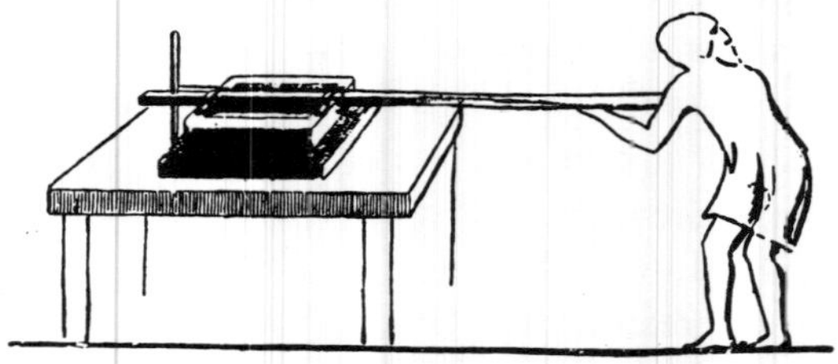

Fig. 33. Greek Grain-rubber

to and fro by the miller who had to kneel as shown by the Egyptian hieroglyph for "miller". Soon, however, a saddle-shaped lower stone was used to ease the labour of grinding. Kneeling behind such a "saddle-quern" still remained heavy work and therefore we find that as early as the Pyramid Age (2700 B.C.) the saddle-quern was placed on a base, inclining slightly away from the standing miller thus enabling him to grind more energetically. The millstone carried a cup on its further end in which the flour collected. There is no trace of any rotary quern in Egypt before Hellenistic times (300 B.C.) when they seem to have been imported from Mesopotamia [8].

In the Land of the Two Rivers several forms of hand-mills existed alongside the saddle-quern which always remained popular in the household and three forms of which are mentioned (for corn, sesame or dates) [9]. In Palestine the saddle-quern, the grain-rubber and the pestle and mortar remain the only crushing apparatus until the rotary mill is generally adopted in Hellenistic times. In the saddle-quern the grain is fed on the near end of the lower stone and it falls off on the far end. Hence in the Old Testament "the maidservant is behind the mill" (Exodus XI.5). The bolster-shaped upper stone is called the "rider" (Deut. 24.6) and Samson is made to work with it like a slave-girl (Ju. 16.21). On the other hand manna is both ground and pounded (Num. 11.8) like corn (Prov. 27.22).

In prehistoric Europe both forms occur. The grain-rubbers often have a saucer-shaped basin sometimes with a rim to guide the squat and bun-shaped pestle. They were used for corn but certainly for the seeds of wild plants too. Grain-rubbers and saddlequerns, both often indifferently dubbed "mills" or "millstones" by the archaeologists, are

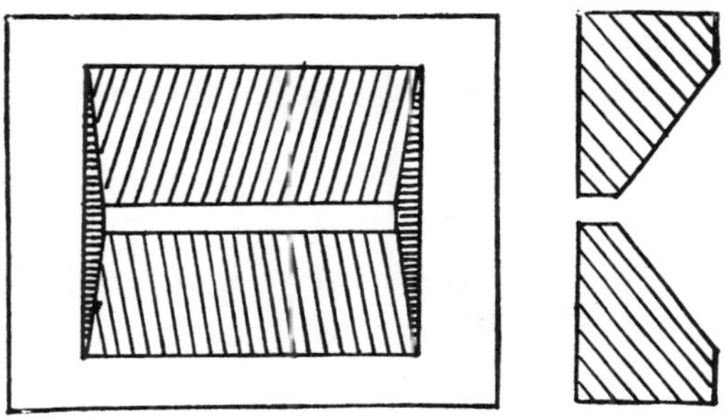

Fig. 34. Section of grain-rubber

found in the Aegean from the Neolithic period onwards in such different places as Knossos (Crete) (19), Tsani (Thessaly) (20), Tsangli near Sesklo (Thessaly), Saratsé (Salonica), Sedes and Magasà (Crete) (21). In Hissarlik (Troy) the saddle-quern is the usual instrument upto the end of the Bronze Age. In the rest of Europe they also disappear by the early Iron Age. The typical American form of the saddle-quern is the "metate" indigeneous in South America, Mexico, Nicaragua and some of the territories inhabited by the North American Indians.

A later development of the saddle-quern returned to the flat stones of primitive times. The upper stone has a hopper plus a slit to feed the grinding surface continuously. This hopper-rubber is pushed to and fro on the lower stone, both surfaces are generally groved which results in a more effective grinding because of the shear-like action of the ribs. VIRGIL refers to them [10] and so they have reached Italy in the first century B.C. In Greece this effect was appreciated much earlier as was the better ejection of the meal from the stones, and they are well attested there from the fifth century B.C. onwards. However, they are also found in the Greek settlements (Tanis and Naucratis) in Egypt and even earlier in Asia Minor (Alishar) and in Tell Halaf (Syria). On the latter site (ninth century B.C.?) the earliest examples of this pushing-mill were found, which has a bar or stick fixed into the hopper-rubber to push it, both stones being placed on a table or pedestal as is clearly shown in a third century B.C. Megaric bowl (22). The Tell Halaf loaf-shaped mill-stones have a deep furrow lengthwise into which a wooden stick fitted by means of which the upper stone was rubbed on a flat nether stone (23). This pushing-mill may therefore have originated in the Near East a few centuries before it came into use in classical Greece, where it never replaced the grain-rubber or the saddle-quern in the household. The pushing-mill called "mola trusitalis" (a term later transferred to rotary mills) seems associated with the production of flour on a larger scale then needed for the home.

b. *The rotary quern.*

We must now discuss the true (rotary) quern, which was not evolved from the saddle-quern but which seems to go back to the grain-rubber and the original primitive mortars. Some very primitive forms are still in use in Southern and Western Arabia. RATHJENS (23a) mentions: "a plate-like understone with a rim of some 7 cm and an opening for evacuation of the flour has a vertical stick around which a cylindrical upper stone is moved by a handle let into its upper rim and having an opening to introduce the cereal to be ground. The flour produced remains in the lower dish to be collected". Some of these old mortar have the form of a slightly concave lower stone and a convex upper stone (24). Some of the grain-rubbers are round or oblong stones with a rim to guide the globular runner, examples have been found as far apart as Egypt, Troy, Central Europe and Scandinavia. The rotary quern owes its invention to concentration on the rotary movement made by the runner in these primitive crushing apparatus. It is very important as "the first major application of rotary motion since the invention of the potter's wheel and the lathe in the remote Oriental Copper Age and it led to the invention of geared machinery and the water-wheel, hence to the first employment of inanimate motive power" (25). The evidence on the earlier forms is still preponderantly archaeological except for a few philological hints [9].

At Ras Shamra (Ugarit) (Syria) strata earlier than 1200 B.C. yielded "two hemispherical stones, the nether stone having a tenon in the middle which fits into a mortise of the upper one, which is also held by a raised collar round the nether stone" (26). At Tell Halaf "there were also round mill-stones (ninth century B.C.?) that have a prong at the middle fitting into the other stone; this has a little hole in its side into which a wooden stick was thrust by which the stone was turned on the mill-stone both stones were grooved" (23). At Gezer a rotary mill was found, the upper stone of which had no peg or handle and which could therefore be moved efficiently to and fro only in semi-circles by the hands of the operator (27). Other sites in Palestine have also yielded small rotary appliances dating back to the end of the second millenium B.C.

The early rotary mills are quite small and seem to have served to grind pigments and the like. They may well have evolved from the special mortars to grind coloured stones and ores, such as the "basalt mills" of the ancient Assyrians [11]. The earliest mills had a semi-circular to-and-fro movement until a peg was added. They certainly spread from the Ancient Near East to the Aegean where a round quern appears in an early Bronze Age stratum at Saratsé near Salonica (21). On Crete true millstones were found at Miamù and Megasà, the upper stone fitting into a hollow in the lower. It seems therefore that the rotary quern adopted to the grinding of corn diffused slowly into the western Mediterranean basin and drifting with other farming appliances into Europe, where two schools of rotary querns can be distinguished, the Iberian quern with a vertical peg and the Central European with the horizontal handle of its Eastern ancestors (25). It should also be noted that these early rotary querns appear in the period when the professional miller comes to the fore and its evolution may well be related to the production of flour on a larger scale than needed for home use only.

The classical authors have many legends about the invention of the rotary mill which is in turn ascribed to Myletas, King of Lacedemonia, Myles the Lelege, the Telchine Mylas of Rhodes or even the godess Demeter (28). Pliny is even more specific: "Varro is again our authority that millstones have been invented at Volsinii (Bolsena) and we find in the records of prodigies several instances of these stones moving on their own accord." Nor can we derive the rotary hand-mill from the donkey-mill, a thesis that could be derived from literary evidence alone but which can not stand in the light of archaeological evidence (29). It was formerly believed that the Homeric poems mentioned the rotary mill (30), but the passage from the *Odyssey* (XX.129—131, trans. W. Cowper):

> "Twelve maidens day by day toiled at the mills
> meal grinding, some of barley, some of wheat,
> marrow of man. The rest (their portion ground)
> all slept."

does not refer to the rotary mill, which may be suggested in VII. 123—124:

> The rapids mills
> these turning, pulverize, the mellow'd grain."

The confusion is increased by the indiscriminate use of the terms "mulé" and "mola" by the classical authors [12].

Three fifth-century rotary querns from the Greek world (Syracuse, Motya and Olynthos) are still hotly debated. They still seem fairly rare in Greece about the third century B.C. when the pushing mill was still in favour with the saddle-quern and the donkey-mill was emerging. There is some doubt about the statement that the rotary mill was a devolution of the much larger donkey-mill as it was adopted by the farmer to rural needs (29). The early Greek rotary quern spread north of the Alps, where we can trace it throughout the area of the Celtic La Tène civilisation (second and first centuries B.C.) even as far as Moldavia. It has a hopper in the upper stone which has a lateral socket for radial horizontal handles like Mediterranean examples found in Algeria and Delos. It must also have spread to Spain where a distinct Iberian type with a slightly convex lower stone and a concave upper one with a vertical handle was certainly in use by the Roman conquest (second century B.C.) and probably introduced two centuries earlier. They may represent the "Spanish mill" referred to by Cato which he recommends as the equipment of a 240 acre oliveyard together with a donkey-mill and a pushing mill (31). It may have been brought by sea to England as it seems to be the ancestor of the Scottish brochs, just like the Celtic mill reached southern England in the first century B.C. Excavations at Bolle (Denmark) show that the rotary quern reached Denmark about the birth of Christ. The movement was probably provided by a handle attached to a wooden band fitted round the upper stone as still common in Karelia (31a).

The spread of the classical portable rotary hand-mill with its two flat stones seems intimately connected with the armies of Greece and Rome. Already XENOPHON makes Cyrus say: "We ought to take handmills for grinding, those are the lightest machines for the purpose" (32). The soldiers of classical armies were supposed to grind their own corn, hence in order to help Scipio to organize his conquest of Spain "the cantons of Etruria provide hand-mills" (33) which form a common feature of all Roman army-camps. In the army one "molae manuariae" should be provided for each group (contubernium) of 5—10 men, so the Roman strategists claim who insist that "each man carry his flour for thirty days" (34). Still northern Germany and Scandinavia did not know the rotary quern until the third century A.D.

The hand-mill was used for corn but also for herbs and even for pigments like white lead (35). Special types of mills were developed such as the small wooden pepper-mills ("buxea mola") and the ancestor of our coffee-mill, so well-described by PLINY with these words: "Etruria pounds the ears of emmer, after it has been roasted with a pestle shod with iron at the end, in a handmill that is serrated (fistula serrata) and denticulated inside with grooves radiating from a centre, so that if people put their weight into it while pounding the grains are only splintered up and the iron is broken" (37).

c. *The donkey mill.*

The larger type of rotary mill was called the "mola asinaria" (jumentaria) because it was driven by blindfolded horses, mules or donkeys as well as by slaves. It represents the first step towards mechanisation of the mill and certainly does not antedate the professional miller. It has a conical lower stone with a slope of 35—40°. The hour-glass shaped upper stone turn on the spindle of the lower one from which it is separated by an iron bridge, the rynd, resting on top of the spindle at the narrowest opening between the two stones. Though the slope of the stones serves no practical purpose (but represents a relic of the saddle-quern) the top of the upper stone served as a hopper [13].

By metonomy the upper stone is called "donkey" in Greek and from the date of the earliest references we can conclude that the donkey-mill was known in Greece about 300 B.C. (38). ARDAILLON believes that they were evolved to grind ores as they were found in the Laurium silver-mines (400 B.C.) and then adapted to corn. As roller-mills for olives of the trapetum-type of the same date were found at Olynthus this definitely puts back the rotary quern in Greece before that date, that is in the fifth century B.C.

The donkey-mill always has grooved surfaces and it was moved by pushing the handle or pole projecting horizontally from the waist of the mill and attached to the upper-stone. The stone used for the mill was often lava. It should be hard and have large grains, Vesuvian stone being often used (39). Its introduction in Italy dates from the first century B.C. when OVID speaks of the "cava machina" (40) and CATO prescribes as the necessary apparatus for a vineyard of 100 jugera "three mills worked by asses and one hand-mill" (41). This is probably the type of mill at which the Roman poet PLAUTUS worked (42) and it long remained the typical mill of the millers of Rome who resisted the introduction of the water-mill. It also spread from Greece to the East where Renan found the first Roman donkey-mill in Phoenicia many decades ago (43).

The first definite reference to a rotary hand-mill on the Roman country-side dates from the same century, when the poet VIRGIL tells us that the farmer grinds his corn in one and uses a mortar (mortarium) for mashing herbs (44).

d. *Mechanisation of the rotary mill.*

The evolution of the water-driven corn-mill during the Roman Empire simply meant the adaption of the water-wheel with the help of gear-wheels to the ordinary pair of millstones which go to make up the rotary quern. This quern was not changed and hence its mechanisation really forms part of evolution of prime movers which no longer belong to the development of farming operations. The corn mill, either water- or wind-driven, belonged to the miller or the lord, not to the farmer.

However, apart from this very important development there was an evolution of the rotary quern, which benefited the farmer or soldier. It is concerned with the rotation of the upper stone and the development of the handle. The crossbar handle was usually let into the upper stone, it is clearly derived from the original side peg. Not until after the close of the Roman period we find the vertical handle in a vertical socket near the outer edge of the stone thus facilitating rotation.

The handle was sometimes extended to form a long bar which could be fixed to the ceiling and rotated describing a cone. This form is well-known in the Middle Ages, but the claims that it dates back to the Roman period (45) are not substantiated. In the larger handmills the difficulty of rotating the runner singly is often solved by having two people continuously passing on the vertical handle as the stone has completed a semi-circle. The possibility of translating the to-and-fro movement of the operator or prime mover into rotation by means of a crank was unknown in Antiquity, it seems to have been invented in the early Middle Ages.

The Romans of the Imperial period also had "molae machinariae", large fixed mills with a rider 75 cm in diameter attached to a spindle which bore near its end a gear-wheel probably engaging another wheel moving in a vertical plane and operated by a slave (45).

Certain tribes of east and south-east Asia now use cranks on their handmills attached to very long bars, so that the operator has to make only a short to-and-fro movement. In Europe we find fairly late that a double crank is built into the spindle of the handmill which has a fixed point on the ceiling of the mill-house. This crank is then moved by the hand of the operator. It is not depicted before 1430 (46). Some fifty years later a system of two cranks above each other is shown (47) one of which carries a counterweight. LEONARDO DA VINCI's notebooks contain a solution of the type still used in Asia (48). The spread of the rotary quern to Asia is still largely unknown. Two clay models found in China can be assigned to the Han dynasty, that is beginning of our era (49). They were first used for corn, then also for ores, etc.

e. *The roller mill.*

It is not yet quite clear whether the roller mill was derived from the saddle-quern or from the rotary-quern, but it is certain that the earliest roller-mill was devised in the period when rotary motion was introduced into grinding. The story of the roller-mill is intimately bound up with that of the third of the agricultural mass-products of Antiquity, corn, wine and olive-oil.

The production of olive-oil involves two stages. In the first one the olives are bruised to avoid crushing the kernels and to get rid of most of the bitter juice, called amurca by the ancients. After the kernels have been extracted from the crushed olives the rest of the oil and juice is obtained by pressing the pulp. The earliest bruising was obtained by pounding or treading. As the Old Testament has it "thou shalt tread the olives" [14] and the best quality oil is kātīt (beaten or pounded) (50). There is no trace of a roller-mill in the Old Testament, they begin to appear in Jewish law in Hellenistic times only (51).

The earliest form of roller-mill was simply a trough (canalis) in which a mill-stone (solea) was rolled to and fro. Remains of such presses were found in Algeria and other sites (52). A variant has a slightly curved trough and the stone revolves on an axis which turns from the centre of curvature of the trough. We do not know whether the Assyrian roller-mill [9] was of this type for actual finds have not been published but it would rather seem to be one of the second type.

The second stage of the roller-mill was the rotary one called "mulè" or "mola olearia" by the ancients (53). It consisted of two cylindrical millstones, rotating on a horizontal axle, which was carried by a vertical beam, that turned round also, placed in the middle of the flat circular trough on which the grinding took place. Actual remains of such oil-mills have been found and mills of this type still exist in southern Europe (54). A sarcophagus at the Palazzo Rondanini, Rome (55) shows a type of olive-mill that is rather a precursor of the mola olearia than an intermediate stage between this mill and the later trapetum. In this olive-mill the axle turns on a spindle in the middle of the crushing vat but the distance of the two millstones and this vat is controlled by the operator who both turns and raises the vertical beam at will. Sometimes these mills have only one millstone and a counter-weight on the other side of the beam (56).

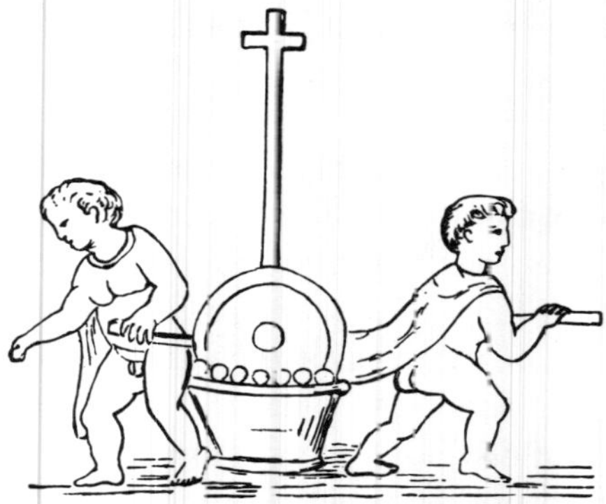

Fig. 35. Roman mola olearia (Pompeii)

It would seem that an early mill of this type existed in Olynthus (57) about 400 B.C. but practically all our knowledge of ancient oil mills is derived from the study of Roman mills, the earlier Greek mills are never properly described by the excavators. Still the mola olearia was the only form of olivemill known in the eighteenth century, the Roman improved version seems completely forgotten until the excavations in Italy revealed their construction. The Roman agronomists (58) discuss various variants of this improved mill called "trapetum". The first two examples were recovered at Stabiae in 1779/80, that of Bosco Reale dates of 1891 and others have since been found.

The Roman trapetum, reputed to have been invented by Aristaeus of Athens (Pliny, *Nat. Hist.* 7.199), consists of a large basin of lava (mortarium) in the middle of which stands a solid column (miliarium) a few cm higher than the lip of the basin (labrum). On top of the miliarium there is a square hole holding an upright pin (columella) fastened with lead. A wooden beam (cupa) fitted over the columella and rested on the mill in a horizontal position; on its arms two millstones (orbes) were threaded which were flat towards the centre and convex on the outer side. They were kept in their places by a system of wedges and washers, described in great detail by the classical authors (56) at a distance of one Roman inch (1.8 cm) from the bottom and the sides of the basin, for the stones of the olives should not be crushed. Still many Roman agronomists prefer the more adjustable mola olearia (59) where no fixed distance between orbes and mortarium existed.

Though this general form of trapetum remained constant in Antiquity we can trace some development in details such as the orbes (56). The orbes of the Catonian trapetum had a big superfluous curve above the labrum. In a later trapetum from Nauplion this part is cut away, the orbes of a Pompeiian trapetum is again more fully curved but it is so narrow that the full curvature is used in crushing the olives. The trapetum is the form of olive-mill introduced in Palestine and elsewhere in the Near East by the Romans [15], it is the most elaborate form of roller-mill known to them.

Pounding

a. *Mortar and pestle.*

Mortar and pestle, the natural offspring of the primitive pounding stone, were already known to the Natufians, the mesolithic inhabitants of ancient Palestine. During pre-classical Antiquity a differentiation in high and low mortars, each for a special purpose took place. In Egypt the mortar was not only used for dehusking corn [6] but also for many technological and pharmaceutical operations [16] and the same holds good for ancient Mesopotamia [17]. Here again the classical legend that "the name 'Pilumnus' belonged to the inventor of the pestle for corn-mills, 'Piso' came from 'pounding' corn and again families were named Fabius or Lentulus or Cicero according as some one was the best grower of some particular crop" (60) does prove nothing but that the proud Roman nobility descended from a strong race of farmers.

Many of the dehusking mortars and pestles were made of wood and the mortar was sometimes placed high on a stand. Small pottery mortars were made by incorporating chips of quartz in the clay before baking, they were used by all ancient peoples. This simple "mortarium' was still in use in Greece and Rome during the first century A.D.

We have many examples of simple mechanisation of the pestle (61 It is suspended from the branch of a tree or some other form of elastic suspension by primitive tribes all over the world. The only classical passage on working the pestle with a rope may refer to it (62). Antiquity never knew the hammerform of the pestle, which is attached to a long pole and worked like a hammer. This type of pestle is still used

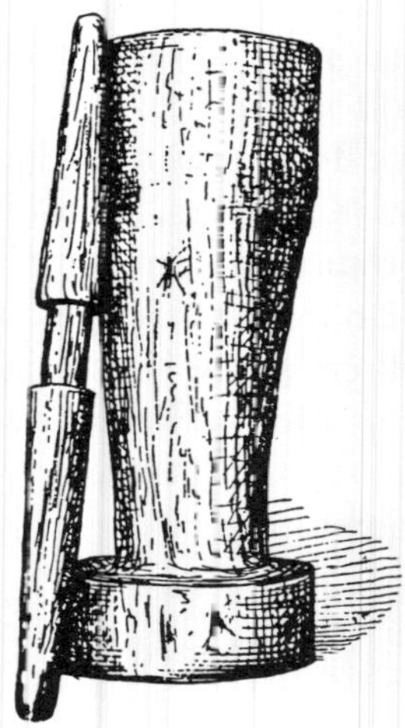

Fig. 36. Primitive mortar and pestle

in the Far East to pound rice and ores (63) and in the Alps. The pole can also be made to hinge so that the end (sometimes counter-balanced) is worked by hand or foot as some farmers in Galicia and Poland still do, and as can still be seen in China and Japan. In mountainous countries the end of the pole often has a vessel that is continuously filled by the water of a brook, lifts the pestle when it is full and then spills its contents to rise to its original position. Thus a simple natural power resource is turned to work the pestle and this may well be the ancestor of the hammer- or stamp-mill which became popular as the water-mill became a prime-mover in the Middle Ages.

Mortars and handmills were turned to use by the ancient miners who wanted to crush their ores, iron pestles being favoured in these cases (64).

b. *Treshing.*

Treshing is another form of crushing by impact which is intimately related to the history of agriculture (65). The methods known to the ancients are very ably summed up in this passage: "The ear itself when reapened is beaten out with treshing sledges on a treshing floor, in other parts by being trodden on by mares, and in other places it is thrashed out with sticks" (66).

Indeed the most common procedure was to spread the corn on a mudbrick or stone threshing floor and to drive oxen, asses or mules over it. These animals and their drivers treading the corn is a favourite subject of the Egyptian painters. The practice was taken over by the Greeks and Roman who preferred horses and mules because they were more tractable.

Beating the corn with sticks was resorted to in certain cases. Ruth "beat out that she had gleaned" and Gideon in secret "threshed wheat by the winepress" (67). The classical authors also refer to the use of sticks and cudgels (68). No classical passage mentions the flail unquestionably and the earliest reference is found in ST. JEROME's *Commentary on Isaiah* [18]. It would seem from the present evidence that the flail was an invention made in Gaul in the fourth century A.D. which very slowly displaced the older stick during the Middle Ages and which is not yet common in the East.

A more elaborate threshing instrument, the threshing sledge, was developed in Antiquity. The ancient Egyptians never knew it but it was common in Palestine and in Mesopotamia [19]. It consisted of a board, sledge or beam studded with flints or iron nails which is driven over the threshing floor by oxen, sometimes loaded with stones and always carrying the driver. This is the Greek "tribola, tribolos" and the Roman "tribula, tribulum" of the classical authors (69). It is still in use in many parts of the Mediterranean basin and Asia (70). Its action on the corn is used as a simile for utter destruction in the Old Testament where Gilead was "threshed with iron threshing sledges" (Amos 1.3) and many other passages (71) and the prophet Isaiah promises "I will make thee a new sharp threshing sledge having teeth; thou shalt thresh the mountains and beat them small and shalt make the hills as chaff (41.15)".

Apart from the threshing sledge the classical agronomists mention an instrument called "plostellum poenicum", adopted from the Carthaginians, which consisted of axles with toothed dises driven over the corn by a driver seated on this cart-like vehicle. The Romans found it in eastern Spain (72). We do not know any details about the "traha" (trahea) which is also mentioned as a threshing instrument (73).

Fire-setting

Fire-setting was a disintegration process commonly used by the ancient miners from the Stone Age onwards. "The miners meet with flinty rocks which they break up by heating them and pouring vinegar on them or more often (for the steam and smoke make the air in the galleries unbreathable) they hew them out with battering machines fitted with irons rams weighing 150 pounds and they bear the debris on their shoulders" (74). This vinegar, still used by some and sometimes mentioned in the accounts of Hannibal's crossing of the Alps, was added because it was believed to make the water extra cold by evaporation. Fire-setting survived in many places as the method of disintegrating rocks which resist the miner's pick.

Notes

[1] Greek "expiezo", Latin "primere, exprimere".

[2] Greek "trapeo", Latin "calcare", "calco".

[3] Greek "embola", "sphenes", Latin "cunei".

[4] The Sumerian for pounding is ÀR, GAZ (-GAZ), (ḫašalu) hence the mortar záGAZ (erettu) made either of stone (zá) or wood (giš), the pictograph of which clearly shows how little mortars have changed in the course of the centuries. With the stone or wooden pestle gišGAZ-ZI-GAZ (kak madâkti, ḫašlu) originally shaped like a club, the miller lúGAZ-ZÌ-DA (hasil qêmi) makes the coarse flour. Pounding *and* grinding form part of his work for the term actually means "he who pounds and grinds", compare MA_5, (qamû), to grind.

[5] The one type of flour is called ZID, ṭênu, (qâmu); hence "grinding to flour" KA-ZID (ṭênu ša qêmi) is the work of the "kazidakku" (miller). Texts of the Kassite period (2000 B.C.) mention this profession for the first time, the mill (ZID-KA, GAZ, ḫašlu) is already mentioned in Lagaš tablets. In contrast to the simple combination of grinding and bolting often simply indicated by "ṭênu" the ancient texts use the term "samâdu" for the complex operations leading to NIG-ḪAR-RA (samîdu), fine flour (Compare Arab. samîd - wheat, Pers. šamad, Sanskrit samitâ, but also Greek semithalis, Latin simila, similago - wheat, OHG. semala, German Semmel - bran). Starting from barley three different grades of flour (SIG,UŠ,DU) are made in the hand-mill NA.ḪAR (UR_5) (erû) by the lúḪAR-ḪAR (lúARA) (ararru) which word later denoted the

professional miller. The words "grinding" and "sieving" form a very common pair in Sumerian and later texts.

[6] The female miller "nḏwt" (II.370.14) (These figures refer to volume, page and line of ERMAN-GRAPOW's *Wörterbuch der Aegyptischen Sprache* where the correct hieroglyphic notation can be found) grinds her corn on the "bnwt" (millstone) (I.458.13). The maid-servant, whose main task seems to have been grinding corn is the "nḏ.tj" (II.370.15), she makes "nḏ", flour ("the ground", II.370.13).
In Egypt too we often find the term "ḥm", to pound (from pestle, "ḥm". IV.215.9) combined with "to sieve" or "to grind" denoting the two types of flour made from different cereals.
Only in the New Kingdom period do we read of a "nḏ", miller (II.370.11) or even later of a "bnw" (miller, I.458.15).

[6a] TLB I, 131, 3 and Chagar Bazar nos. A 974, 982, 987, 988, 989, 993 and 995.

[7] The É-ÀRA (bît erî, bit ararru) usually led by a "gugallu" (inspector or temple-official) later made place for the free "ararru" or "kassidaku". Large mills were sometimes built by the state (Lagaš III) and then opened to the public by the head of the state.

[8] The Egyptians speak of "the (lower) millstone and his son" (s3ś, the runner or rubbing stone (III.422.6) the texts speak only of one type of special mill on which fruit are crushed and ground ("tjšš". V.502.8) The millstone is sometimes called "the pulverizing stone" (bnwt. wgm, IV.76.11 from "wgm", pulverize (I.377.9) and "wgm", powder (I.377.10)).

[9] The ordinary saddle-quern consisted of the lower ("female") stone, "erittu", and the upper rubbing stone, "narkabu". Then we have several mills for different types of flour, basalt mills (aḪAR-AD-BAR, erû adbari) and hand-mills aḪAR-ŠU, erî kalî) (erû ḫabisi, baker's mill). There were also larger mills such as the crushing mill (aḪAR zi-bu-um, erû zibi), a roller revolving on a floor to crush grain and moved by a donkey or mule. The aḪAR-DUK-KA-BUR (erû pahari, potter's mill) is sometimes suspected to be only a potter's wheel but it may well be a crushing mill for potter's ingredients as still in common use.

[10] "lapis incusus", *Georgics* I. 275.

[11] The special mortar aNA-ZA-GÌN-NA is used to crush ultramarine. We have no proof yet that the hand-mills mentioned in [9] are rotary querns, though these are known in Assyrian times.

[12] Cato uses "mola" for presses and roller mills, for THUCIDYDES VI.22) "mulon" is the space in which several saddle-querns are housed (the later "mola", "pistrinum" or "moletrina"). The Homeric "mulè" is probably the saddle-quern. "Mule", "mola", "molere" can be derived from an Indo-Germanic root *mar = to grind. Both "mulè" and "mola" first seem to denote grain rubbers or saddle-querns, they are then used for rotary querns and even for roller mills. Our modern terms for mechanical mills such as mill, Mühle, molen, moulin, muileann are derived from a late-Latin (fourth century A.D.) "moli-

na". The quern was dubbed "hand-mill" in the eighteenth century only, the word "quern" is related to the Celtic "bró" and the Welsh "breuan" and it belongs to a North-European class of words like "corn" and "grind" all related to the production of flour from cereals There is also constant confusion between the mola trusitalis (cheiromule) (pushing mill) and the rotary quern (mola versatilis).

[13] The lower stone is called Greek "mulè", Latin "meta", the upper one Greek "onos" (donkey), Latin "catillus".

[14] Micah 6.15 has "dārākh" (to tread) but the Syriac version gives "'asar'" (to press). In Arabic "daras": threshing with animals "or" crushing olives in a mill" hence it refers to crushing by impact.

[15] In the "oil-press-house" (bīt hab-bad) the olive mill "reḥájim" (later called miṭḥān) was installed. Some texts speak of an "upper" and a "lower" stone, meaning "upright" and "base", they could be taken to denote the mola olearia should excavations prove their existence in ancient Palestine.
When the Mishna speaks of the basin as "'ām" (sea) or "'adāšā" (lens) and of the mill-stone as "māmēl" (grinder) it clearly describes the Roman trapetum. At present primitive olive-mills of the "mola olearia" type are in use in Palestine and Egypt.

[16] The mortar (šd, IV.566.11) and pestle (ḥm, IV.215.9) are used to crush mineral ingredients like salt (an operation called "tmtm", V.309.7), to crush corn for brewing (tš3, V.329.17), to crush herbs dry or in a liquid (ḥbk, I.488.3) and to pound corn for baking (dḏw, V.502.8). Certain herbs were crushed with a thorn (tjtš, V.330.5).

[17] Apart from the saddle-quern (which originally also was a mortar and pestle) the herb mortar made of wood (gišGUM, ursu) or of stone and pestle (záNA-ZAG-ḪI-LI- (ŠAR), elît urṣi) were used and to crush (SÚD, zâku) or pound (ḪUM, ḫamâšu) herbs and other compounds.

[18] "virga excutintur et baculo quae vulgo flagella dicumtur". The German Flegel and the English flail both go back to this late-Latin flagellum.

[19] The Akkadian "narpasu" (from "rapâsu", to trample). The Old Testament term is "morāg" (Isa. 41.15) or "hārūs, hārīs" (Hiob 41.22). In the Mishna (Para XII.9) it is explained as "ṭurbāl" (the Greek "tribolos") and it is now common in Egypt as naurag and in Palestine as "nōraǧ".

Bibliography

(1) Horwitz, H. Th., *Beiträge zur aussereuropaeïschen und vorgeschichtlichen Technik* (*Beiträge Gesch. Techn. Ind.*, Vol. 7, 1917, 169—189)

(2) Vickery, K. F., *Food in early Greece* (Urbana, Ill. 1936, 52 & 58)

(3) *Annals Brit. School Athens*, Vol. 8, 1901, 308

(4) *Annals Brit. School Athens*, Vol. 11, 1904, 276—277; vol. 8, 1901, 295, 334; *Rendiconti Accad. Lincei*, Vol. 16, 290

The "oil press" mentioned in A. Evans, Palace of Minos, Vol. I, p. 378; Vol. II, p. 543 is wrongly identified

(5) Renaudin, *Vases préhelléniques de Thera*, *Bull. Comm. Hell.* 1922, 113—159

(6) Bosanquet, R. C., *Excavations at Praesos*, *Ann. Brit. School Athens*, Vol. 8, 1901, 264

(7) Bethge, K., *Aus der Zeit der alten Weinpressen* (*Beitr. Gesch. Techn. Ind.*, Vol. 14, 1924, 210—216)

(8) Cato, *De Agri Cultura* chap. 10—13, 14—18 (edit. Brehault, New York 1933)

Pliny, *Natural History*, XVIII, 317 (edit. Rackham, *Loeb Classical Library*)

Vitruv, *De Architectura* VI, 9,3 (edit. Granger, *Loeb Classical Library*)

Hero, *Mechanics*, III, 13—21 (edit. Nix & Schmidt, Teubner, Leipzig 1900)

(9) Beck, Th., *Cato der ältere*, (*Civilingenieur*, Vol. 33, 1887, 418—438)

Hörle, J., *Catos Handbücher*, Paderborn 1929

Paton, W. R. & Myres, J. L., *On some Karian and Hellenic Oil-Presses* (*Journal Hell. Studies*, Vol. 18, 1898, 209—217)

Drachmann, A. G., *Ancient Oil Mills and Presses* (Copenhagen 1932)

(10) Brønsted, J., *Recherches à Salone*, Vol. I, 1928, 110 & fig. 103

Egger, R., *Forschungen in Salona*, Berlin 1926, Vol. II, 9

(11) Drachmann, A. G., *Heron's screw-cutter*, *Journal Hell. Studies* 1936, 72—77

(12) Hamilton, R. W., *Note on chapel and a wine-press at 'Ain el Jedîde* (*Quart. Dept. Ant. Palestine* 1935, 111—117)

(13) Gsell, S., *Les monuments de l'Algérie*, Vol. I & II, Paris, 1901

(14) Dalman, G., *Arbeit und Sitte in Palästina* (Gütersloh 1935, Vol. IV, 206 & 221)

(15) Mau, A., *Pompeii in Leben und Kunst* (2° edit. Berlin 1908) plate 1x & fig. 185 showing such presses from the house of the Vettii, Pompeii and from Herculaneum

(16) Boer, W. den, *Hesiod's Mortar and Pestle* (*Works and Days*, 423—426) Mnemosyne ser. IV, vol. IX, 1, 1956, 1—10

Landsberger, B., *Zur Mehlbereitung im Altertum* (*Or. Lit. Ztg.*, Vol. 25, 1922, 337—344)

(17) SAN NICOLO, M., *Ein Mühlenbaurecht des Tempels Eanna in neubabylonischer Zeit* (*Arch. Orient.* 1935, 367—371)
(18) HORWITZ, H. TH., *Die Drehbewegung in ihrer Bedeutung fur die Entwicklung der materiellen Kultur* (*Anthropos*, Vol. 29, 1934, 99—107)
(19) EVANS, A., *The palace of Minos*, Vol. II, p. 13
(20) WACE and THOMPSON, *Prehistoric Thessaly*, page 146
(21) VICKERY, K. F., *Food in early Greece* (Urbana 1936)
(22) ROSTOVTZEFF, M., *The Social and Economic History of the Hellenistic World*, Oxford 1941, Vol. I, page 176 & Plate XXV
(23) OPPENHEIM, M. VON, *Tell Halaf*, London 1932, page 205
(23a) RATHJENS, C. and WISSMANN, H. VON, *Vorislamische Altertümer*, 95
(24) FOUQUÉ, *Santorin et ses éruptions*, Paris 1879, pags. 103 & 112
(25) GORDON CHILDE, V., *Rotary querns on the Continent and in the Mediterranean Basin* (*Antiquity*, Vol. 17, 1943, page 19)
SANKALIA, H. D., *Rotary Querns from India* (*Antiquity* XXXIII, 1959, 128—130)
(26) SCHAEFFER, CL. F. A., *Les fouilles de Minet-el-Beida et de Ras Shamra* (*Syria*, Vol. X, 1929, p. 286—287; Vol. XII, 1931, pag. 2; Vol. XV, 1934, page 106)
(27) MACALISTER, S., *Excavations of Gezer*, London 1912, vol. I, pags. 96, 369, 392; vol. II, page 36 & Fig. 228
SELLIN, E. & WATZINGER, C., *Jericho, Ergebniss der Ausgrabungen*, Leipzig 1913, page 153 and fig. 41
SCHUMACHER, G., *Tell-el-Mutesselim* I, Leipzig 1908, page 62 & fig. 32
(28) PAUSANIAS, III.20.2
PLINY, *Nat. Hist.* 36, 135—136
(29) CECIL CURWEN, E., *Querns* (*Antiquity*, Vol. XI, 1927, 133—151)
CECIL CURWEN, E., *More about Querns* (*Antiquity*, Vol. XV, 1941, 15—32)
DESTEXNE-JAMOTTE, J., *Communication sur les meules omaliennes de la Hesbaye Liègeoise* (*Bull. Soc. Préh. Franc.* nos. 9—10, 1951, 474—478)
(30) LINDET, L., *Les origines du moulin à grains* (*Rev. Arch.* 1899, 413—427; 1900, 17—44)
GLEISBERG, H., *Geschichte der Getreidemühle* (*Abh. Ber. Dtsches Museum* 24, 1956, Heft 3)
(31) CATO, *De Agri Cultura* X.4
(31a) STEENSBERG, A., *Farms and watermills in Denmark* (Copenhagen 1952 297)
(32) XENOPHON, *Cyropaedia* 6.2.31, see also *Anabasis* I.55
(33) LIVY, XXVII, 45
(34) FRONTINUS, *Strategems* IV.1.6
(35) DIOSCORIDES, *Herbal* V.103
(36) PETRONIUS, *Fragm. trag.* (edit. BURMAN) 74
(37) PLINY, *Nat. History* XXVIII, 97
(38) XENOPHON, *Anabasis* I.55
ARISTOTLE, *Probl.* 35.3
ALEXIS (350 B.C.), *Amph.* 1 & *Pyraun.* 4
(39) VARRO, *De Re Rust.* I. 55

Ovid, *Fast.* VI, 318 & 470
(40) Ovid, *Fast.* VI, 383
(41) Cato, *De Agri Cultura* XI.4
(42) Aulus Gellius, III.3
(43) Renan, *Mission en Phénicie*, page 93, plates 1 & 5
(44) Virgil, *Moretum* 19, 30—39
(45) Jacobi, H., *Römische Getreidemühlen* (*Saarburgjahrbuch*, Vol. III, 1912, 81)
Winniczuk, L., *Le travail du meunier et du boulanger dans la Grèce et Rome antique* (*in Polish*) (*Bibl. popularna Meandra* VI, Warzawa, 1951)
(46) *Münich Cod. Lat.* 197 (Hussitencodex) fol. 18 b & 42 b
(47) *Mittelalterliches Hausbuch der Familie Wolfegg*
(48) *Codex Atlantico*, fol. 381 rb
(49) Laufer, B., *Chinese Pottery of the Han Dynasty*, London 1916, pags. 15—16
(50) Exod. 27.20; 29.40; Lev. 24.2; Num. 28.5; Ki. 5.25
(51) Dalman, G., *Arbeit und Sitte in Palästina* (Gütersloh 1935, Vol. IV, pags. 206 & 221)
(52) Hörle, J., *Trapetum*, *Pauly-Wissowa*, Vol. VI.A.II.2187 ff
(53) Blümner, H., *Technologie und Terminologie der Gewerbe und Kunste bei Griechen und Römern*, Leipzig 1912, pag. 337
(54) Brønsted, J., *Recherches à Salone*, Vol. I, 1928, page 112, fig. 108
(55) Blümner, H., *Arch. Ztg.*, Vol. 35, 1877, page 53
(56) Thouvenot, R., *Elements de pressoir à huile trouvés à Sale* (*Publ. Serv. Antiq. Maroc*, vol. X, pags 227/30)
Camps-Fabrer, H., *L'olivier et l'huile dans l'Afrique romaine* (lger, 1953)
Drachmann, A. G., *Ancient Oil Mills and Presses*, Copenhagen 1932, 7
(57) Robinson, *Olynthus*, Vol. VIII: The Hellenic House, page 338
(58) Columella, *De Re Rust.* XII. 52.6; Cato, *De Agri Cultura* cap. 20—22
(59) Columella, *De Re Rust.* XII, 52.6; Palladius, XII, 17.1
(60) Pliny, *Nat. History*, XVIII.10
(61) Maurizio, *Histoire de l'alimentation végétale*, Paris 1932, page 305
(62) Polybius, *World History* I.22
(63) *Mining & Metallurgy*, May 1938, page 244
(64) Forbes, R. J., *Metallurgy in Antiquity*. Leiden 1950; Studies Vol VII (1963)
Rickard, T. A., *Eng. Min. J.*, Vol. 122, 1926, page 650
(65) Löwe, P., *Das Dreschen einst und jetzt*, (*Beitr. Gesch. Techn. Ind.*, Vol. 18, 1928, 139—142)
Tritton, W., *The origin of the threshing machine*, (*Lincolnshire Magazine* 1935)
(66) Pliny, *Nat. Hist.* XVIII. 298
(67) Ruth 2.17; Ju. 6.11
(68) Columella, *De Re Rust.* II.20.10 "baculis et fustibus"
(69) Varro, *De Re Rust.* 42.1
Columella, *De Re Rust.* II.21
(70) Crawford, O. G. S., *A primitive threshing machine*, (*Antiquity*, Vol. 9, 1935, 335—339)
(71) 2 Sam. 12,31; 24.22; 1 Chron. 20.3; 21.23; Hiob 41.23
(72) Varro, *De Re Rust.* 42.1
(73) Columella, *De Re Rust.* II.20.4
(74) Pliny, *Nat. History* 33.71

CHAPTER SIX

SALTS, PRESERVATION PROCESSES, MUMMIFICATION

In discussing the salts known to the ancients we will confine ourselves to those produced in sufficient quantity and applied on a fairly large scale, e.g. common salt, natron, natural alkali and alum. However, we have to add a few remarks on saltpetre and sal ammoniac, because these salts are often wrongly mentioned in translated texts due to the complicated ancient nomenclature (see Table XVII).

Common Salt

People living on a diet of meat get all the salt they need in their food. The appetite for free salt was wetted with the increase of the vegetable component in food and hence the rise of salt production in prehistoric times coincides with the establishment of settled agriculture. Salt consumption amounts 1 kgr per head per year. Cato allows a modius (8.75 l) a year for every slave on the farm, as they live practically on a vegetarian diet.

Hence the ancients have to produce salt or as Pliny has it (1): "By Hercules, salt is an essential to civilised existence, and so necessary is this substance that the word which denotes it has come to be used also of pleasures of the mind; these are called sales, and no other word can better sum up all the grace of life, the height of merriment, and recreation after toil.

Even in military awards it finds its place, and the word salarium (salt-money) is derived from it. It was held in high honour among the ancients, as is clear from the salaria via, a road so called because along it the Sabines were permitted to import salt. King Ancus Marcius gave six thousand modii of salt as a largess to the people, and was the first to open salterns. Varro also tells us that our ancestors used salt as a seasoning and it is clear from the proverb that they ate it with bread. It is in sacred rites, however, that it admittedly achieves the highest importance, for no offerings are perfect without salted spelt."

Salt and incense have been proclaimed the chief economic and religious necessaries of the Ancient World. The quest for salt from the earliest times onwards is reflected in the "salt-routes" which together with the trade routes of amber, flint and other valuable merchandise form a network covering the whole of Europe and the Mediterranean basin stretching beyond the Ancient Near East into Asia. Unfortunately little is known about the actual production of salt in prehistoric times apart from these trade-routes along which cakes of salt have been found. Such cakes were used as money and they often served to pay imposts, as still customary among primitive tribes (2). It seems, that both rock-salt deposits and salines were worked, salt obtained by evaporation of the water of saline springs and certain spots on the Atlantic and North Sea were famous for their salterns. Place names compounded with "hal" (such as Halstatt) or with "wich" (such as Droitwich) refer to old salt production which is often contemporary with the beginning of iron metallurgy. Now and then short passages in the works of classical authors enlighten us on this point and we have a fairly long passage in PLINY (3), which (omitting the medical applications of salt) runs thus:

"Salt is of two kinds, that wich is prepared by man and that which occurs in nature. In each case there are several varieties, but two ultimate causes, the condensation and the evaporation of moisture. In the lake at Tarentum the water is evaporated by the summer sun, and the whole pool, which is rather small and nowhere more than knee-deep, turns into salt. The same thing occurs in Sicily in Lake Cocianus and in a lake near Gela, but in these cases only the edges of the lake dry up. This happens also in Phrygia, in Cappadocia, and at Aspendus, where evaporation covers a wider area, as much as half the lake. Another remarkable feature in the latter case is the fact that the salt removed by day is restored by night. Lake-salt is granular and never occurs in large masses.

A second kind is produced spontaneously from seawater, when spray, left on the rocks and on the upper reaches of the shore, is concentrated by the sun. The salt found on the rocks has a sharper taste than other salt.

There are three further variations of naturally occurring salt. In Bactria there are two vast lakes, one towards Scythia, the other towards Ariana, which seethes with salt, just as at Citium in Cyprus and around Memphis. The salt is drawn from the lake and dried in the sun. Again, the surfaces of rivers solidify into salt, beneath which the rest of the river flows as beneath a sheet of ice. This happens in the case of the "salt-rivers" near the Caspian Gates and among the Mardians and the

TABLE XVII

Ancient Nomenclature of the Common Salts

ENGLISH	EGYPTIAN	SUMERIAN	ACCADIAN
SALT (SODIUM CHLORIDE)			
salt	hmȝ.t (III.94.1) hmȝj.t (III.94.6)	MUN	ṭâbtu (Hebrew mélaḥ)
(stone of the blood)		(^{a}MUD)	(aban dâme)
rocksalt, halite	—	MUN-KUR	ṭâbat šadî
sal gemma	—	MUN-KÙ-GA	ṭâbtu ellitu
red sal gemma	—	MUN-Ù-MU-UN	ṭâbat amâni
river salt	—	MUN-EME-ŠAL-LA(LIM)	ṭâbat emesalli
NATRON (NATURAL CARBONATE OF SODA)			
natron	nṯrj (II.366.8)	(Hebrew nèthèr)	nitiru, nitru
sal murale ("crust of the wall")	—	SAḪAR-ÚR	eper assurê
crude (?) natron	ḥsmn (III.162.11)	—	—
granular natron	bḫḫ (I.471.15)	—	—
red natron	ḥsmn dšrt	—	—
natron from Wadi Natrun	šrp (IV.528.4)	—	—
natron for purification	bd (I.486.5) (refined ?) bsn (I.475.11) św'b (IV.67.4)	—	—
NATURAL ALKALI VEGETABLE			
vegetable alkali (Salicornia)	—	^{ú}NAGA	^{ú}uḫûlu (Hebrew: gasûl)
"horned alkali"	—	^{ú}NAGA-SI	^{ú}uḫûlu ḳarnânu
plant ashes used as alkali	—	—	^{ú}uḫûlu ḳalâti (Hebrew: kali, borith)
SALTPETRE (POTASSIUM NITRATE)			
nitrate of potash	—	^{zá}AN-NE (IZI)	mil'u
SAL AMMONIAC			
sal ammoniac ("sublimate of scrapings")	—	IM-KAL (-LA)	aklu (ḫaṣbu, ḫilṣu)
"soot from dung"	—	SAḪAR-SIS	iṭru, iṭranu
ALUM			
alum	ibnw (I.63.8) imrw (I.87.19) (?)	IM-SAḪAR-ZÁ-KUR-RA	gabû (Hebrew: seriph)
white alum (refined ?)	—	IM-SAḪAR-BABBAR-KUR-RA	annuḫaru
black alum	—	IM-SAḪAR-GE-KUR-RA	kitmu
alunite, alum stone	—	^{a}DÙ-ŠUB-BA	^{a}aban šikkati
(" lichen of the tamarisk")	—	—	(^{ú}kamun bîni)

Armenians. Moreover, the Bactrian rivers, Ochus and Oxus, carry down particles of salt from the hills over against them and certain lakes in Africa are actually turbid with salt. Hot springs too are sometimes salt-bearing, witness those at Pagase. So much for the varieties of salt which are spontaneously produced from water.

Mountains of salt are found, like Oromenus in India, where it is quarried like stone and renews itself, and kings derive a greater proportion of their income from salt than from gold and pearls. In Cappadocia it is dug out of the earth, where it has clearly been formed by the condensation of moisture, and may indeed be hewn like lapis specularis (mica). The lumps are of great weight and are popularly known as micae.

At Gerrhae, a town in Arabia, walls and houses are made with blocks of salt cemented together with water (3a). King Ptolemy also found salt near Pelusium, when he was camping there, and later it was similarly discovered when the sand had been removed, in the parched districts between Egypt and Arabia, and in the thirsty lands of Africa as far as the oracle of Hammon, where it grows with the moon of nights. For the country round Cyrene is famous for the salt of Hammon, so called because it is found close to the altars of that deity. It resembles alumen schiston in colour, and occurs in long opaque pieces, unpleasant to the taste but useful in medicine. The more transparent it is, the better, and it should have a rectilinear cleavage. It is said to have this remarkable quality, that, though very light in the mines where it is found, it increases in weight to an extent which is scarcely credible when brought to the light of day. The reason is obvious; the moist vapour of the mines renders the miners an assistance like that of water. It is adulterated with the Sicilian salt which we have named Cocanicum, and with Cyprian salt which is marvellously like it. Salt is mined also, in almost transparent lumps, at Egelesta in Hither Spain, and most doctors have long given this variety the palm over other kinds of salt. Every place in which salt naturally occurs is barren and brings forth no fruit of any description.

There are various kinds of artificial salt, most of it being made by the common process of leading the sea into salterns with streams of fresh water. Rain-water, however, is the most helpful, and a hot sun is indispensable — otherwise the brine does not evaporate to dryness. Africa rears its heaps of salt like hills near Utica, and when they have been hardened by the sun and moon, water cannot dissolve them and even iron can scarce cut them. Yet salt is prepared in Crete without any addition of fresh water by leading the sea into salterns, as well as in Egypt, where the sea washes itself up into land sodden, I understand, by the Nile. Again, salt is prepared by driving well-water into salt deposits. In Babylon, the first product to separate out by condensation is a fluid and oily bitumen, which is used for lamps — this once removed, the salt is found underneath. In Cappadocia, too, they drive well- and spring-water into the deposits. In Chaonia they boil spring water, which on cooling deposits a salt which has neither transparancy nor savour.

In Gaul and Germany, salt water is poured on burning logs.

In a certain part of Spain, the salt water is drawn from wells and called muria. The Spaniards indeed consider the nature of the wood to be a matter of importance. Oak-wood is best, for its ashes, even when not thus treated, have a saltiness of their own; elsewhere hazel-wood is praised. So, when the salt water is poured on, even the charcoal is turned to salt. Salt made with wood is always black. I find in Theophrastus that the Embri used to boil down the ashes of reeds and rushes with water, until the liquid had been reduced to a small bulk. Why, salt can even be recovered by heat from brine used for pickling; when the liquid is all gone, the salt is found unchanged. Most people prefer the brine used for menae for this purpose.

The best sea-salt comes from Salamis in Cyprus, while the best lake-salts are the Tarentine and the Phrygian which is known as Tattaean,.... The driest varieties taste most salty. Tarentine salt, which is the whitest of all, is also the blandest, and, for the rest, the whitest salts are the most brittle. All are sweetened by rain, while dew gives a blander salt. Salt is deposited plentifully during northerly gales, and not at all if the wind is south. Flower of salt is produced only when the wind is northerly. Neither Tragasaean salt nor Acanthian (named after that city), nor spray salt from any source, nor finely-divided salt crackles or leaps in the fire, while Agrigentine salt, which is unaffected by fire, leaps out of the water.

Variations in colour occur, salt being red at Memphis, reddish near the Oxus, and purple at Centuripae, while near Gela, which is also in Sicily it glistens so as to present a reflecting surface, and when mined in Cappadocia, it is saffron-coloured, translucent, and very pleasantly scented. For medical use our ancestors held Tarentine salt in the highest esteem and after it any sea-salt, especially that deposited by the spray....

All the best kinds for seasoning food deliquesce easily, and therefore are moister, for these varieties, like Attic and Euboeic, are less bitter. Dry and bitter salt, such as Megarian, is more suitable for preserving food, it excites the appetite and stimulates it so that one easily picks out its flavour amid a multitude of condiments, and it is this same flavour which attracts those who eat garum (fish-sauce). Why, it is particularly effective in giving even sheep and cattle and baggage-animals such an appetite for pasture that they give a much more plentiful supply of milk, which furnishes cheese of a far more pleasing quality.

Pits that furnish pure salt have this chief distinguishing characteristic, that they produce favilla salis (ash of salt) which is really the finest and whitest part of salts. (here follows a discussion of flos salis (flowers of salt) a substance which seems to have nothing to do with salt and which can not be identified).... Besides these there occurs in salt mines what some call salsugo, others salsilago (brine). This is entirely liquid, salter than sea water and differing from it in efficacy."

Pliny rightly distinguishes three different base materials for salt production: rock-salt, brine waters and sea-water. It would seem that the quarrying of rock-salt is the oldest form of salt production and that man then turned to concentrated brines from wells or saltmines and finally produced "solar salt" from sea-water in salterns on the shores of the sea and ocean.

In prehistoric Europe the rock salt mines of the eastern Alps play an important part. The mines of Salzburg, Hallstatt, Dürrnberg and Hallein were worked on a scale which far transcended local needs at an early date (4). Galleries were driven as far as 350 M. into the mountains. Picks, wooden shovels and wedges were used for the production of salt. Stones to grind the picks were found in the galleries as were torches stuck in staves about 1 M. long and held by two rings made of lime-bark. A certain amount of timber work was necessary to prevent the galleries from caving in and bronze tools of the ancient carpenters were found too. The lumps of rock-salt produced were broken up with the help of wedges and hammers. The form of the tools suggests that these mines were certainly operated during the later stages of the Bronze Age (from say 1400 B.C. onwards) and may be even during the earlier stages. Exploitation was carried on at Hallstatt until it was seemingly interrupted by the invasions of the Celts about 400 B.C.

However, during the Early Iron Age the miners seem to have abandoned the mining of rock-salt and to have concentrated on the brine recovered from the sumps in the mines, which they concentrated in salterns in the meadows in front of the mines. These and brine-springs now constituted the base materials of an industry, the extent of which is demonstrated by the rich Hallstatt cemetries of the Iron Age. The concentration of such natural brines (or even artificial ones produced by washing the salt strata with water) was effected by heated stones or artificial structures of clay bars and pedestals erected over a fire, over which structure brine trickled from clay troughs. The concentrated brine mingled with the ashes to form a black mass sold in cakes or lumps. We have seen PLINY's report on this ancient method and TACITUS (5) when discussing the land of the Cattians, tell us that "according to the creed of those savage nations, that part of the world lay in the neighbourhood of the heavens and thence the prayers of men were wafted to the ears of the gods. The whole region was by consequence peculiarly favoured; and to that circumstance it was to be ascribed, that the river and the adjacent woods teemed with quantities of salt, not, as in other places, a concretion on the seashore formed by the foaming of the waves, but produced by the simple act of throwing the water from the stream on a pile of burning wood, where by the conflict of the opposite elements, the substance was engendered. For this salt a bloody battle was fought (between the Hermundurians and the Cattians)".

This burning and briquetage of salt also took place in the Saale valley near Halle and Magdeburg and in the Saale valley, east-north-east of Nancy. When later sea-water was concentrated certain regions in the north where more rains fell, this was usually carried on the last stages of concentration on structures as described above with the help of artificial heat. Such reddish burnt soil and quantities of briquetage of Hallstatt-inspired industries dating back to the Iron Age A were found on the Lincolnshire coast and also near LaPanne in Belgium. This method was not only still used in Roman times but it is mentioned in a Frisian deed of 1258 (6) though peat was then used instead of wood and "Frisian salt" is mentioned upto the nineteenth century. It is still in use in Transsylvania and Moldavia. PLINY makes it clear that the salt water from the bitumen seepages of Mesopotamia was also used for the production of salt.

The salt produced as rock-salt or by the concentration of brine derived from salt-bearing strata is often very pure or contains but few impurities, thus identifying each type of salt by the taste imparted to it by its few impurities. Producing salt from sea-water is much more complicated a process, for the waters of the sea have dissolved many different salts. Generally speaking, if we evaporate a solution of different salts like sea-water, the least soluble salt will be precipitated first as its saturation point is reached. Hence we can expect the following order of crystallisation in saltpans: calcium carbonate, calcium sulphate (gypsum), sodium chloride (salt), magnesium sulphate, carnallite (potassium magnesium chloride), magnesium chloride. Hence the calcium salt will separate from the solution before the salt crystals appear, but the magnesium salts are the most soluble and may be included in crude salt to impart a bitter taste to it.

True this simplified picture is complicated in practice by the simultaneous and overlapping crystallisation of some of the salts, but we can certainly divide salt-making from sea-water into three phases:

a) the separation and removal of the calcium salts and other less soluble impurities, b) the concentration and crystallisation of the salt itself and c) the removal of the mother liquor or bitterns from the crystallised salt or the separation of the magnesium salts by leaching the crude salt. These three phases are usually preceded by an evaporation of the bulk of the water by solar heat in salterns, the total area of which is ten times that of the crystallisation ponds in which the latter stages take place.

We find these different stages in the earliest reports on the production of salt from sea water, not only from Chinese sources but also in classical texts (7). The first stage is the wholesale evaporation of the greater part of the water. The sea water drawn up by means of Archimedean screws or introduced by opening a canal towards the sea is now divided over a series ponds connected by ditches and left there to evaporate by solar heat, until the colour turns red.

As the concentration of the brine approaches saturation, the "brine-worms" (or "clearer worms") and algae die, the specific gravity of the brine approaches the value 1.21 and it becomes pinkish in colour because of the growth of certain bacteria. The salt-maker takes this change of colour as an indication that the brine is ready to be trans-. ferred to the crystallisation ponds. Salt water is not at all sterile and the formation of the "red water" was a phenomenon well-known to the ancients (8). The colour is not due to the presence of slight amounts of iron oxide which have but a slight influence but to that of pink, red and purple bacteria such as "codfish" bacteria, red yeasts and purple sulphur bacteria, depending on the kind of organic material or impurities present. Certain of these bacteria contain a green pigment which upon decomposition yields a brown water-soluble product.

These bacteria are the red organisms discolouring the salt of certain pre-classical sites and of those mentioned by PLINY in the passage we quoted above. Many desert lakes along the Mediterranean shore are called the "Red Lake". Similar phenomena have been noticed elsewhere, e.g. in Searle's Lake, California. In certain cases plants may be the cause of the red colour or rather chlorophyll-bearing organisms such as Dunaliella salina. There is good evidence that this was sometimes the case in Antiquity too. When PLINY mentions "pleasantly scented" salt from Cappadocia, this may be due to the formation of ionon by the decomposition of the carotin of these organisms.

The oldest Chinese treatise on pharmacology, the Pen ts'ao kang mu gives instructions which differ little from those mentioned by PLINY, even the tests are very similar. In China the south wind blowing with force during summer and autumn may make the salt "grain" over night, but if it does not come all the profits are lost. PLINY's remarks on the winds are probably also indications on the speed of evaporation in the salt-works. No hydrometers were known yet, and the specific gravity of the brine was measured in China with a hen's egg or a lotus seed, tests which are equivalent to those given by CATO and other classical authors. PLINY (9) gives what is surely one of the earliest estimates of the solubility of salt, four sextarii of water dissolving one sextarius of salt. The sextarius is a volumetric unit and taking the density of salt to be 2.174 we arrive at a solubility of less than 54.3 grams of salt in 100 grams of water. We can not calculate an exact figure for all depends on how much air space his solid salt contained. The true concentration is 34.5 grams per 100 grams of water.

The "red water" being led into the much smaller crystallisation ponds increases in specific gracity from 1.21 to 1.25, when the salt would begin to settle. As the "hoppers begin to corn" the liquor is now led to the "bitterns", where sulphates and calcium salts (notably in pit salt or brines from wells) have to be removed.

The sulphates are decomposed by anaerobic bacteria and combine with any iron compound present to form a black mud of clay interspersed with hydrous ferrous sulphide. When exposed to the air this mud gives of the evil-smelling hydrogen sulphide and hence in many languages the words for "salt" and "stench" are etymologically connected. The "briner" has to "harvest" his salt with flat shovels without disturbing this "slutch as black as the cuttle-fish". This is called the "purification by *harvesting*". The calcium salts can usually be removed by *clarification*. In certain older recipes such as that of Agricola this is accomplished by adding one part of blood to 1500 parts of brine and some strong beer to hasten the crystallisation of such impurities. Usually, however this clarification is combined with the earlier first stage of evaporation and achieved by the "clearer worms", which the ancients do not mention but which appear on the Arab menu and which were used by the old English briner.

As the specific gravity of the brine in the salterns (crystallisation ponds) rises from 1.25 to 1.275 fine and coarser qualities of salt crystallize and are removed with shovels. Then the mother liquor is transferred to the bitterns where crude salt and qualities only suitable for pickling, etc. can be produced. As this mother liquor contains nearly all the magnesium salts which are very bitter, this final product and even those of the earlier stages sometimes have to be purified by *leaching*. The salt then looses most of the magnesium salts; for instance by exposing a salt pile to the rains, its bitter taste almost disappears and its hygroscopity is reduced.

In certain cases the ancients helped themselves by buying crude salt and refining it at home. CATO (10) gives us a recipe for this: "Make white salt as follows: Take a clean amphora with the neck broken off, fill it with pure water and set it in the sun. Suspend in it a little bag of common salt, shake it and fill it up from time to time. Do this several times each day until the salt has for two days ceased to dissolve. This will be the sign: put in it a small dried fish or an egg; if it floats it will be brine such as that in which you preserve meat or cheese or pickled fish. Pour off this brine in pans or shallow dishes and set it in the sun. Keep it in the sun until it has dried. In this way the best of salt is made. When the weather is cloudy and at night set it under a roof; by day, when the sun shines, set it in the sun".

The salt production of ancient Egypt fairly large, but we have few technological data on this subject. In Egypt natron, the natural sodium carbonate, had absorbed the religious and magical importance, which salt enjoyed in other civilisations. This purely practical meaning of salt to the ancient Egyptians is clearly reflected in its very simple nomenclature. For though the papyrus Ebers and other medical writings mention salt (11) as in ingredient in their recipes, they have no separate terms for the "mine salt", "sea salt" or "salt of the north", which they mention. There are several salt deposits in the Western desert, but HERODOTUS is wrong in saying (12) that 'the ground is coated with salt, in somuch that the very pyramids are wasted thereby!". We get the impression, that salt was mainly produced from sea water in the lakes of the Delta. PLINY apart from a "lake near Memphis", mentions the "salt pans of Pelusium", which also occur in HERODOTUS' narrative, where the centre of the Royal monopoly of salt production was in Ptolemaic times. Now this centre has shifted to Lake Mareotis in the north-west corner of the Delta. These salterns ensured an abundant supply of salt, which was used for gold refining, for the manufacture of glazes and in medical recipes. A curious use is that of salt and oil in night lamps (13), in which the salt no doubt dessicated the oil and coloured the flame. The main application of salt, however, was the seasoning of food and the salting of fish, to which subject we will revert later on. To obtain pure ricinus (or kiki) oil the Egyptians mixed the seeds of the castor oil plant with salt before expressing them.

Salt was traded in ancient Egypt in the form of lumps or bricks, many examples of which have been found. Two bricks, dating from about 1500 B.C., had the following dimensions: 20 × 11 × 5 cms and 19 × 9 × 4 cms. Down to our oldest analysed sample (VIth dynasty) this salt proved to be very pure, which again points to salterns as the main source of salt supply.

A certain amount of salt was, however, also produced in the Oasis of Ammon. This was the Hammonic salt mentioned by PLINY, whose story is corroborated by STRABO(14), ARRIAN(15) and HERODOTUS(16). This was not the modern "sal ammoniac" but real salt which is here found in the form of rock-salt in gypsum, with a salt content of some 10—20%. It seems that the priests of the famous temple of Ammon have extracted the "many beds of salt still to be found there and jets of salt water rising to some height" on which Strabo reported, to which account ARRIAN has the following details to add: "There are natural salts in this district, to be obtained by digging; some of these salts are taken by priests of Ammon to Egypt. For whenever they are going towards Egypt, they pack the salt into baskets woven of palm leaves and take them as a present to the king or to someone else. The grains of this salt are large, some of them have been known to be more than three finger's breadth; and it is so clear as crystal. Both the Egyptians and others who are particular about religious observances, use this salt in their sacrifices, as being purer than the sea-salts."

This salt seems to have been traded as far as Persia. HERODOTUS in the same passage (16) mentions rock-salt deposits further west on the North African coast in Fezzan and the country of the Garamantians. STRABO too has a few passages on rock salt quarried by the Aethiopians and the Arabians (17).

ARRIAN is wrong when he claims that this salt was used in the Egyptian temple for the ancients themselves were aware of the fact that the Egyptians preferred natron to salt in ritual. PLUTARCH (18) reports that sea salt was called "foam of Typhon (Seth)" in ancient Egypt and that the Egyptian priests avoided it. They may have believed the rock-salt of Ammon to be a kind of natron as mined in the other oases, but this is not confirmed by any text.

Salt played a much larger part in the Semitic world (19). If we call Egypt the land of natron, Mesopotamia is verily the land of salt, where natron, though known, is of minor importance. Many different types of rock salt were recognized, e.g. "mountain salt", sal gemma and red sal gemma (the andarânî of India). Large deposits were known near Ali Dagh, north of Tuz Khurmatli, near Koh Tuz not far from Mardin and near Vihan and Sert, but they do not figure largely in our documents. Brine springs were numerous in Mesopotamia, Persia and Phrygia, the well-known bitumen seepages of Hit producing large quantities of saline water. However, the table salt for everyday use was "impure river salt" derived from river water by simple evaporation. This mixture of crude sodium chloride and certain quantities of magnesium salts is often referred to as "the salt that broadens, the tongue", "salt from the middle of the river" or "salt of mankind". This and the purer desert salt (ṭâbtu) were sold in rough lumps (kirbanu) at the bazar and when used crushed to powder in the mills (sahle) also used for darnel and other herbs. The Assyrians carried salt in small pouches called "tukkânu".

The best quality, desert salt, was used in the service of the gods, for the offerings had to be seasoned with salt in the same way as the Jews were ordered to salt theirs. "Thou art salt, produced in a pure place and destined to Enlil for eating by the great gods. Without thee no meal is taken in the temple." It seems that this first quality salt was refined by crystallisation. Medically it is frequently used, e.g. as an emetic. It figures in recipes for glass and glazes. Its magical purifying powers were used practically to preserve food. As early as the Agade period we hear of fish and salt dispatched together, though we can not infer from this evidence that this meant pickled fish. Later texts mention, that fish "in salt thou shalt preserve unto sunrise" and that "meat has been brought thee in salt". In chemical texts and recipes salt sometimes occurs under the cover-name of "stone of the blood".

The use of table salt became of course imperative as soon as mankind no longer consumed its meat raw or roasted. Boiled meat, fish or vegetables need seasoning by extra salt or spices and therefore we find this custom in all the large sedentary civilisations in the Near East (20). As in Mesopotamia salt was a necessity in baking bread in Palestine. To eat somebody's salt was identical with eating his bread. Salt was indeed considered to be one of the "principal things for the whole use of a man's life" (21) in the world of the Old Testament. Fish is cooked and eaten with salt. "Cook fish in its brother (salt), put it in its father (water), eat it with its son (juice) and drink with it its father (water)."

Salt has a definite religious meaning in Palestine like in ancient Mesopotamia. The Old Testament does not only refer to the "Covenant of Salt" (22), but it prescribes the use of salt in offerings (23), even when the sacrifice consists of a slaughtered animal (24).

We hear, that this salt was mainly rock salt from Khirbet Qumrān near the Dead Sea (25). The salt from salterns near Ostrakine on the Mediterranean coast was considered inferior quality. In Hellenistic times salt seems also to have been produced at Magdala, from the water of Lake Tiberias for the curing of fish (26). The Temple of Jerusalem had storehouses for salt (salt-chambers, liškat ham-mélah) on the north side of the central court, which were supervised by a special official (27). It was probably traded in lumps or cakes, for we read that salt was crushed in wooden mortars. Apart from the seasoning of food and the curing of fish salt was used in oil lamps in ancient Palestine in analogy of Egyptian custom. This was believed to produce a brighter light and to improve the life of the wick.

We have no very early data on salt production in Asia Minor, but in classical times there were several centres. Salt was produced in salt pans on the sea-coast such as the Tragasaean "where salt is naturally caused to congeal by the Etesian winds" (29), the salt works of Athena Polias of Priene, protected by the father of Julius Caesar (30), on the mouth of the Halys (31) and near Aspendus. The most famous brand, however, came from Cyprus (the neighbourhood of Salamis) (32) which Pliny praises and from Lake Tatta in the interior, which was "a natural salt-pan; and the water so easily congeals round everything that is immersed in it that when people let down into it rings made of rope they draw wreaths of salt, and that on account of the congealing of salt, the birds which touch the water with their wings fall on the spot and are caught thus" (33).

Cicero tells us (34) that the salt-pans of Attalid Asia Minor were in the hands of publicani being leased as sources of public revenue.

Roman Syria had a sufficient though not abundant supply of salt (35) and once the introduction of the camel had made trans-desert trade possible the salt of Palmyra, a local monopoly (36), became an important factor in the economy of this famous town. Further north salt was produced from Lake Urmia which had "a harbour Capauta, in which salts effloresce and solidify" (37).

Arabia was known to have several deposits of rock-salt and "the soil near Gerrha contains salt and the people live in houses made of salt; and since flakes of salt continuously scale off owing to the scorching heat of the sun, and fall away, the people frequently sprinkle the houses with water and thus keep the walls firm" (38). Further east in India salt was produced too, PLINY informs us that this was an important source of income for the Indian kings along the sea coast and in Rajputana. By a chance reference in STRABO (39) we know that Alexander the Great had a special mining engineer and prospector (metalleutes) on his staff during his great expedition. This Gorgus investigated the mineral resources of the kingdom of Sopheites (near the modern Lahore) and found not only rich veins of silver and gold but also "a mountain of mineral salt sufficient for the whole of India". Like PLINY STRABO held that this rock-salt filled up again in time (40).

Greece had no deposits of rock salt and domestic supplies were obtained from sea water and brine wells. Third-century Greece had to import fairly large quantities of salt notwithstanding salt-works in Attica (Gephyra), Megara, Euboea and Crete. HOMER may have called salt divine (41) and the poets may have referred to it as "the holy ice of Aigaion" (42) but it played no prominent part of religion. Large quantities were imported from Olbia from salt-works at the mouth of the Borysthenes (Dnjepr) known to HERODOTUS (43) and in the Tauric Chersonesus (44). Salt production in those regions was essential for the exports of pickled "Pontica salsamenta", an essential part of Greek diet (45) and in Byzantine times even a necessity the lack of which might cause serious domestic trouble (46). STRABO (47) also mentions salt-works in the Illyrian area, where "the salt was made to crystallize out of water which in the springtime flowed at the foot of a certain mountain glen; for if they drew off the water and stowed it away for five days the salt would become thoroughly crystallised". In the early days salt seems even to have been exported to be sold "among such men as know not the sea, neither eat meat savoured with salt" (48).

In the Hellenistic period salt monopolies seems to have been common in most Hellenistic states who may have acted on early attempts of this kind by the Persian financial administration. Salt was of course a product that lent itself very well to monopolistic control, it belonged to the many raw materials for industrial production which the state manipulated. The salt was extracted in the Delta from sea-water, marshes and even the desert soil, and also from lakes near Memphis, from Mount Casius and Paraetonium. These salt pans and mines belonged to the government and they were worked in the same way as other mines and quarries. We have few data to establish the precise relation between the crown and the salt-workers. Only once do we find that women were assigned as a liturgy to the salt-workers of Hermopolis (49). It looks as if the wholesale trade was not free, it was supplied to dealers by government officials, the price for retail trade being fixed by royal decree. The dealer had to pay for his licence (50), which payment was often made in advance (51). Some groups like the priests, the army or officials acquired it directly from the state.

Only once, in this case for the Fayum province, is a broker of the salt sellers recorded (52) whose duties were unknown but who may have purchased the wholesale supplies of the district after he and his colleagues had submitted bids to the government official, the "strategus" of the district (53). Furthermore every inhabitant of Egypt (except a few privileged groups) paid the salt tax (halike) apart from paying for the salt he consumed. As to the latter we do not know whether citizens were required to take off a minimum for neither private household bills nor the papyrus informing us of a cargo of salt to be shipped (54) give any such detail There is, however, definitely a tax on the sale of salt (emponoin halos) (55), a kind of purchase tax apart from the salt tax (halike) of the third century B.C., which latter was a real capital tax. Women paid less than men, slaves pay half the tariff and children were exempt. Freedom was sometimes alotted to prominent officials and victors in the games, but even priests had to pay it (56). The money of this hated salt tax was spent in the province where it was levied (57). The rate was high and it weighed heavily, it was probably reorganised during the second century B.C. Still this form of poll tax lingered on in the Arsinoite nome even in Roman times. The tariff on salt, the purchase tax, was much lower, it amounted to 3 oboles for an artaba of salt in the second century A.D. (58), 4 drachmae on a camel-load a generation later (59) and one drachmae for a measure of salt in the middle of the third century (60).

Salt production was organised on similar lines in Hellenistic Palestine and the "halike" was no less unpopular. Like in other

Hellenistic countries the salt-pans were private possessions of the kings. In the books of the Maccabees and in Josephus' Antiquities it figures as an important source of revenue for the crown. The salt-tax was possibly regarded as the people's contribution to the management of the salt-pans but in addition to this tax they received a certain allowance of salt from the government on payment of a certain sum of money every year. In Seleucid Syria and Babylonia this method of collecting taxes on salt was virtually the same.

In the Roman world salt was more prominent in religion. The Romans always added salt to the barley or flour for their offerings (61) and used sea-water or salt solutions for lustrations. Salt also enters into Roman love-spells (62). It was "bred from the purest parents, sun and sea" (63) or even called "that from the sea" (64). We have already reported that fact that the Roman soldier originally received a salt ration which "salarium" was later paid out in money, and then acquires its present meaning.

The first salines on both sides of the river Tiber near Ostia are reported to have been opened by King Ancus Martius (65) and there was a salt monopoly which can, however, hardly have been profitable for during the second Punic War the state sold six pounds of salt for one as (66). There is some evidence of a salt tax in Sardinia at this very period (67). Polybius does not mention any contract for the salt monopoly which was probably more of the nature of an organisation for the purpose of insuring a regular salt supply. The censors of 204 B.C. had reorganised this as so to insure distributing stations in all towns with fixed prices scaled according to the distance from the source of supply. To manage this business some capital was needed and a number of agents but only a fair interest seems to have been taken. During the later republic even a small town like Miturnae contained publicans, as the inscriptions tell us, who were engaged in farming the revenues of the neighbouring salt-pans, but we have no data to assess the yield of these revenues.

The conquest of Sicily opened up a new source of supply for rock-salt was found near Centuripae (68) and Agrigentum (69). We have only evidence of three salt-farms on this island, one near Gela (70), at Pachynum (71) and at Lake Cocanicus near Agrigentum, as Pliny tells us.

In Spain and Portugal salt was found on many places. The celebrated solar works at Setubal are supposed to have been founded by Hasdrubal. Rock-salt deposits are mentioned by many classical authors (72), in particular those between Seville and Cadiz (73) about which Strabo tells us: "they have salt quarries in their country and not a few streams of salt water; and not unimportant either is the fish-salting industry that is carried on, not only from this country but also from the rest of the seaboard outside the Pillars and the product is not inferior to that of the Pontus," and which were probably worked before the fifth century B.C., and also a large mine at Cardona near Barcelona which certainly worked in CATO's days (74). Many of the brine wells were also used for their health-giving qualities and the Romans claim that they taught the natives of Spain to bathe in hot water (75). The Portugese rock-salt "is red, but when crushed it is white" (76).

The pork-exporting industries in Gaul needed much salt. STRABO mentions (77) that in the middle of the "Stony Plain (now Plaine de la Crau) stands water and salt springs and also lumps of salt". Much salt was used in the country of the Sequana (78) whence "the finest of salted hog-meat is brought down and shipped to Rome".

In Britain there were many coastal salt-works, though "in the Cassiterides tin and lead were exchanged for salt, pottery and copper utensils" (79). During the Roman occupation of Britain they seem to have declined as brine-pits of inland Britain were opened up at Droitwich, Northwich and other places.

The early salts-pans were traced in the many "Red Hills" on the Essex coast of the Thames near Goldhanger. Another group was found on the south shore of the river Crough near Canewdon. They were structures consisting essentially of clay floors heated by flues, their date is confirmed by Romano-British pottery. Numerous objects made of briquetage or rough clay (fire-bars and fire-supports) were found (80). Further works were discovered on the north coast of Kent and on the Channel coast near Dymchurch (81), in east Anglia near Norfolk, in Somerset, the Brue district and on the north coast of Wales

Salt was not only an invaluable ingredient in ancient diet, but as PLINY tells us it has a stimulating effect on grazing animals, a point which several other ancient authors make (82). His remarks on the changes in taste of salt through leaching and refining can be compared with the well-known passages on the "salt of the earth" in the New Testament (83). Salt was also a valuable refining agent in metallurgy (84), the action of salt breezes and brine on metals was well-known (85) and it played its part in soldering and in dyeing (86).

Nowhere in the West did the salt industry attain the degree of sophistication achieved in China during Antiquity. There apart from the usual types of solar evaporation, drilling for salt was applied in the province of Szechwan. A fourth-century geography of the area records the drilling of twenty salts wells in 67 B.C. in this area and inscriptions state that during Han times gas from "fire wells" (natural gas) was used for evaporating the brine. These wells were drilled with derricks, the brine hauled up with the aid of a windlass if it did not flow from itself, poured in a hopper and led through bamboo pipes to evaporation pans. An oven held five such pans and it was heated by natural gas from gas wells which was brought to the site in bamboo pipes too. Not only do reliefs in Han tombs depict this industry, it is also described in detail in the T'ien kung k'ai wu, a Chinese book on industrial technology of 1637. This salt, like that obtained from saltings, played a large part in ancient China's economy (86a).

Natron

Carbonate or bicarbonate of soda never played a large part in the technology of ancient Mesopotamia. The sal murale (87) represents an impure carbonate of soda, which efflorescence, like the sajji matti of the Indian dyers, is collected and used in dyeing with tumeric. The purer nitiru is also mentioned in some dyer's recipes, but never in texts on glass manufacture.

However, natron (the nitron or litron of the classical authors) is far more important in ancient Egypt, where its use eclipsed that of common salt, even as a preservative (88). This natron is a natural compound of sodium carbonate and sodium bicarbonate with varying percentages of sodium chloride and sodium sulphate. This natural product contains from 22—75% of carbonate, 5—32% of bicarbonate, 4—26% of salt (in a few cases upto 60%), 0.8—39% of sodium sulphate and 0—16% of insolubles. The absence of potassium compounds is so typical, that this can give one a clue to the use of natron or plants ashes as an alkaline component in ancient materials. There were three centres of production of natron, all mentioned by Strabo and Pliny (89) though no "artificial natron" was produced from the Nile as Pliny claims.

The most important of these centres was the oasis in the Western desert called Wadi Natrum to this day. Its oldest Egyptian name "st.p.t" became "šrp" (90), which word also came to be used for natron itself. Water from the Nile seeps into this Wadi in the flood season forming twelve little lakes, which gradually dry up as the Nile retires.

The riddle of the formation of crusts and layers of natron from this seepage water is not yet entirely solved. The second centre is near Barnugi (Beheira province) (91) near the ancient merchant port of Naucratis. Finally natron is found in some five localities near El Kab in Upper Egypt, which is referred to in ancient Egyptian texts as "natron from nḫb". The product of these centres, especially that of Wadi Natrun, which continued upto the present day, was an important State monopoly in Ptolemaic times.

The many forms and varying composition of this natron is the root of the many ancient Egyptian terms for his product. The term "ḥsmn" seems to refer to the crude product, it is often said to be red and the word did not only come to mean "purify oneself" (92), but it is used of old for the production of natron. The purified product ready for use was dubbed "the pure" (93), a word philologically connected with that for god (94) and incense (95) in the ancient Egyptian language. Surely in the Egyptian mind natron, the pure product and incense, "that which purified", were acceptable to the gods, the pure ones (96) and they would serve to consecrate their statues and their temples.

Not only were both burned to please the gods, natron and incense were often mixed as aromatic ingredients. This may also be the case in ancient Palestine, where perfume and incense are said to be "a confection after the art of the apothecary" (97). Here salt is certainly not used, but natron, which seems to have been imported from Egypt, whence other aromatic substances came too and may have been used in the way the Egyptians did.

The sacredotal character of both natron and incense in ancient Egypt was enhanced because both were stored in the "house of Natron". Like aromatic resins and incense natron was produced in granular form. We have a later term "bḫḫ" denoting this granular natron which shows some similarity with the general term for resin of the same Greek period (98). Otherwise natron seems to have been sold both in lumps and in granular form. It was certainly mostly used in solid form. This is shown by the use of terms which from "to sow, to scatter" come to mean "to sprinkle natron all around a temple" or which also mean "purifying with granular soda by sprinkling in buildings" (99).

Indeed so intimately are the concepts purification and natron linked, that not only do names for qualities of natron for purification purposes come to mean "purify with natron or incense", but the reverse happened in the case of a term (100) originally "to purify" but later used for "natron". Natron is used by the believer to purify his mouth, either by chewing (wš') natron or by rinsing it (swr) with a solution of natron often referred to as natron lye (101). This solution and the solid natron used as desiccating agents in mummification too. Analyses of samples of ancient incense have proved that actual mixtures with solid natron were used.

Apart from this use for religious purposes, which absorbed large quantities we find natron applied in ancient Egypt for the manufacture of glass (replacing alkali), glazes and the blue and green frit used as pigments. It occurs frequently in medical recipes; it is used to cook such vegetables as radishes; linen is bleached with natron and mixtures of natron and clay were probably used as soap in the same way as the fullers of ancient Palestine used "nether" imported from Egypt.

The production of "nitrum" in the desert west of Alexandria where later the monks and anachorites settled continued until far into the Roman period as Strabo and Pliny inform us, though we have no detailed information on their operation except that Jewish workmen were sometimes employed there (102). The production belonged to the royal monopolies and as the main offtake went to the textile industry it was thus partly controlled too. The government also seems to have controlled the distribution as the yarn, nitre and kiki-oil for washing cloth was apparently furnished to the weavers by the government. As soda and castor oil were used as soap mainly by the fullers and laundry-men these artisans paid a special tax (nitrike) for the right of buying soda from the crown. In 117 B.C. a contractor of the nitron tax in Cerceosiris asked the special protection of the influential Amenneus, the royal scribe (103). A passage in another document suggests that the washing was also done by the linen-weavers in their own establishment, kiki-oil and nitre being supplied by the government (104). This system of distribution per province had its difficulties for we observe in one of the Zenon papyri (105) that a linen cleaning establishment is on the point of closing down for the lack of nitrum in its nome and now tries to get it from another province. We have many bills for payment of the nitrike by bleachers, fullers and weavers, and a late document tells us about a purchase tax on nitrum (106).

Forms of soda more or less causticised were used for soap and dyeing in Asia Minor. They were obtained from Philadelphia in Lydia, Magnesia on the Maeander and from Lake Ascania near Nicaea in Bithynia (107). From the fairly long passage which Pliny devotes to nitrum it is clear that this is natural soda and not saltpetre (108):

"We must not postpone an account of the character of nitrum, a substance rather like salt, and one which should be described all the more diligently because it is clear that the physicians who have written about it were ignorant of its true character, and that the most precious information was given by Theophrastus. It is produced in small quantities under the name halmyrax, in Media, where the valleys whiten in the dry season, and in still smaller amount in Thrace near Philippi, contaminated with earth, and known as "wild nitrum". The quantity made by burning oak-wood was never great, and the practice has long since been entirely abandoned. Nitrum-containing waters are found in several places, but they are not strong enough to repay concentration.

Clitae in Macedonia furnishes the best and most plentiful supply, to which the name Chalastrian is given; it is white and pure, very like salt. There is a nitrum-bearing lake, in the midst of which wells up a little fount of fresh water. There nitrum is formed for nine days about the rising of the dog-star, next disappears for as many days, and again it appears on the surface and then vanishes. It is clear from this that its production depends on the nature of the soil, for it has been ascertained that, when it vanishes, neither sun nor rain are of any avail. This too is marvellous that, though the gushing fountain ever flashes up, the lake does not rise, although it has no outlet. Rain, however, if it comes on those days on which the nitrum is being produced gives a salter product, while an inferior nitrum is obtained when the wind blows from the north because it stirs up the mud too strongly.

So much for nitrum which occurs as such. In Egypt, however, it has to be prepared; the quantity is much greater but the quality poorer, for it is dark-coloured and stony. It is prepared in almost the same way as salt, except that the sea is turned into salterns, the Nile into nitrum-pits. The latter dry up as the Nile retreats, but remain moist with the nitrum-bearing liquid for forty days on end, instead of yielding intermittently as in the case of Macedonia. If it rains during this period they add less river-water, and the nitrum is hastily collected as soon as it begins to be deposited, for fear it should dissolve back into the nitrum-pits.

In this case also its properties include an oiliness which makes it a remedy for itch in animals. When piled in heaps, however, it becomes hard. It is a curious fact that, in the case of Lake Ascanius and certain springs near Calchis, the surface waters are fresh and potable, though the deeper waters hold the nitrum in solution. The best nitrum is exceedingly light — it is this quality that gives to "foam of nitrum" its superiority — but for some purposes, such as dyeing cloth with purple and other dyestuffs, the impure substance is useful. Its use in large quantities for the manufacture of glass will be set forth in the proper place.

In Egypt, nitrum-beds used to be found only in the neighbourhood of Naucratis and Memphis. The latter are inferior, for there the heaps of nitrum petrify, and many mounds have thus turned into rocks from which vessels are made. Often too, the substance is melted and heated with sulphur. Again, nitrum is used for mummifying bodies. Some of the nitrum-beds of this country furnish also a nitrum red by the surrounding earth.

The ancients considered that "foam of nitrum", a substance of the highest reputation is formed only when the dew falls, and when the nitrum-beds, though pregnant, are not yet in travail, and that accordingly none is formed when they are at the point of delivery, even though the dew should fall. Others have come to the conclusion that it is formed by the fermentation of the heaps.

Physicians of the next generation taught that aphronitrum (foam of nitrum) is collected in Asia, where it drips down in humid caves, called collogae, and is dried in the sun. Lydian is considered the best, the criteria being low density and great friability, combined with an almost purple colour. It is imported in tablet form, while the Egyptian kind comes in vessels pitched to prevent deliquescence, vessels which are finished by drying in the sun.

The qualities required of nitrum are lightness, sponginess and porosity. In Egypt it is sophisticated with lime, an impurity which is detected by the tongue, for, when pure, nitrum dissolves immediately, but when adulterated, it burns by reason of the lime, and if sprinkled with water, gives a strong smell. Nitrum is heated in an earthen vessel, with a lid to prevent spitting; apart from this, it does not crackle in the fire. It neither produces nor supports life, while vegetation grows in salterns and the sea teems with so many animals and so much seaweed.

But the greater bitterness of nitrum (as compared with salt) is clear, not from this evidence only, but also from the fact that the nitrum-pits cause rapid deterioration of shoe-leather, although on the other hand they are healthy and good for the eyes. Opthalmia is unknown in their neighbourhood, and ulcers brought to this district heal very quickly, though those formed locally mend slowly. Nitrum acts also as a sudorific and softens the body when used with oil as a liniment. The Chalastaean variety is used in bread-making, to replace salt; the Egyptian in cooking radishes. It renders them more tender, while it disimproves fish and bleaches them, and gives vegetables a greener colour."

This passage shows that PLINY does not distinguish his nitrum (soda) from potash (which is potassium carbonate) derived from plant ashes nor do others (109). Potash was the "natural alkali" obtained by the ancients from the ashes of certain plants which may contain upto 30% of this salt. This distinction was of course not made until many centuries later. Pliny's "aquae nitrosae" were just alkaline liquids like most of the mineral waters are. If their soda content in high enough they can indeed be used as soap like the waters of Lake Ascania. Soda was often used as a detergent and the careless husband who forgot to bring litron home, forgot his soap (110).

Natron is often mentioned in medical recipes, even by PLINY (111) it was useful when dyeing with certain organic dyes such as madder, alkanet and kermes because it dissolved them and it entered in recipes for making glass (112). PLINY's remarks on the use of natron to keep vegetables green during cooking are perfectly correct and they were communis opinio in Antiquity (113).

NATURAL ALKALI

Alkali (potash), apart from natron, was available to the ancients in the form of the ashes of certain plants. Sometimes plant-ash was used as table-salt (114). We have no proof, that this "vegetable alkali" was ever used in ancient Egypt. There is no specific term which we can identify with it, nor it is obvious from the analyses of ancient Egyptian glazes or glass, that some component containing mainly potassium carbonate was used. For both glass and glazes natron was used. Neither did the Egyptians use natural alkali to make soap, for which they seem to have relied on mixtures of natron and clay.

In the Semitic world, however, the ashes of certain plants rich in carbonates were used. The fullers of ancient Palestine obtained "borith" or "kali" by burning the soda plant "gasûl" (Salsola Kali). The Bible (115) mentions these "cinders of borith" as fuller's soap. The ancient texts from Mesopotamia mention "uḫûlu" or alkali, derived from Salicornia, e.g. two species of the alkaline Chenopodiaceae (glasswort). The ashes of these plants, common in Mesopotamia and abounding in soda, for the alkaline component of many glass-recipes. In some cases the adjective "ḳalâti" (burnt) is added, in which word we recognize the root of our term alkali. Curiously enough the glass recipes do not give the amount of ashes to be used, but seem to mention the weight of the raw dried plant, which may indicate, that the plants and not the ashes were sold. Vegetable alkali does not play prominent part in classical technology.

Soap and detergents

A few words should be devoted to the problem of soap in Antiquity. Notwithstanding the great cleanliness of the ancient Egyptians and the frequent ablutions and washings prescribed for their priests we have no sign that soap as such was known to them. An Old Kingdom picture shows a square object with a bowl, jug and towel, which has often been taken to be a cake of soap. It is more probably a cake of natron, so beloved for its purifying character. We have a Coptic term: "ⲁⲛ ⲩⲓⲣ" which is usually translated "soap", an hieroglyphic equivalent of which occurs in later magical papyri. However, the common detergents used by the ancient Egyptians were natron, fuller's earth and may be pounded lupins, which are still used in that country (doqáq). Some medical recipes (Ebers Papyrus, etc.) prescribe the boiling of oils and fats with large quantities of alkaline substances but the soap formed is never mentioned as such.

Nor was soap known in ancient Palestine, where "nether", soda and "borit", vegetable alkali were used for washing, sometimes combined with urin, fuller's ashes and other similar ingredients. The Hittites dissolved plant ashes in water to clean their hands.

In Mesopotamia, however, some kind of soap was manufactured, certainly as early as the Ur III period, when the Sumerians boiled oil and alkali together. Various recipes mention the use of palm-oil, castor-oil, potash, soda, resin and salt to compound this soap. Still soap as such is not separated from the mixture and we have no special term for soap, In washing wool the use of beech-ash is strongly recommended and textiles in general are known to have been washed with "soap", soda, vegetable alkali and alum. In some cases the lye is obtained by burning rue. In general we can therefore state, that though mixtures containing soap were known and used, soap as such was unknown, but many detergents were in use.

The classical world had no better detergents and used bran, pumice-stone, natron, vegetable alkali and the like. Real soap comes much later, it is mentioned for the first time by THEOKRITOS (116) but more in detail much later by PLINY (117) and GALEN (118). However, this is a soap made by boiling animal fat with potash made from beech-wood or from ashes of seaweed, which give a soft and a hard soap respectively. PLINY claims no more than that this invention of the Gaul is used to dye their hair. GALEN who first refers to the use of soap for washing the human body and clothes expresses preference for the softer type of German soap. Sammonicus, who in the third century A.D. recommends it for washing the body as part of the treatment of certain illnesses does not imply in his poem that the use of soap was anything like common in his days. During the Imperial period there lived a "negotiator artis saponariae" at Lyons (119) and at Grand (Vosges) a basrelief was found which seems to depict the workshop of a soap-manufacturer dedicated to Juno Saponaria (120).

SALTPETRE, NITRE

The frequent identification of the ancient "natron" and nitre forces us to say something about this salt, thta had no practical importance in Antiquity. Though sodium nitrate, as a white efflorescence, occurs in large areas of Upper Egypt, where it is now used as a fertilizer, neither potassium nor sodium nitrate were known or used in ancient Egypt as far as our evidence goes. Neither does it seem to have been used in ancient Palestine. The ancient inhabitants of Mesopotamia, however, knew and used it. They do not seem to have imported mined potassium nitrate from the deposits of Elburz and Azerbijan in Iran. In ancient Mesopotamia, like in modern India, it was obtained as an efflorescence of the soil in certain places where organic matter decayed (cattle yards and stables). The mixture of salt and saltpetre was then "washed", that is separated by fractional crystallisation. It was dissolved in boiling water, the solution was then strained and boiled down for one day, after which crystals of saltpetre could be separated from the lye. Hence the Accadians distinguished different kinds of mil'u, such as "white, black, male, female, washed and unwashed", all of which are mentioned in the texts on glass technology and in a few medical recipes.

In very few cases does the context of classical texts allow us to translate "nitrum" by nitre, but in the greater majority of instances soda or natron is really meant.

Sal ammoniac

Ancient technology had no particular use for ammonium chloride, but the Accadian medical recipes use a product "aklu", the meaning of which word is literaly "sublimate of scrapings" and which judging from its use is most certainly sal ammoniac. Another term "iṭtru", lit. "soot from dung fires", probably denotes the same substance though, this second term is sometimes loosely used to denote any efflorescence.

Alum

Though we are certain that alum was produced in large quantities in ancient Egypt, we have only circumstantial evidence for its production in pre-classical times. Pliny assures us, that the Egyptian alum was the best quality known in his days (121) and he refers to its use as a mordant for dyers and as an ingredient in medical recipes. The alum was produced in the oases of Dakla and Kharga, west of the Nile valley, both of which are honeycombed with ancient workings. Surface sherds at Kharga indicate very active production in Roman times and the Greek papyri point to the same for the Hellenistic period (122). Herodotus tells us that after the destruction of the temple of Delphi the Egyptian king Amasis "gave them a thousand talents (over 25 tons!) of alum and the Greek settlers (in Egypt) twenty minae" (123). Also late-Assyrian texts mention imports of Egyptian alum into Mesopotamia. If we add to this evidence, that Caton Thompson and Gardner, in their survey of the oases, tell us that "miles of the outlying foothills are riddled with shallow workings", we can safely suppose that alum was mined many centuries before Pliny wrote.

Alum was not only used by dyers but possibly also by leather workers. Two Egyptian terms, which may be identical, denote alum, this is proved by their use in medical texts, where the astringent qualities of alum are put to use. Alum is also mentioned in magical incantations.

In Mesopotamia alum was generally used by the cloth merchants as a mordant, but also by the tanners (124). It also occurs in some glass recipes. If not imported from Egypt it was won from the deposits at Shap Ma'dan (near Kara Hissar), from the region of Tuz Khurmatli or from Hamairan on the Persian Gulf. Alunite was known and used for seals, but alum was derived from it by boiling with water as some medical recipes tell us. The different Accadian terms for alum indicate that it was refined by crystallisation and that different qualities were recognized. Its alchemical "cover-name" was "lichen from the tamarisk".

Cyprus seems to have produced "feathered alum" for exports to the Near East in late pre-classical times. In Palestine alum was known and produced from deposits near the Dead Sea, a second quality alum came from the town of Machairus in Peraea. The Talmud occasionally mentions alum mines (125).

In Greco-Roman Egypt alum was produced in the cases of Kargeh and Dakhlah. These deposits were evidently controlled by the state for we have a number of reports dating from the third century A.D. which give five-day surveys of the production, presumably by officials in charge of the workings (126). The overseers of the Little Oasis mines sent a cargo of alum to the Fayum and the camel-driver had to pay the "comptrollers of the alum in the Arsinoite nome" (127). Apart from this wholesale tax on alum there was also a purchase tax such as retail dealers had to pay at the Serapeum of Oxyrhynchus (128). At Arsinoë the tariff in 140 A.D. was 1½ drachme per talent of alum imported (129).

Pliny gives a fairly long passage on the virtues of alum (130): "Of no less importance, nor indeed very dissimilar, is the use of alumen, which is believed to be a salt exudation of the earth. There are several varieties of it. In Cyprus you find a white kind and one rather darker, the difference in colour being slight, but the difference in employment great, for the white, liquid variety is used especially for dyeing wool bright colours and the darker sort when dark and somber hues are required. The latter is used also for cleaning gold.

All alumen arises from water and slime, and is a natural exudation from the earth. It is washed into a hollow in winter, and brought to maturity by the summer suns. The portion which separates first is less coloured than the rest. It occurs in Spain, Egypt, Armenia, Macedonia, Pontus, Africa and in the islands of Sardinia, Melos, Lipara and Strongyle. The best quality is found in Egypt, and the second best in Melos. The latter is also subdivided into liquid and solid alumen. The test for the liquid kind is that it should be clear and milky, not gritty when rubbed between the fingers, and with some spark of colour. This is called phorimon. Adulteration is detected with pomegranate juice, which does not darken the alumen if the latter is pure.

Another kind belongs to that variety which is pale and rough and coloured by adding oak-galls. This, therefore, they call paraphoron. Liquid alumen has astringent, hardening and corrosive properties....

One kind of solid alumen is called schiston by the Greeks, from the habit of dividing into white hair-like threads, a property which has caused some authorities to call it trichitis. It forms on the mineral from which copper is smelted (chalcitis by name), and may be considered as an exudation of the mineral which has soldified into a surface scum. This kind of alumen is less dessicative and less potent in checking excessive perspiration....

There is another alumen of a less active type called strongyle. It also comprises two varieties. The first resembles a fungus in appearance, dissolves readily in very small amounts of liquid, and is in complete disrepute. The other and better kind is like pumice in appearance, with tubular openings like a sponge, and occurs in globular form. It is more nearly white than the former variety, possesses a certain richness, is free from grit and friable, and does not give dark colours in dyeing. It is roasted by itself on clean coals until it is reduced to ashes.

The best kind of all is that which is called melinum from the island where it occurs....

The characteristic property of every variety of alumen is astringency — hence the Greek name...

Attention has already been drawn to its importance to the non-medical aspects of life, by reason of its power to stain leather and wool".

Both in this passage (in which we have omitted the lines on the medical applications of alum) and two less important ones (131) it is difficult to identify the different alums belonging to the family of true alum (a double sulphate of aluminium and potassium) but containing iron, manganese or magnesium sulphates. Some of these give darker colours when used in dyeing, but the ancients took them all to be variants of one single substance.

Some alum seems to have been imported from the Mauretanian side of the African frontier for we have a custom's tariff for alum from Zaraï (Africa) (132).

FOOD PRESERVATION PROCESSES

Leaving aside the protection of materials against corrosion by coating with paint and bitumen, which will be dealt with elsewhere, we will now deal primarily with the preservation of food. Hoarding foodstuffs for use in times of shortage began in the food-collecting stage. It became even more important in the food-producing stage of man's history, when transport of food over fairly large distances and storage followed by distribution became part of the social activities of towns and tribes. Preservation of staple food became an essential part of the technology of an ever-growing population.

The processes available in pre-classical days were few. The growing knowledge of the biological causes of decomposition in the eighteenth centuries led to many new methods of preservation of food, e.g. sterilization of food, e.g. sterilization by heat (PAPIN, APPERT, 1810), dessication of meat (LIEBIG and VON PETTENKOFER, 1850), evaporation of milk (BORDEN, 1856), refrigeration by cold air or cold brine, deep-freezing and finally the addition of chemical preservatives. None of these methods were available to the ancients. From the earliest days onwards and for many centuries to come preservation processes remained purely empirical. Drying, smoking, curing or salting by application of a dry granular salt and pickling (immersion in a salt solution or brine) or combinations of these processes were applied to foodstuffs. Pickling in vinegar was theoretically possible but we have no data to show that this method was used. HERODOTUS (133) refers to honey as a means of preserving bodies, but we have no further texts confirming this usage.

Apart from pickling all these methods are based on desiccation. Nature's own method of preservation. All such natural products as nuts, which contains less than about 10% of water, can be kept indefinitely. *Smoking*, which is still applied to fish and meat, was known to the prehistoric inhabitants of Europe. This process not only dries the food but it also changes its taste by decomposition of the fats and so often avoids the use of spices. It was used by the German tribes and even by the Romans in historic times. Pope Zacharias (VIIIth cy. A.D.) warned Boniface to stick to boiled or smoked bacon and pork during his travels amongst the heathen tribes. Smoking was, however, not practised in the ancient Near East, as far as we know, for the lack of cheap fuel was always at the background of technological processes in these regions. In a few cases drying by heat was necessary, for instance when drying certain drugs and plants. The hieroglyphic notation of the Egyptian verb "to dry drugs" (134) shows the brazier sign. The preparation of a few other ingredients for medical recipes also seems to have involved a combined drying and roasting process. This is proved by two Egyptian words "to dry cereals" (135) and "to dry dates, grain or bread" (136), both of which seem connected with the term "the blaze of a fire" (137). The custom of slightly roasting cereals in order to improve the separation of chaff and grain during threshing and to improve storage stability was practised only in prehistoric Europe and the world of Greeks and Romans.

However, *drying* on a large scale generally meant relying on sun and wind only in the Ancient Near East. Desiccation by burying in the hot desert sand was not common practice. This was the common procedure for such fruit as dates, figs and grapes. We have one representation only of the making of raisins (138). Dried figs (139) and raisins (140) were known in ancient Palestine and Mesopotamia. Medical plants and drugs were also preserved by simple drying (141). Meat, which was not yet consumed on a large scale, was generally dried (142) both for household and mecidal purposes. The store-rooms of the houses of the rich are shown to have held a fair amount of pieces of dried meat. Only in the first millennium B.C. terms for smoked beef (143) and even pickled beef (144) crop up now and then in the texts. Egyptian reliefs show us how this dried meat was marrowed by beating with stones. Salting meat was slightly less unusual in Mesopotamia. In certain cases even human bodies seem to have been preserved there by "putting them into salt" (145), a custom that was also common amongst some Spanish tribes according to Valerius Maximus. The Assyrian king even ordered to send him the corpse of the slain king of the Elamites "preserved in salt", probably as a check on battle reports.

In the case of fish, fowl and birds, which were consumed in great quantities, drying (often combined with salting) was resorted to. "Many kind of fish they eat raw, either salted or dried in the sun. Quails also, and ducks and small birds, they eat uncooked, merely salting them first. All other birds and fishes, excepting those which are set apart as sacred, are eaten either roasted or boiled" (146). The birds were of course first plucked, and the extent of their consumption can be measured from HIPPARCHUS' remark (147): "Nor did I care for the life that the Egyptians lead, forever plucking quails and slimy magpies".

Salting (148) fish and fowl is essentially a desiccation process. An old process of producing dried salted fish still common in the east is probably identical with that by which the "māliāḥ" of Magdala (the ancient Tarichéai) (149), Palestine or the dried, salted fish exported from Egypt to Syria and Palestine were produced. The modern Egyptians make this "fissikh" of preserved fish by gutting fresh fish on a cemented slope and washing it with water. Coarse salt is then rubbed into the gills, mouth and scales. Alternate layers of salt and fish are covered by dry matting. After standing from 3—5 days the pile is turned over to stand for a similar period. During this drying the body fluids drain away and salt solution penetrates the fish. After this drying they are firm and hard, though in some cases left to dry in the air somewhat longer.

This is essentially the same process depicted in various stages and variations by the ancient Egyptian reliefs. Some fish were cut in half and suspended on ropes for the purpose of drying in the sun, the passing current of air being found to accelerate the process; sometimes the body was simply laid open with a knife from the head to the tail,

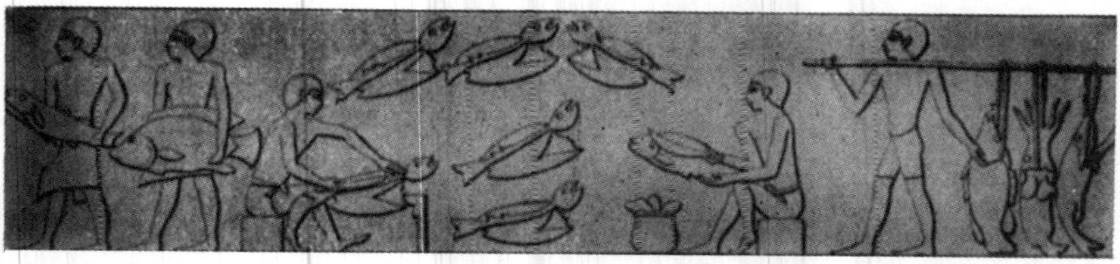

Fig. 37. Preparing and drying fish. (After Lepsius)

the two sides being divided as far as the back bone. Many were contented with taking out the intestines and removing the head with the tip of the tail, exposing them, when salted, to the sun. The roe (151) is collected and stored in pots as a special delicacy. This process of drying, sometimes combined with salting according to the species of fish treated, remained unaltered all throughout the long history of Egypt. Similar methods of salting were common in Palestine and Mesopotamia though there pickling was also used at least in the first millennium B.C. We do not know how long the fish or ducks thus preserved kept well. The large stores shown in pictures of ancient houses and the fact that Wen-Amon and others tell us of exports of cured fish to Syria go to prove the efficacy of the process.

We also notice the intimate relation between salt-production and the preservation of food. The easy availability of salt in coastal districts in contrast to inland regions is still reflected in the different ways of treating butter in northern and southern Germany and certainly the Celts of Spain and other prehistoric inhabitants of Europe who had easy acces to salt could store their surplus more safely than the tribes inland. This certainly is the main factor behind the extensive prehistoric salt-trade in these regions. The ashes of salt-bearing plants such as Salicornia might form a substitute for salt as they did in ancient Palestine and Mesopotamia, they could never be produced in sufficient quantities to cover the full demand for salt, or any preservative compound.

In the classical period salting, the invention of which process is often ascribed to the Median tribes, was wide spread even among the barbarian peoples. Diodor tells us that the "locust-eaters" of Africa salted their catch. Sallust and Valerius Maximus (152) stress the common practice of salting in Spain and tell us the gruesome story that

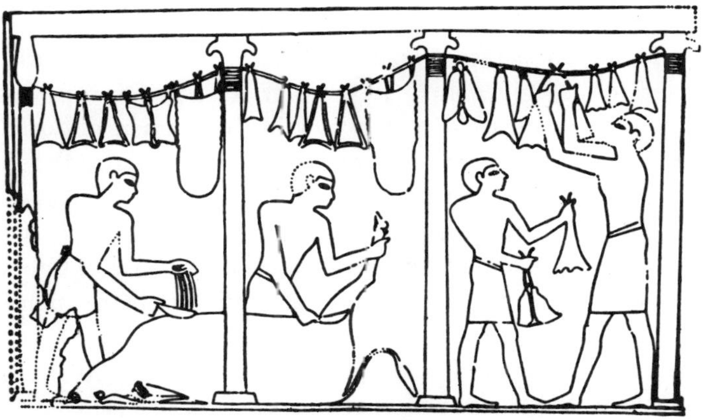

Fig. 38. Drying meat at the butcher's

the Callaguritans when besieged by Pompey killed their spouses and children as they had no cattle and ate them but pickled the surplus to feed the soldiers. Athenaeus firmly believed that there was once a time when salt was unknown. "When later mankind liked salt with its food, they still kept to their old customs when offering food to the gods."

Salted, dried and pickled fish was the staple food of the Greeks, salted or dried meat was rarely consumed. The demand for pickled and salted fish was such that large quantities were imported from the Pontic regions. Pickled olives were served at meals. There is even a saying, which paraphrases the instability of wealth, running: "The salt cargo returns whence it came." (153).

The term used by the Greeks when referring to the embalming of animals and men and to the pickling of fish "taricheio". SUIDAS (154) explains it by saying "tarichos is meat strewn with salt." "If there is no meat one has to be content with tarichos. A tarichos costs one obol but what goes with it two." The technique of salting fish differed little from that of pre-classical days, it is described in detail by several authors, e.g. in the Geoponica (155). XENOPHON even mentions salted dolphins (156). We have already mentioned the important salted fish industries of Spain and southern Russia, and CATO the Elder claimed that no city could exist where fish had become more expensive than meat.

In the Roman world the use of sal nativum (rock-salt) and sal factitum (sea-salt) for pickling and salting attained even larger dimensions. The trade (and probably the preparation) of pickled wares was in the hands of the salsamentarii. In certain cases salt pickled with spices was used (sal conditum). Columella mentions the use of salt when preparing cheese from goat's milk. CATO (157) preserves "green olives in brine" and gives adequate instructions how to preserve olives. Much attention is devoted to the pickling of ham and pork, large quantities of which were produced in Gaul and Spain. Strabo informs us that excellent ham came from the present Burgundy (158) and ATHENAEUS (159) says: "In Spain there is a town called Pompelon where excellent hams are made which can compete with those of Cantabria." In fact CATO has a detailed instruction on "salting of hams and of small pieces as are put up at Puteoli" (160) which runs thus:

"Hams should be salted in the large storage jars or in the smaller jars in this way: When you buy the hams cut off the feet; take for each ham a half-modius of Roman salt ground in a mill, sprinkle the bottom of the large jar or of the smaller one with salt, then put in a ham, skin side down, and cover completely with salt. Then put a second on top, cover in the same way, take care that meat does not touch meat. Cover them all in the same way. When you have placed them all, cover above with salt so that the meat will not show. Make the salt level. When they have been five days in the salt take them all out, salt and all. Place on the bottom those that were on top, and cover and arrange in the same way. After twelve days in all, take the hams out, wipe off all salt and hang them in the wind for two days. On the third day wipe them off well with a sponge, rub them thoroughly with olive oil and vinegar mixed, and hang them up on the meat rack. Neither moths nor worms will touch them."

MUMMIFICATION

We have had occasion to cite methods in preserve human bodies by some curing process (161). This intimate connection between the curing of fish and the preservation of the human body is well illustrated by the classical authors. HERODOTUS (162) and DIODORUS (163) use the same Greek word "taricheio" for curing and for embalming. ATHENAEUS does so more than 60 times in his passage on fish in ancient Egypt (164). The verb means "to embalm, pickle, salt, preserve shrink, age", thus proving that the principle of mummification in ancient Egypt was desiccation, like that of curing fish and fowl.

It is important to bear this link between curing and mummification in ancient Egypt in mind, for in no other country in the ancient Near East, nor in prehistoric Europe (as far as we know) were any large scale attempts made to preserve the human body after death. We cannot go into the religious and philosophical background prompting the ancient Egyptian to mummify his king and his nobles during the earliest periods of his history, which custom later spread to all classes. We must needs limit our discussion to the technical processes employed to preserve the body, which processes, contrary to general belief, show a striking evolution and degeneration.

We should also constantly bear in mind, that mummification was a magico-religious act. In order to prepare the human body was proper receptable for the returning soul every act from the moment the body was placed on the special table (165) for evisceration up to the final "Opening of the Mouth" (166) ceremony, that prepared the mummy magically for its task every act was minutely regulated by the Ritual of Embalming. Copies of these papyri describe the ritual and incantations as well as minute instructions on the swathing of head, back, hands, legs, etc. In the early days the embalmer's chamber was a temporary affair, a tent or booth set up for the seventy days necessary for the whole process. However it certainly had the character of a shrine. It is called the Beautiful House (167), the House of Purification (168) or the Tent of the God (169). This letter expression not only stresses its temporary character, but also refers to the hall in which Anubis embalms Osiris and expands this concept to the dead man, who hopes to be one of Osiris' band. On other occasions it is simply the Embalming Tent (170), the Bandaging Place (171) or the Embalming Place (172). Only in the first millennium B.C. (XXIst and XXIInd dynasties) does this embalmer's hall become more permanent. We then find a term (173) connected with "grave" and with "chapel, temple chamber", indicating a permanent building in the necropolis.

In prehistoric times the Egyptians buried their dead in contracted position (like the child in its mother's womb), wrapped loosely in an animal skin or folds of linen in a shallow desert grave. The heat of the sun and the sterile porous sand formed perfect means of desiccation and kept the body in a dried mummified state. This phase is still echoed in the oldest portions of the Pyramid Texts, where the limbs and the flesh are summoned to shake off the desert sand. These circumstances so favourable to preservation were no longer present when in early dynastic times, after the Union of Upper- and Lower Egypt by king Menes so dominant in Egyptian philosophy, deeper pits lined with sun-dried bricks were dug into the desert sand for the burial of kings and nobles. The closer wrapping of the dead body evolved in the first three dynasties, which gradually became an elaborate separate swathing of each limb and a second bandaging of the whole also helped preservation. The ancient Egyptians became perfectly aware of what would happen if decomposition of the fleshy parts (174) were not stopped. Their term for burial (175) is closely connected with that for bones (176).

However, religious tenets demanded that the body should be preserved as a receptacle, an envelope, to house the descending soul, should it want to contact the world of the living. It was imperative that the exterior forms of the individual body be preserved. From this strong urge the whole elaborate ritual of embalming arose in a frantic effort to keep the mortal remains intact from decomposition. Hence also the strongly religious character of this ritual in which the embalming (177) was performed by craftsmen headed by the chief embalmer (178) a man of priestly rank equal to the ceremonial priest (hrj.ḥb) also present and assisted by the "wt inpw", personifying the god Anubis, the patron of the embalmers, and reciting the correct incantations for each stage of the process.

Our information on the details of this process depends on the meticulous but difficult examination and analysis of actual mummies begun by PETTIGREW early in the nineteenth century and supplemented by the reports from classical authors. A fairly good description is given by HERODOTUS (179), who visited Egypt in 449 N.C. and certain details can be added to this from DIODOR's account (180) some four hundred years later. From these reports it would seem that there were three "classes" of mummification in Herodotus' time. The most costly and elaborate treatment involved: a) the removal of brain, abdominal and thoriac viscera except heart and kidneys, b) cleaning the viscera with palm wine and spices, c) filling up the body cavities with myrrh, cassia and other aromatic substances and sewing up the embalming incision, d) treating the body with natron and washing it afterwards, and finally e) anointing the body with cedar oil and other ointments, rubbing it with myrrh, cinnamon and other fragrant materials and wrapping it in bandages. A second and cheaper method was the substitution of an injection per anum of cedar oil for the operations a) and b) then followed by the treatment by natron, etc. The third and cheapest method also removed the viscera by solution, but in this case the expensive cedar oil was replaced by some cheaper, less efficient oil. We miss in these descriptions details of what the dissolving action of these injected oils were and also no detail is given on what was the fate of viscera removed in the more elaborate operation.

From these data and the host of essays on this subject we now have at least a knowledge of the outlines of this intricate process and its evolution, which is rather different from the picture drawn by HERODOTUS, which is just a phase of mummification as practised during the Persian occupation and domination of Egypt. Mummification is not really identical with embalming (lit. to preserve in balsam). As cold storage and the injection of germicidal and antiseptic fluids into the blood vessels were still unknown, the only means of preserving the body open to the ancient Egyptians was desiccation. This was a difficult job, for the human body consists of no less than 75% of water. Drying in the sun would be too slow and insecure, artificial heat was never used probably for economical reasons. The only dehydrating agents available were salt and natron, as quick-lime was never used in Egypt before the Ptolemaic period, however abundant limestone was in that country. The preservative powers of salt were well-known, fish and birds being cured with it. We must however remind the reader of the purifying sacred nature of natron according to Egyptian tenets. Hence the choice of the dehydrating agent was not difficult, it was to be natron, not the cheaper common salt.

This is proved by a large array of facts, all unequivocal evidence, that natron was the dehydrating agent. After the treatment with natron the body is so desiccated, that no further drying is needed. There is no evidence that soaking the body in a bath of a solution of natron ever played any part in Egyptian mummification. However, there is a small amount of circumstantial evidence, that at least in some instances the body was not specially dried after the washing following up the dehydration operation. Certain mummies must have been damp when wrapped up. In analogy with the curing methods of fish and fowl already discussed the desiccation must have been effected by treating the body with dry granular natron. The use of the same word "taricheutes" for embalmer and curers of fish and fowl in Greek literature on Egypt supports this evidence of the mummies themselves. The operation has been tried out in birds and fowl with the same result already known from excavations. Dehydrating the body with dry natron in wooden boxes or mats was the basic operation in mummification.

During the Old Kingdom (—2250 B.C.) the ancient Egyptians could not yet preserve the body but they were experimenting. They had already started to remove the intestines. An albaster box was found containing four compartiments in which the viscera of Queen Hetepheres (the mother of Cheops) were immersed in a 3% natron solution after having been wrapped up in linen bandages. This custom was the first phase of the preservation of the viscera in the four Canopic jars, placed at the four corners of the sarcophagus in later Old Kingdom graves. In order to preserve the features of the dead person and counteracting their distortion by decomposition of the tissues linen strips soaked in resinous materials were moulded on the shrunken body to reproduce them. Sometimes resins were used in paste form. The abdomen and other body cavities were stuffed with linen, limbs and external organs accurately moulded in the resinous linen under the outer bandages. Signs of careful bandaging were already present in a Second-Dynasty mummy according to ELLIOT SMITH. The heart was treated separately, from the VIth dynasty onwards it was removed and a stone substitute placed in the body. Bodies disturbed by tomb-robbers were carefully rewrapped and re-buried.

However, during the Eleventh Dynasty (2100—2000 B.C.) some mummies show no attempt to open the abdomen, all the organs are still present. Attempts were made to preserve at least the surface of the bodies, as they were still soft when bandaged. In general no incision of the body was found, but in some cases attempts seem to have been made to remove the viscera partly through vagina and rectum by first introducing some "dissolving" agent and draining the cavity. Desiccation with natron was practised, after which treatment the body was swathed in linen covered with the resinous mixture of aromatic ingredients, though this impregnated layer may follow the linen bandages next to the body. In some cases the bodies of soldiers or other attendants must have been buried temporarily in desert graves before the honorary mummification and burial with their chief.

During the Twelfth Dynasty (200—1780 B.C.) this treatment was elaborated, the incision in the flank grew more common and the viscera were generally removed. Liver, lungs, stomach and intestines are preserved in the four Canopic jars. The heart was removed, washed and bandaged to be put back in the body together with the heart amulet in the form of a scarabaeus. The body cavities were stuffed with bandages soaked in resinous mixes.

During the New Kingdom e.g. practically down to the Twenty-First Dynasty (1546—1055 B.C.) we find an entirely new state of affairs. Solid natron in definitely in common use to stop the decomposition of the body surface. The brain was carefully extracted as were the viscera. The heart was returned to the body after treatment but the

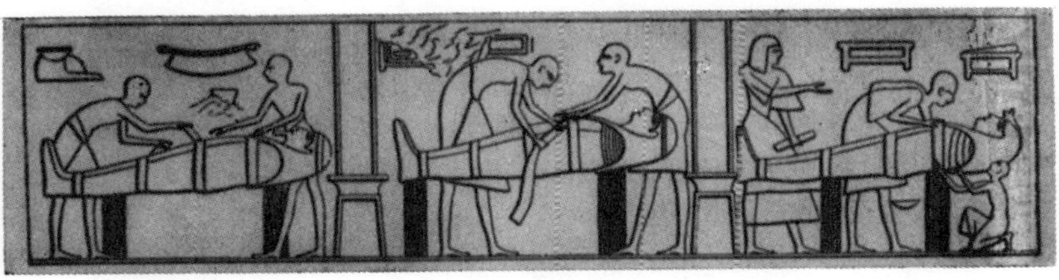

Fig. 39. Some phases of mummification

heart amulet was wrapped into the outer bandages of the mummy. The abdominal and chest cavities were carefully filled with linen impregnated with resins, sometimes hot resinous mixes were poured into them. Some mummies were covered with a layer of beeswax before swathing. In certain cases limbs show the rise of "mud-packing", that is the filling of cavities between the skin and the bones with sand to replace the shrunken muscle-material. Here again members of a family must have been buried first in desert graves until the last member died, when the whole family was embalmed to be buried ritually.

During the Twenty-First Dynasty (1085—945 B.C.) a great change took place. Henceforth the body cavity was filled with linen bags full of natron or chaff, lichen and sawdust impregnated with natron. In this mass the organs were placed after washing and swathing together with wax images of the "Canopic deities". The Canopic jars disappeared from use. Mud and sand were now regularly used to "pack" the skin. Mixtures of butter and natron wrapped up in linen were inserted in mouth and cheeks, the brain was extracted and the cavity filled up with resin. Then the body was washed and swathed.

Gradually the bandages of organs, limbs and other parts of the body acquire separate names and a host of these pervade the later embalming rituals.

For as the dynasties roll by degeneration of the careful embalming practices sets in and ritualistic intricacy seems to have been resorted to where actual preservation methods were neglected or even for-

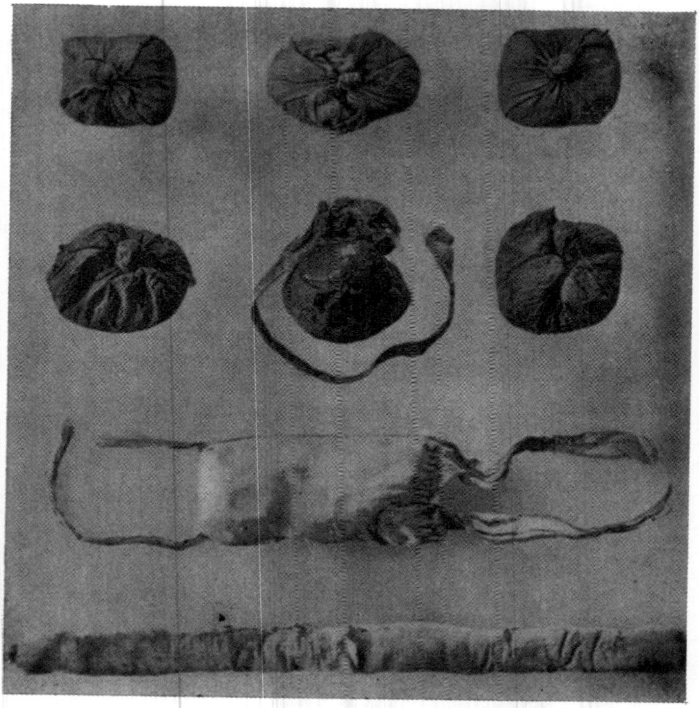

Fig. 40. Bags of natron used in making a mummy. (After WINLOCK) (161)

gotten. In these later periods the elaborate and intricate series of bandages in many cases cover nothing but a dead body just covered with pitchlike material without any further treatment. Sometimes the skeleton is made into a human form by moulding pitch and resins onto it. In some cases bodies must have been robbed, for the mummies are nothing but a jumbled collection of bones passed off as a human body by careful swathing. This bundle is then enclosed by a cartonage case on which a portrait and other decoration form the substitute for the carefully preserved and swathed body of earlier generations.

The materials used by embalmers of different dynasties need not be deduced from the mummies only. We have found several caches of their surplus materials, which were carefully wrapped up and buried after the ceremony was over because they were sacred and unclean.

Mummification has proved to be a desiccation process of the human body supplemented with certain operations to preserve the shape and features of the living body and the vital organs in order to provide the soul with a magically endowed receptable. Both the process and its detail vary with the dynasties and even within a certain period involved and less elaborate operations were practised. Its evolution is dominated by the development of religious thought in ancient Egypt. The darker side of this mummification craft is well illustrated by the following passage of Papyrus Sallier II: "The embalmer, his fingers are foul, for the odour thereof is that of corpses. His eyes burn from the greatness of the heat. He is too weak to stand up against his own daughter. He spends the day cutting up old rags, so that clothing is an abomination to him."

BIBLIOGRAPHY AND NOTES

(1) PLINY, *Nat. Hist.* XXXI, 88—89

(2) HEHN, V., *Das Salz* (Berlin 1891)
BUSCHMAN, J. C. VON, *Das Salz* (Leipzig 1906—1909, 2 vols.)
NENQUIN, J., *Salt, a study in economic prehistory* (Brugge, 1961)
EINZIG, PAUL, *Primitive Money* (London 1949)

(3) PLINY, *Nat. Hist.* XXXI, 73—92

(3a) CARPENTER, R., *Houses built of salt* (AJA LXI, 1957, 167—177)

(4) KYRLE, G., *Der prähistorische Salzbergbau am Dürrnberg* (*Jahrb. f. Alter-t.kunde*, Vol III, 1913, page 5)
HOFMAN, E., & MORTON, F., *Der prähistorische Salzbergbau auf dem Hallstätter Salzberg* (*Wiener Präh. Z.*, Vol. 15, 1928, pags. 82—101)
BEIERLEIN, P. R., *Neues über die ältere Geschichte der Salzquellen zu Altensalz* (*Freib. Forsch.* 1962, D 39)
BENOIT, F., *Les voies du sel* (Revue Archéol. Centre Vol. I, 1962, 158—159)

(5) TACITUS, *Annals* XIII.57

(6) *Oorkonden Boek van Holland*, Vol. 11 (1258)

(7) BAAS BECKING, L. G. M., *Historical Notes on Salt and Salt Manufacture* (*Scient. Monthly* 1931, pags. 434—446)
LI CH'IAO-P'ING, *The Chemical Arts of Old China* (Easton 1948, pags. 55—65)
SCHROETER, J., *Das Salz in der Vorgeschichte und in der Antike* (*Ciba Z.* 1943, No. 90, pags. 3154—3161)
BLOCH, R., *The History of Salt Technology* (*Actes du VIIe Congrès Int. d'Histoire des Sciences*, 1953, pags. 221—5)
RIEHM, K. *Prehistoric salt-boiling* (*Antiquity* XXXV, 1961, no. 139, 181–191)

(8) PLUTARCH, *Symposion* 1.4.3

(9) PLINY, *Nat. Hist.* XXXI.67

(10) CATO THE CENSOR, *On Farming* (*De Agricultura*) (transl. E. BREHOUT, New York 1933) 88; see also *Columella* XII.55

(11) "hm3.t" (III.94.1), sometimes written "hm3j.t" (III.94.6)

(12) HERODOTUS, II.12

(13) HERODOTUS, II.62

(14) STRABO, I.3.4. cap. 49

(15) ARRIAN, *Anabasis* III.4.3

(16) HERODOTUS, IV. 181—185

(17) STRABO, XVI.4.21. cap. 779; XVII.2.2. cap. 822

(18) PLUTARCH, *de Iside et Osiride*, cap. 32; *Quaestiones conviv.* v.10.1

(19) LÖW, J., *Das Salz* (*Jewish Studies dedic. to G. A. Kohut*, 1935, pags. 429—462)

(20) FREYDANK, H., *Das Salz und seine Gewinnung in der Kulturgeschichte* (*Kali*, Vol. XXIII, 1929, pags. 145—151; 161—168; 177—181)

(21) Ecclesiast. 39.20
(22) 2 Chron. 13.5
(23) Levit. 2.13; Mark 9.49
(24) Ezek. 43.24
(25) Ezek. 47.10—11; Zephaniah 2.9; Joshua 15.62
(26) STRABO, XVI.2.45. cap. 764
(27) Ezra 6.9; 7.22
(28) Job 6.6
(29) STRABO, XIII.1.48. cap. 605; ATHENAEUS, *Deipn.* III.73 d
(30) Inschriften van Priene 111, 11.112 ff
(31) STRABO, XII.3.12. cap. 546; XII.3.39. cap. 561
(32) DIOSCORIDES, V.109; see also C. V. BELLAMY, *A Description of the Salt Lake of Larnaca* (*Quart. J. Geol. Soc.* London, vol. 56, 1900, page 745)
(33) STRABO, XII.5.4. cap. 568; DIOSCORIDES, V.109
(34) CICERO, *De Imp. Pomp.* 6.16; *Pro Leg. Man.* 16
(35) Bab. Kethub. 79 b
(36) C.I.S. II.3.1. 3913
(37) STRABO, XI.13.2. cap. 523
(38) STRABO, XVI.3.3. cap. 766; see also (3a).
(39) STRABO, XV.1.30. cap. 700
(40) STRABO, V.2.6. cap. 224
(41) HOMER, *Iliad* IX.214
(42) LYCROPHON, *Alexandra* V.135
(43) HERODOTUS, IV.53; DIO CHRYS., XXXVI.437 M 25; KADEEV, V. I., *L'industrie du sel en Chersonèse à basse époque antique, Ier-IVe ss. de notre ère* (Arxeolog Ukrain. S.S.R. 13, 1961, 89—94)
(44) STRABO, VII.4.7. cap. 312
(45) ATHENAEUS, *Deipn.* IX.366 c; DIO CHRYS., *Oratio* 35. par. 25
(46) NICEPHOR, *Gregor. Hist. Byzant.* IX.5.6 & XIII.12.17
(47) STRABO, VII.5.11. cap. 318
(48) HOMER, *Odyssey* XI. 122—123; XXIII, 269—270
(49) P. Ryl. 92
(50) P. Tebt. 732
(51) O. Tait. I Bodl. 52; W.O. 341
(52) P. Fay. 23
(53) P. Mich. 123 R VII.27: XXII.27; XXI. 40; 128.11
(54) P. Hibeh 152
(55) P. Petrie III.121 b
(56) W.O. 1227
(57) P. Petrie II.4 (11)
(58) S.B. 7365
(59) P. London 1169
(60) P. London 1170 V.
(61) PLINY, *Nat. Hist.* 28.2 & 31.89; VIRGIL, *Aeneid* II.132—133; OVID, *Fastes* I.128, 337, PLAUTUS, *Amphitr.* V.740
(62) LUCIAN, *Hetear.* IV.4
(63) DIOGENES LAERTIUS, *De Clarorum philos.* VIII.1.35
(64) PLUTARCH, *Quaest. conv.* IV.3.638 F

(65) Livy, I.33
(66) Livy, 29.37
(67) C.I.L. I.2.2226
(68) Solinus, 5.18—19
(69) Solinus, 5.18—19; Augustinus, *De Civ. Dei* 21.5
(70) Pliny, *Nat. Hist.* 31.86
(71) Solinus, 5.18
(72) *Columella*, 6.17; Vegetius, *Ars Veter.* 4.22; 4.27; Sammonicus, *de Med.* 65; Solinus, 23.4; Sidonius, *Epist.* 9.12
(73) Strabo, III.2.6. cap. 144
(74) Gellius, *Noctes Att.* 2.22.29
(75) Justinus, 44.2.6
(76) Strabo, III.3.8. cap. 155
(77) Strabo, IV.1.7. cap. 182
(78) Strabo, IV.3.2. cap. 192
(79) Strabo, III.5.11. cap. 175
(80) *Proc. Soc. Antiq.*, *ser.* ii. vol. XXII, page 164; vol. XXIII, pags. 66—96; vol. XXX, pags. 36—54)
(81) *Archeol. J.*, *Vol.* VII, pags. 70, 175
(82) Aristotle, *Hist. Anim.* 8.10.59a, 16—26; Virgil, *Georgics*, 3.394—397
(83) Luke 14.34; Matthew 5.13
(84) Pliny, *Nat. Hist.* 33, 109; 33, 84; 34.106
(85) Pliny, *Nat. Hist.* 33.63; 33, 157
(86) Pliny, *Nat. Hist.* 9.133; 34.106
(86[a]) Forbes, R. J., *Studies in Early Petroleum History* (Leiden, 1958, 173 ff.)
Rudolph, R. C., *Han tomb art of West China* (Figs. no. 91 & 92)
Balasz, E., JESHO III, 211
Gale, E. M., and Ch'en Sung-ch'iao, *China's salt administration* (*J. Asiat. Studies* I, 1958, 137—217)
Encyclopaedia Sinica, 1917, 495
Rudolph, R. C., *A second-century Chinese illustration of salt-mining* (*Isis* 43, 1952, 39—41)
(87) eper assurê, lit. dust of the wall
(88) Lippmann, E. O. von, *Das Natron im alten Aegypten* (*Naturwiss.* 25, 1937, 592)
Steuer, R. O., *Zur Kenntnis des Natrons im alten Aegypten* (*FuF* 14, 1938, 54—55)
Levey, M., *The early history of detergent substances* (*J. Chem. Educ.* vol. 31, 1954, pags. 521—524)
(89) Strabo, XVII.1.23. cap. 803; Pliny, *Nat. Hist.* 31, 109—111
(90) šrp (IV.526.3)
(91) Coptic per.nḏj: Greek Nitria
(92) ḥsmn (III.163.3 & 6)
(93) nṯrj (II.366.8), compare the Accadian nitiru, Greek litron, nitron, Latin natrum; Gibbs, F. W., *On "nitre" and "natron"* (*Annals of Science*, Vol. III, 1938, pags. 213—216)
(94) nṯr (II.358.1), Coptic ⲛⲟⲩⲧⲉ
(95) snṯr (IV.180.7)

(96) Bissing, F. W. von, *Versuch sur Bestimmung der Grundbedeutung der Wortes NUTR fur Gott im Altägyptischen* (*SBAW*, phil. hist. Klasse 1951, Heft 2)
(97) Exodus 30.35; Sirach 49.1
(98) bšš (I.478.15)
(99) stj (IV.347.2) Coptic ⲥⲓⲧ and bsn (I.475.11)
(100) św'b (IV.66.1)
(101) mw nw ḥsmn (II.51.4)
(102) S.E.G. VIII. 366
(103) Teb. 40
(104) Teb. 703, 99
(105) P. Cairo-Zenon 59304
(106) P. Lond. inv. 1562
(107) Dioscorides, V.133; *VitaGallien.* 6. Aristotle, *peri thaum.* 53.834.a. 31
(108) Pliny, *Nat. Hist.* XXXI. 106—115
(109) Varro, *R.R.* 1.7.8; Theophrastus, *Hist. Plant.* 3.7.6
(110) Theocritus, 15.16; Plautus, *Truc.* 5.10; see also Palmer, *Hermathena* 1882, page 8
(111) Pliny, *Nat. Hist.* 35, 177, 181, 185
(112) Pliny, *Nat. Hist.* 36, 191—194
(113) Apicius, 3.1; Martial, 13.17.1
(114) Hornung, V., *Ueber Salzpflanzen und die Verwendung von Pflanzenasche an Stelle von Kochsalz* (*Kali*, Vol. 31, 1937, pags. 131—135, 141—144, 156—157)
Levey, M., *Gypsum, salt and soda in ancient Mesopotamian chemical technology* (*Isis*, 49, 1958, 336—341)
(115) Malachi, III.2
(116) Theokritos, *Idyll.* XV.30
(117) Pliny, *Nat. Hist.* XXVIII.191
(118) Galen, XII.170, 180
(119) C.I.L. XIII.2030
(120) Jullian, *Rev. Etud. Anc.*, Vol. XIX, 1917, page 199;
Bossert, H., *Zur Geschichte der Seife* (*Forsch. und Fortschr.* 29, 1955, 208—213)
André, J., *Gaulois sapana, latin sapo, grec sapon* (*Etudes Celtiques* VII, 1955/56, 348—355)
(121) Pliny, *Nat. Hist.* XXXV, 184
(123) Herodotus, II.180
(124) K. 4994; VAT 9722; see also Levey, M., *Alum in ancient Mesopotamian technology* (*Isis*, 49, 1958, no. 156, 166—169)
(125) Pal. Shekal. 5.49 a. 48; Bab. Kethub. 79 b
(126) P.O. 2116
(127) BGU 697
(128) P. Lond. inv. 1562
(129) BGU 697
(130) Pliny, *Nat. Hist.* XXXV. 183—190
(131) Pliny, *Nat. Hist.* XXXIII. 88 & 98; see also Charles Singer, *The earliest Chemical Industry* (London 1948)

(132) C.I.L. VIII.4508
(133) Herodotus, I.93 & 198
(134) 'wg (I.173.8)
(135) w3 (I.244.9)
(136) w3m (I.251.10)
(137) w3w3.t (I.250.4)
(138) wnš (I.325.5)
(139) 1. Sam. 25.18; 30.12
(140) 1 Sam. 25.18; 30.12; 2. Sam. 16.1; 1 Chron. 12.40
(141) wšr (I.374.13); šwšr (IV.76.6)
(142) śšr (IV.295.9)
(143) dg3j.7 (V.500.3)
(144) dr (V.475.2)
(145) VAB VII. 4 & 60
(146) Herodotus, II.77 & 86
(147) Athenaeus, *Deipn.*, 393
(148) Hornung, V., *Konservierung und Würzung insbesondere mit Kochsalz in den Anfangen der Kultur* (*Kali*, Vol. 31, 1937, pags. 54—56; 63—65; 73—74)

Koller, R., *Die Pökelung im Altertum* (*Schlachthofwesen und Lebensmittelüberwachung, Beilage Dtsche Tierärtzl. Wochenschr.*, Vol. 47, 1939, 549—551)

Benoit, F., *Le commerce du sel et les pêcheries, l'économie du littoral de la Narbonnaise en Antiquité* (*Riv. Studi Ligurri* XXV, 1959, 87—110)

Doorman, G., *Het haringkaken en Willem Beukels* (*Tijdschr. v. Geschiedenis* 1956, 371—386)

Higgs, E. S. and Peter White, J., *Autumn killing* (*Antiquity* XXXVII 1963, no. 148, 282—289)

(149) Strabo, XVI, 2.45. cap. 764
(150) ḏ'wt (V.535.5)
(151) śwh.t (IV.73.6)
(152) Valerius Maximus, VII.6. exter. 3
(153) Cercidae, V.106
(154) Suidas, *de Aristophanus*, *Ranae* 558
(155) *Geoponica*, XIX.9
(156) Xenophon, *Anabasis* V.4.28
(157) Cato, *On Farming* 7.3; 117
(158) Strabo, IV.3.2. cap. 192
(159) Athenaeus, XIV. 657
(160) Cato, *On Farming* 162
(161) Kraemer, C. J. and Spencer, F. A., *New Light on the taricheutes in Augustan Egypt* (*Trans. Proc. Amer. Phil. Assoc.* 1934, xlv)

Dawson, W. R., *References to Mummification by Greek and Latin Authors* (*Aegyptus*, Vol. IX, 1928, pags. 106—112)

Engelbach, R. & Derry, D. E., *Mummification* (*Ann. Serv. Ant. Egypte*, Vol. 41, 1942, pags. 233—269)

Sethe, K., *Zur Geschichte der Einbalsamierung bei den Aegyptern* (*Abh. Preuss. Akad. Wiss.* 1934, pags. 211—239)

SAUNERON, S., *Rituel de l'Embaumement*, Pap. Boulaq III (Cairo 1952)

DAWSON, W. R., *Making a Mummy* (*J. Egypt. Archaeol.*, Vol. XIII, 1927, pags. 40—49)

LUCAS, A., *The Use of Natron in Mummification* (*J. Egypt. Archaeol.*, Vol. XVIII, 1932, pags. 125—140)

LUCAS, A., *Preservative Materials used by the Ancient Egyptians in Embalming* (Cairo 1911)

WINLOCK, H. E., *Materials used at the embalming of King Tut-ankh-Amun* (New York 1941)

HERRMANN, A., *Einbalsemierung* (*Reallex. Christ. Antike* IV, 1959, 798—821)

LAUER, J. PH. et ISKANDER, Z., *Données nouvelles sur la mommification dans l'Egypte ancienne* (ASAE 53, 1953, 167—194)

SANDISON, A. T., *The histological Examination of Mummified Material* (*Stain Technology*, Geneva N.Y. vol. 30, 1955, 3, 277—283)

SAUNERON, S., *Rituel de l'Embaumement*, *Pap. Boulaq* III, *Pap. Louvre* 5, 158 (Paris, 1952)

BAUMANN, BILL B., *The botanical aspects of ancient Egyptian embalming and burial* (*Econ. Bot. Vol.* 14, 1960, No. 1, p. 84—104)

(162) HERODOTUS, II.85 & 88; IV.53

(163) DIODORUS, I.3

(164) ATHENAEUS, III. 116—121

(165) '.t nm.t (II.264.8)

(166) wp.t r3 (I.300.6)

(167) pr-nfr (I.517.11)

(168) w'b.t (I.284.4)

(169) sḥ - nṯr (III.465.2)

(170) s'ḥ (IV.52.17)

(171) ḥm3g.t (III.94.8)

(172) wt (I.380.2) possibly connected with wt (I.379.4), bandage, and with wḥ3t (I.347.12), the copper kettle in which the resinous mixes and unguents were heated

(173) ḥ3j.t (III.16.6), vide ḥ3.t, grove and h3j.t, chapel

(174) nkbt (II.236.13)

(175) krś (V.63.11)

(176) kś (V.68.2)

(177) k3t.wt (I.378.7)

(178) wt (I.379.9)

(179) HERODOTUS, II.86—88

(180) DIODOR, I.7

CHAPTER SEVEN

PAINTS, PIGMENTS, INKS AND VARNISHES

Introduction

Colouring agents and protective coatings were used from the dawn of history onwards. Their decorative value was not the main factor leading to their use. We must be fully aware of the religious and magical meaning attached to colours (and hence to pigments and dyes) by the ancients and this aspect of their use should always be in our mind when discussing them. Chemistry arose when scientists and philosophers became interested in the phenomena of colouring, dyeing and colour change and started to study them. Blood-red, white and black colours play a large part in white or black magic. We still wear black, dark red, brown or white according to our religion when we mourn over our beloved dead as did the ancients. In ancient Egypt colours, scenes and their composition in the tombs and temples were fixed in all details in ritual. In classical times red was especially valued and used in rites on the principle of sympathy, because of its equation with the sun, its relation to the spirit of life, blood, and because of its effect on the human soul (1).

The ancients had only vague ideas about the origin of painting, and this is what Pliny has to say (2):

"The origin of painting is obscure, and hardly falls within the scope of this work. The claim of the Egyptians to have discovered the art six thousand years before it reached Greece is obviously an idle boast, while among the Greeks some say that it was first discovered at Sikyon others at Corinth. All, however, agree that painting began with the outlining of a man's shadow; this was the first stage, in the second a single colour was employed, and after the discovery of more elaborate methods this style, which is still in vogue, received the name of monochrome."

In fact the oldest paint support was probably the human body. The samples of red ochre found in graves from Cro-Magnon (Upper Palaeolithic) times onwards, are sometimes layers of pigment encasing the dead body, added may be as a life-giving substance because of its ressemblance to clotted blood. In some cases, however, it would seem that the ochre was used less abundantly and was originally applied as war-paint or body-decoration by the living man. Tattooing the skin with red, yellow and blue patterns seems also to have been practised at a very early date.

The skeletons of a triple sepulchre in a cave of Grimaldi were found embedded in red ochre. In Indian graves in Maine (U.S.A.) in every case a quantity of red ochre was placed on either side of the head of the skeleton (3). Red ochre has also been applied to bone ornaments from a Neanderthal grave of Spy (Belgium) and others of Acheulian date.

Prehistory

From the start we should make a clear distinction between dyes and pigments. A *dye* is any substance used for tinting fabrics, the word "dye" is derived from an Old English word "deag" meaning colour. In a few cases dyes are used in painting, but in general painters will use *pigments*, e.g. dry colour powders mixed with a medium or thinner to make them sufficiently fluid for application in the painting ground. The word "pigment" (from the Latin pigmentum) is also sometimes used in the more general sense of "colouring material" as derived from plants and animals, but we will use it here in the stricter sense of powdered colouring agent to be used by the painter.

Generally speaking mineral pigments and the paints made from them resist corrosive agents such as air and humidity much better than dyes. Coloured natural mineral (mostly iron) oxides have been used since Palaeolithic times and evidence of their use is abundant not only in such cases as mentioned above but in real paintings.

Pliny was not quite correct in his hypothesis on the origin of painting. In fact painting starts in Aurignacien times with the imprints of hands pressed on a background covered with fat and then delineated by red ochre blown onto them (4). Such silhouettes first received red, then black shadings. Then come tracings with fingers dipped in colours These tracings of curves and wavy lines develop into patterns and pictures of animals. Later brushes of spliced wooden sticks or feathers were used and the help of plastic art was invoked enhance the resemblance to the object depicted. The fact, that the ancient Sumerians regarded most of their mineral pigments as some kind of clay (5), speaks for itself. Unfortunately the lack of analytical data on prehistoric paints contrasts shrilly with the host of books and essays on the religious and magical meaning of the Aurignacian and Magdalenian (Upper Palaeolithic) cave drawings and the later Neolithic rock-drawings, as well as their artistic aspects. The only exceptions are the cave-drawings of Altamira and Lascaux, discussed in two publications (6) at some length.

The basic pigments used were natural iron or manganese oxides, that is the fundamental colours are yellow, red and black. In Lascaux a "coal-black" and a "dark-nigger" manganese oxide were used. The lumps of earthy iron oxide were sometimes cut into pencils ranging from reddish-brown to straw colour. A natural peroxide of iron used has now turned violet red and mauve. At Lascaux there is no trace of white paints, but in other caves kaolin seems to have been used. In some cases calcined bones were the source of the black pigment used.

TABLE XVIII

TECHNIQUES OF WALL-PAINTING

Techniques of wet support	
Al-fresco and buon fresco	Crete 2000 B.C.
Casein tempera	Pompeii
Stuccu-lustro	Hellenistic
Sgrafitto and later techniques	Post-classical
Al-secco techniques on dry support	
Water colours (adding honey or gum)	Egypt 3000 B.C.
Pigments with glue (size)	Egypt 3000 B.C.
Casein colours	Upper Palaeolithic
Lime/glue technique	Greece 600 B.C.
Egg tempera	Egypt 1000 B.C.
Encaustic (wax) technique	Greece 300 B.C.
Lime/casein (blood) oil paints	Neolithic
Waterglass colours	XIXth century

These pigments were finely ground and stored in naturally hollowed stones or shoulderblades. The paint was prepared by mixing this powder with urine (as still used by primitive man) or more commonly hot animal fat or grease. The outline of the final drawing was sometimes traced in thin lines with a flint graver. In some cases it was outlined by a series of coloured dots covered by the subsequent filling in. In

Altamira the sweeping "bones of the drawing" must have been traced with a pointed brush dipped in hot paint.

The heated grease-paint was brushed in a fairly thin form to reinforce and supplement the engraved outline. A sliced end of a stick or brushes with real tufts of hair together with pads of lichen, moss or may be soft leather then served to dab on the hot paint. Pads of this kinds served well to work in colours, graduate them or wipe them off. Only after cooling could the colour be scraped off. The coating of surfaces generally required less of a thicker liquid. In Altamira the dark outlines and more salient characters were painted with a well-pointed brush dipped in very hot paint of a full black or some other strong colour.

In some cases a "vaporizing" technique as still used by some Australian tribes was applied. The powdered pigment was blown onto the surface covered with hot grease. Finds of hollow bones filled with ochre confirm this.

It should be remembered that we know next to nothing about the binding medium used as such materials escape our analysis in most cases (7). The above-mentioned grease paints would not be water-proof, they would be suitable for cave-drawings only. The water-proof rock-paintings of Eastern Europe may have been made with grease paints to which blood or milk may have been added. Blood was used in Neolithic times to harden mud floors. The Neolithic in-crustations of white paint in deeply incised lines is said to contain lime, but this would imply that lime burning was already known, of which we hold no certain proof. In some caves stone saucers have been found still containing slight traces of pigments. They have probably served to mix the ground pigments with water, grease or whatever medium was employed.

Pigments

Our knowledge of the pigments used by the civilisations of the Ancient Near East is considerably larger for here analytical data and documents are fairly profuse though not as detailed as we would wish them to be. This pertains more particularly to data from ancient Meso-potamia, where the humidity of soil and climate have destroyed prac-tically all ancient wall-paintings, documents written on papyrus and parchment, textiles and similar less stable remains of these civilisations. A pot in a furnace of the Uruk/Jemdet Nasr period contained some

	Produced from	Egyptia
Red Ochre	—	ṯmś (V.369.
Burnt Red Ochre	—	—
Nat. ferric oxide	red clay, haematite	ḫntj (III.301.
Red Lead	litharge burnt	djdj (V.421.
Cinnabar, Vermilion	mercury sulphide	—
Realgar	red sulphide of arensic	—

plum-coloured paint and a red paint was also found but neither were analysed (7a). Here we have to rely more strongly on texts than in Egypt where most of the tomb-paintings are nearly as fresh as on the day they were painted many centuries ago.

During Antiquity the scale of natural pigments was increased with several artificial ones or as PLINY has it (8):

"When we contemplate the number and variety of colour known, we are overcome by admiration for the early masters. The greatest artists Apelles, Aetion, Melanthius and Nichomachus used four colour only for those immortal masterpieces — melinum as a white pigment, Attic sil among the yellows, Pontic sinopis as a red and the black atramentum — and yet towns lavished their whole resources on a single picture. To-day when purple has made its appearance on our walls and India contributes the slime of her rivers, the blood of dragons and elephants, no noble paintings are produced.

So inferior resources produced a higher standard of achievement. This, as I have said is the result of our concern about the value of materials used rather than the genius of the artist."

Or in another passage (9):

"Pigments may be divided into the subdued and the vivid, examples of both classes being afforded, now by nature, now by the mixing bowl. The vivid pigments comprise those which are supplied to the artist by his patron: minium (cinnabar, for red-lead is "secundarium minium") Armenian stone (azurite), cinnabar (dragon's blood resin), chrysocolla (malachite), Indian blue (indigo) and Purpurissum (an earth dyed with Tyrian purple). All other pigments are classed as subdued.

ts

Sumerian	Accadian	Hebrew	Greek	Latin
·KA, IM-SA$_5$	ŝarŝerru	siḳra	sinopis	rubrica
-MAL-LI-GUG	kalgugu	—	tektonike	
IM-SA$_6$	ŝarŝerru	—	—	haematitis
ªZA-TU-BE	sâsu	ŝâŝer	sandarakè	syricum (minium) (sandaraca)
GUG	sându	—	kinnibari, miltos	minium, cinnabaris
IM-GUŠKIN	lêru, ŝindu	—	sandarakè sandyx	sandaraca

Pigments may be classified differently - into the natural and the artificial. The natural pigments are sinopis, rubrica, paraetonium, melinum, Eretrian earth and orpiment (auripigmentum, arrhenicum). The remainder are artificial, and include, first and foremost, those described in our accounts of the metals, and also the cheaper pigment ochre, ceruse, roasted ceruse, sandarach, sandyx, syricum, and atramentum."

The pigments available in Imperial Rome were practically the same we find in use in the Far East during that period (10).

Antiquity was particularly rich in *red pigments* such as ochre, red lead, cinnabar and sandarach.

Red ochre was the most widely used red mineral pigment from Predynastic times until a very late date. Though several analyses report "burnt ochre" it is doubtful whether the Egyptians really burnt yellow ochre to obtain their red pigment. Natural supplies were plentiful near Aswan and in the Oases of the Western desert. Egyptian red ochre had a good reputation amongst classical authors (11). Red ochre was also used in Mesopotamia, in Asia Minor and Palestine, both for pottery and wall-paintings.

Ochres are natural earths consisting of silica and clay and owe their colour to anhydrous or hydrous iron oxide. Pliny discusses the different qualities known to the classical world (12):

"Sinopis was first found in Pontus, and derives its name from the Pontic city of Sinope. It occurs also in Egypt, the Balearic islands, and Africa, but the best kind is mined from caves in Lemnos and Cappadocia. The material close to the rock is the choicest. The interior of the lumps is uniform in colour, but on the surface they are speckled.

This was the material which the old masters used to produce "glow" in their pictures.

There are three kinds of sinopis—bright red, dull red and an intermediate shade. The best costs two denarii a lb, and is used for brush-painting and for colouring wood. The African variety, which they call cicerculum (chicken-pea), costs eight asses, and, being a brighter red than the rest, is more in demand for colouring wall-panels. The very dark variety, called pressior, sells at the same price, and is used for colouring the lower parts of the panels....

Some authorities have expressed the opinion that sinopis should be regarded as a *rubrica* of second quality, the premier place being given to Lemnian rubrica. The latter is inferior only to minium and was famous among the ancients as the island where it is found. Every piece sold had to be officially sealed hence the name sphragis (a seal). It is used as a foundation of minium paint and for the adulteration of minium (rubrica is the general name for red ochres corresponding with the Greek miltos)....

Of the other kinds of rubrica, the most suitable for craftsmen are the Egyptian and African, since they are the most readily absorbed by plastered walls (al-fresco painting). Rubrica is found also in iron mines. It is moreover prepared artifically by igniting yellow ochre in new vessels luted with mud...."

Dioscorides mentions that Spanish ochre "was being burnt and turned into rubrica" and Vitruvius mentions ochre from Spain and the Balearic isles too. It was later rivalled by Spanish cinnabar (13). Sinopia was later also used as a ground for gilding under the name "leukophoron" and true Armenian "bolus" was also sold as "poliment" (14).

Haematite was certainly used in certain cases in preclassical times, it was identified as one of the pigments used in the tomb of Perneb (15). Then there were cinnabar, already used in colouring the famous oracle bones of ancient China (16), realgar and red lead. These are the pigments often referred to by classical authors as "sandyx" or "serikon". They were used as a base for rouge in cosmetics. The use of cinnabar as a pigment during this early period is still doubtful. Red lead was known in ancient Mesopotamia and prepared by heating lead, ceruse and dross in an oven to form litharge which was then ground and heated to give red lead. Its introduction in Egypt is due to the Romans, the earliest evidence for its use are finds at Hawara. The Egyptian term then applied to red lead is much older and seems first to have indicated some natural form of bole occurring near Elephantine.

The difficulties which beset the ancients when trying to identify these different red pigments will be clear from the garbled account which PLINY has given us (17):

"Another thing found in silver mines is minium, still one of the most valued pigments and formerly held not merely in honour but in veneration by the Romans. Verrius gives a list of authorities who inspire confidence, to prove that it was customary on festive occasions to paint with minium the face of the image of Jove himself, and that of the bodies of triumphing generals were similarly stained, a custom followed by Camillus in his triumph. Through the sense of this sacredness it was also added to the unguents used at a triumphal banquet, and to make a contract for painting Jove was one of the first duties of the censor.

Why this is I wonder, and yet it is known that minium is still in demand by the Aethiopian peoples, that their chieftains dye themselve with it from head to foot, and that is the colour they use for the images of their gods. For this reason we shall the more diligently investigate all the facts.

Theophrastus relates that the original discovery of minium was made ninety years before the archonship of Praxibulus (that is, in the three hundred and forty-ninth year of our city) (405 B.C.), by Callias, an Athenian, who hoped at first that gold could be extracted by roasting from the red sand which occurs in silver mines. He adds that, before his time, a hard and sandy variety had been discovered in Spain, and that it has also been found among the Colchians on a certain inaccessible crag, from which they knock it down by throwing javelins at it. This variety, however, is impure and the best comes from the Cilbian plains beyond Ephesus, where the sand has the colour of the kermesberry. This is ground to a powder, washed and allowed to subside, the deposit being subjected to further washing. Differences of procedure are found. Some, in preparing the minium, wash only once. Others find that this gives too weak a colour and wash a second time to get a superior product.

I am not surprised at the esteem in which this colour was held. For even in Trojan times red earth was honoured, as we learn from Homer who makes his ships agreeable with it, although he rarely speaks elsewhere of paints and painting. The Greeks call the red earth miltos and minium they call cinnabar whence mistakes have arisen on account of the name Indian cinnabar. For this name is given by them to the gore of the dragon crushed beneath the weight of the dying elephants, a substance which in, as we have already related (dragon's blood) the blood of both animals mingled, and which is the only colour which properly represents blood in painting....

Cinnabar was used by the early artists for what are still called monochromata. The use of Ephesian minium, which they also employed was abandoned on account of the difficulty of preservation. Besides that, both colours were deemed too vivid. So they had recourse to rubrica and sinopis (red ochres). Cinnabar is adulterated with goat's blood or pounded service-berries (sorb-apples, the fruit of Pyrus domestica), the pure material costs fifty sesterces a lb.

Juba related that minium is also found in Carmania and Timagenes that it occurs in Aethiopia, but we import none from either country. Almost our entire supply comes from Spain, from that famous minium mines in the region of Sisapo in Baetica, which is a source of revenue for the Roman people. Nothing is more jealously guarded, for it is illegal to refine and roast it there. The ore is brought to Rome under seal to the extent of about two thousand lbs per annum, and there it is washed. A law has been passed fixing the maximum selling price at 70 sesterces a lb, but it is adulterated in many ways, so much illicit profit to the company. For there is a kind which occurs in almost all silver and lead mines and is prepared by burning certain rocks which are mixed with the main vein of ore — not those rocks whose exudation we call quicksilver for the product obtained by roasting them is also quicksilver — but others found simultaneously. These contain no quicksilver and are recognized only by their lead colour (cerussite) for they do not become red until they have been heated in the furnace, after which they are pounded to powder (evidently this is red lead prepared from cerussite, native lead carbonate and obtaining its colour after roasting (oxidation).

This is a second-rate kind of minium, known to very few and far inferior to the native sands already mentioned. It is used in the company's workshops to adulterate genuine minium. Syricum, the manufacture of which will be described may also be employed at will. A calculation, however, made by weighing one against another reveals a minium that has been treated with Syricum (manufactured from rubrica (red ochre) and sandarach). In another way it is convenient for dishonest painters who repeatedly charge their brushes and then dip them in water. The pigment settles and remains at the bottom for the thieves.

Pure minium should have the brilliancy of kermes, but when the second-rate minium is used for mural paintings it experiences rusting, though it is itself the rust of a metal.

In the minium mines of Sisapo (cinnabar!) the vein of sand is pure and contains no silver. It is roasted like gold (mistaken statement as Pliny is here confusing red lead and cinnabar). It is tested with red-hot gold, for adulterated material darkens, while the pure pigment keeps its colour. I find that lime is also used as an adulterant and that the fraud can be detected in a similar manner using a plate of hot iron if gold is not available.

Sun and moon injure a minium paint. To prevent this, when the wall is dry, hot Punic wax melted with oil should be applied with brush, and then heated with a brazier of oakapple-charcoal till it sweats. It is rubbed with wax candles and finished with a clean cloth, just as marble statues are polished. Minium refiners in a factory envelop their faces with loose bladders which enable them to see without inhaling the fatal dust. Minium finds an application also inscriptions on rolls, and more vivid letters, even in sepulchral ornamentation, have been produced on gold and marble by its said."

From this quotation from BAILEY's technologically correct translation (18) we see clearly that PLINY confuses three red pigments:

1) *Vermilion* or cinnabar, that is red mercuric sulphide, which was one of the first chemical compounds to be synthesized by the early chemists from sulphur and mercury. PLINY calls it both "cinnabaris" and "minium".

2) "Cinnabaris" is also used for *dragon's blood*, the resin of Pterocarpus draco.

3) *Red lead*, the tetroxide of lead made by heating litharge or white lead for some hours at 480° C, is called "minium secundarium" by PLINY and regarded as a kind of second quality vermilion.

A better discussion of the properties of vermilion and red lead is given by VITRUVIUS (19), who too is still unable to distinguish them properly:

"I will now go on to describe the treatment of minium or vermilion. It is said to have been discovered in the Cilbian fields of Ephesus. The material and its treatment is sufficiently wonderful. For what is called the ore is first extracted. Then, using certain processes, they find minium. In the veins the ore is like iron, of a more carroty colour, with a red dust round it. When it is mined, and is worked with iron tools, it exudes many drops of quicksilver, and these are at once collected by the miners.

When the ore has been collected in the workshop, because of the large amount of moisture, it is put in the furnace to dry. The vapour which is produced by the heat of the fire, when it condenses on the floor of the oven, is found to be quicksilver (argentum vivum)....

I will now return to the preparation of vermilion. When the ore is dry it is bruised with iron rammers and by frequent washing and heating the waste is removed and the colour produced. When, therefore, the quicksilver has thus been removed, minium loses its natural virtues and becomes soft and friable.

And so when it is used in the finishing of enclosed apartments, it remains of its own colour without defects; but in open places like peristyles and exedrae and so forth, where the sun and moon can send their brightness and their rays, the part so affected is damaged and becomes black, when the colour loses its strength. Among the many instances of this is the case of the public official Faberius. He wished to have his palace on the Aventine elegantly finished, and had all the walls of the peristyle covered with vermilion. In a month the walls turned to an unpleasant and uneven colour; and so he was the first to let a contract for laying on other colours.

But if anyone proceeds in a less crude fashion and wishes a vermilion surface to keep its colour after the finishing of the wall is dry, let him apply with a strong brush Punic wax melted in the fire and mixed with a little oil. Then putting charcoal in an iron vessel, and heating the wall with it, let the wax first be brought to melt, and let it be smoothed over, then let it be worked with waxed cord and clean linen cloths, in the same way as naked marble statues; this process is called ganosis in Greek.

Thus a protective coat of Punic wax does not allow the brilliance of the moon or the rays of the sun to remove the colour from these finished surfaces by playing on them. The workshops which were in the Ephesian mines are now removed to Rome, because this kind of vein has been discovered in parts of Spain. The workshops are between the temples of Flora and Quirinus.

Minium is adulterated by the admixture of lime. If anyone wishes to test its purity, the method is as follows. Take an iron plate, put the minium on it and set it on the fire until the plate is red-hot. When the colour is changed by the heat and is black, take the plate from the fire, and let the minium on cooling regain its former colour: its purity will be demonstrated. But if it remains black, it shows adulteration."

VITRUVIUS describes the testing of cinnabar better than does PLINY but still the confusion of vermilion and red lead remains in his test (20) which holds good only when vermilion is heated sufficiently to evaporate completely to yield a residue which may show up adulteration by red lead or iron compounds but not lime compounds! There were rich workings at Sizma (Lyaconia) near Laodicea before the Spanish production took the lead (21). This confusion of vermilion and red lead is found in other classical authors too (22).

In the ancient Near East the use of red lead seems to have preceded that of vermilion and the "vermilion" of the Bible (23) was probably red lead. From the passage from PLINY and VITRUVIUS cited above it is clear that the production of red lead from lead compounds such as the natural cerussite or from litharge was well understood. VITRUVIUS is most explicit on this matter in the following passage (24):

"When white lead is roasted in a furnace, under the heat of the fire it changes its colour and becomes sandaraca. This fact was accidentally discovered in a conflagration. A much better result is obtained in this way than from the natural substance which is produced from the mines".

As we have noted earlier PLINY recognizes a similarity between the oxidation of lead to red lead and that of iron to ferric oxide, both changes can easily be produced by heating the metal in air and there is no reason why we should refuse to believe that the ancients were capable of such deductions. In certain passages PLINY confuses red lead and realgar, which he calls sandarach, though further on in the same passage he defines his syricum (red lead) as a distinct pigment (25)

"According to Juba *sandarach* and ochre are found in Topazus, an island in the Red Sea, but our supplies are not derived from the same source. We have already described the production of sandarach, an imitation of which is made by igniting ceruse in a furnace. This substance should be flame-coloured and costs five asses a pound (red-lead of course!).

If this ceruse is ignited with its own weight of rubrica sandyx (red lead plus ochre) is formed, although I observe that Virgil supposed sandyx to be a plant when he wrote the line (see also Propertius 2.25.45): Sponte sua sandyx pascentes vestiat agnos. The price per pound of sandyx is half that of sandarach, and these two pigments are the heaviest in use.

Another artificial pigment is *syricum* (red-lead made by heating pure ceruse), the use of which as a foundation for minium has been already mentioned. It is a mixture of sinopis and sandyx."

Usually sandarach, our realgar, the natural orange-red sulphide of arsenic, is properly described and distinguished from other red pigments:

"An indication has already been given of the nature of sandarach. It occurs in both gold and silver mines, and its excellence is proportional to the depth of its red colour, its sulphurous smell, its purity and its brittleness...." (26).

The most famous sandarach mine was not on the island of Topazus but in Asia Minor according to most classical authors (27) and this is what STRABO has to tell about this mine:

"And in Pontus too a place was proclaimed a city, I mean Pompeiopolis; and in this city is mount Sandaracurgium not far away from Pimolisa.... (this mound) is hollowed out in consequence of the mining done there, since the workmen have excavated great cavities beneath it. The mine used to be worked by publicans, who used as miners the slaves sold in the market because of their crimes; for, in addition to the painfulness of the work they say that the air in the mines is both deadly and hard to endure on account of the grievious odour of the ore, so that the workmen are doomed to a quick death. What is more, the mine is often left idle because of unprofitableness, since the workmen are not only more than two hundred in number but are continuously spent by disease and death". The relation between the two sulphides of arsenic, realgar and orpiment is clearly indicated by Pliny and others (28).

The *pink colours* were compounded by mixing red and white pigments. In classical times pink was sometimes obtained by using an organic red dye (madder) on a gypsum base. An example of Graeco-Roman date has been found in Egypt.

The choice of good *blue pigments* was confined in Antiquity to lapis lazuli, blue frit, azurite and indigo, all of whom are often indiscriminantly called kyanos or caeruleum by the classical authors.

Lapis lazuli was known in the Ancient Near East for many centuries and it was treasured a as semi-precious stone, especially by the Egyptians. It came from the only source known to the ancients, the mines of Badakshan and it is highly dubious whether it was ever used as a pigment. A cake of lapis lazuli pigment is reported to have been found in Sargon's palace of Chorsabad, but lapis lazuli or turquoise if simply ground would make poor pigments. We have no evidence of the refining and washing of ground lapis lazuli in order to prepare ultramarine (free from silica and calcite particles) before the sixth and seventh centuries A.D. in Afghanistan and its use in Byzantine times is established (29) but not earlier.

TABLE XX

Blue and purple pigments

	Prepared from	Egyptian	Sumerian	Accadian	Hebrew	Greek	Latin
Lapis lazuli	lazurite	ḫśbḏ (III.334.1)	^{a}ZA-GÌN	^{a}uḳnû	—	kyanos	sapphiros
Egyptian blue Blue frit	sand, alkali + copper salts	ḫśbḏ (III.334.1)	—	uḳnû	—	kyanos	caeruleum (lomentum)
Azurite	basic copper carbonate	tfrr (V.300.2)	^{a}ZA-GIN-KUR-RA SÍG-ZA-GÌN-GÍG	tâkiltu	—	armenion	armenium ammium
Red purple glaze	sand, alkali + cupro salts	—	^{a}ZA-GÌN-DIR$_5$	—	—	—	—

TABLE XXI

Yellow pigments

	Produced from	Egyptian	Sumerian	Accadian	Hebrew	Greek	Latin
Yellow Ochre	iron oxide	mnšt (II.89.12)	IM-MAL-LI	kalû	?	ochra	sil
Limonite	natural product	ḳnjt (V.52.10)	^{a}KA-SIG$_7$, IM-GUŠKIN	—	?	—	—
Orpiment (King's Yellow)	yellow sulphide of arsenic	×	ŠEM-SAHAR-GUŠKIN	šêpu, lêru	zarniq	arrhenikum arsenikon	auripigmentum
Massicot, litharge	lead oxide	×	—	sândi	?	litharguros	usta, spuma argenti
Napels Yellow	lead antimoniate	?	A-BÁR	abaru	?	—	—

The presence of cobalt compounds in Mesopotamia glazes and glass has been established but this may be due to a fortitious contamination of the real ingredients. Such compounds were certainly never used in Egypt or in classical times.

One of the early blue pigments in ancient Egypt was azurite (or chessylite?), the basic copper carbonate imported from the Sinai mines. This was indeed the most important blue pigment for wall paintings in preclassical times. It is not reported for Roman wall paintings though the classical writers are well aware of its existence (30). In ancient Mesopotamia a special type of mortar and pestle are mentioned for the purpose of grinding such mineral pigments (31).

An artificial substitute was found in Egypt at a very early date (IVth Dynasty), the name of which was the same as that of lapis lazuli like in ancient Assyria. This blue frit, first used as a glaze and then in powdered form as a pigment, was prepared by heating silica, malachite, calcium carbonate (chalk, limestone) and natron for 24 hours between 800 and 900° C. Laurie and his collaborators have established that the critical temperature for the formation of this copper-aluminate is about 830° C (32). The natron of the recipe can be substituted by salt (33) with profit. It would not combine with lime on a wet surface but the pigment could be pressed in with the trowel or it could be applied with yolk of egg in "al secco" fresco painting. Remains of such a frit factory were discovered at El Amarna (Egypt).

The secret of its manufacture was known to the ancient Assyrians about 1500 B.C. They became very fond of it and it was used as a substitute for the expensive lapis lazuli in paints, glass and glazes. Even small objects were shaped from it. The secret of its manufacture was lost between 200 and 700 A.D.

This blue frit was the caeruleum of the ancients, the manufacture of which is described by PLINY in these words (34):

"Caeruleum is a hard substance. Three varieties have long been known—the Egyptian, which is considered to be the best, the Scythian which is easily disintegrated in water, and on grinding yields four shades of colour, the lighter, the darker, the coarser and the finer, and the Cyprian which is, however, superior to the Scythian. To these we may now add varieties from Puteoli and from Spain, where deposits are being worked for the first time. All kinds are dyed, and absorb the colour when boiled with the appropriate herb. The rest of the preparation is identical with that of chrysocolla.

What we call lomentum is made from caeruleum, and prepared for use by washing and grinding. It is lighter in tint than caeruleum and costs ten denarii a lb., while caeruleum costs eight. It can be used on a background of chalk, but is injured by lime. A kind recently introduced is the Vestorian, so called from its inventor. This is made from the lightest part of Egyptian caeruleum and sold for eleven denarii a lb. The caeruleum from Puteoli is used, under the name of cylon, for similar purposes, but it is also employed for windows.

The importation of caeruleum Indicum, at seven denarii a lb. is a recent development. It is used in painting for incisurae, that is the divisions between light and shade. Finally there is the cheapest kind of lomentum, the so-called ground variety, priced at five asses per lb.

The test for pure caeruleum is that it should burn on a hot coal. It is imitated by boiling pansies with water and straining the extract through a cloth into Eretrian earth."

The Vestorius mentioned by PLINY was a Puteoli banker, the friend of Cicero and Atticus who was a sound accountant and who advised Cicero about building but who does not seem to have taken much interest in philosophy as Cicero informs his friend. VITRUVIUS, who did not know how old the blue frit really was, described Vestorius' process in more details but curiously enough left out the chalk (35):

"The processes for making blue were first discovered at Alexandria; afterwards also Vestorius founded a factory at Puteoli. His method and his ingredients are noteworthy. Sand is ground with flowers of soda (nitri flore) to such fineness that it becomes like flour. Cyprian copper is sprinkled from rough files like fine dust so that it combines with the mixture. Then it is rolled by hand into balls and they are put together to dry. When dry they are collected in an earthenware jar, and the jars are put in a furnace. In this way the copper and the sand burning together owing of the vehemence of the fire dry together, and interchanging their vapours lose their properties; and their own character being overcome by the vehemence of the fire, they acquire a blue colour."

Other authors called this blue frit "kyanos" or "caeruleum" too (36) but they gave the name "native kyanos" to the chrysocolla of the copper mines, which is a green pigment really, but which was sometimes stained blue with indigo as we shall see.

PLINY did not seem to know indigo as a dye, being unacquainted with the process of rendering indigo-blue soluble, he applied indigo to a ground or base to obtain a blue pigment of doubtful quality.

The Assyrians were able to prepare a *purple* frit by smelting sand, alkali and copper salts, but is not known whether it was ever ground to be used as a purple pigment. VITRUVIUS (37) mentioned that "ochre of a good yellow colour can be roasted to a bright heat. It is quenched with vinegar and becomes of a purple colour."

The *yellow pigments* were mostly natural iron oxides (ochres or limonite) which were very plentiful near Cairo and in the oases of the western desert. The same holds good for the rest of the Near East. Thus small cakes of yellow limonite were found in a grave at Gezer. In the classical period too the yellows and browns were mostly natural umbers, siennas and ochres about which PLINY reports (38):

"In silver-mines and gold-mines the pigments sil and caeruleum also occur. Sil is, strictly speaking, a mud (best translated ochre). The best variety is made from the Attic mineral and costs two denarii a lb. The next, marbled sil, is half the price of the Attic. The third is the dark variety which others call Scyrian from the island of Scyros. It now comes from Achaia also and is used for the dark parts of pictures. The price is two sesterces a lb. The so-called clear kind, coming from Gaul, costs two asses less, and, like the Attic kind, is employed for high lights. For wall-panels, only the marbled variety is used since the marble in it withstands the bitterness of the lime. It is also mined in the mountains at the twentieth milestone from the city. It is subsequently burned and the dishonest manufacturers say that it is the dark variety, but its counterfeit nature, and the fact that it has been burned, are revealed by its bitterness and the way in which it has been reduced to powder.

Polygnotus and Micon were the first artists to use sil, but only Attic sil. Their successors used Attic for the high lights, Scyrian and Lydian for the shaded parts. Lydian sil used to be purchased at Sardis, but the demand has now failed."

To which VITRUVIUS adds (39):

"First we will describe the colours which are dug up in their natural state such as the yellow (sil) material which the Greeks call ochre. This is found in many places, as also in Italy. What is used to be the best, the Attic, is not available now, for the following reason. When the silver mines at Athens were worked, shafts were dug underground to find silver, but when a vein of ochre happened to be found they worked it no less than silver. Hence the ancients used a large amount of yellow in their frescoes."

This ochre also appeared in recipes for the preparation of a ground for gilding, PLINY mentions the following composition (40):

"If half a pound of Pontic sinopis is mixed with ten pounds of clear sil and two of Greek melinum and the whole triturated for twelve days, the resulting substance is leucophorum, and is the cement used when a veneer of gold is applied to a wooden surface."

Orpiment, the natural sulphide of arsenic, was found in a small bag in King Tutankhamun's tomb, in wall-paintings of the Theban necropolis and it was fairly generally used from the XVIIIth dynasty onwards. As the mineral does not occur in Egypt it must have been imported from Persia, Armenia or Asia Minor. Its use in Mesopotamia is beyond doubt, cakes were found in the palace of King Sargon II.

This yellow sulphide of arsenic was known to the classical painters as "arsenikon" or "auripigmentum" and it was produced mainly in Mysia, Pontus and Cappadocia (41). The ancients knew the relation between orpiment and realgar quite well as will be clear from the following passage from PLINY (42):

"Arrhenicum is another derivative of the same substance. The best kind is coloured a fine shade of gold; specimens which are paler, or which resemble sandarach, are thought to be inferior. A third variety exists, in which the golden-hued substance is mingled with sandarach. The latter kinds are flaky, while the first-mentioned is dry and pure, and divided into slender pieces along the cleavage lines which transverse it."

Orpiment was the object of one of the earliest alchemical experiment for PLINY tells us (45):

"Hope of obtaining gold, which he coveted exceedingly, induced the Emperor Gaius to order a great quantity of orpiment to be roasted and he certainly obtained some excellent gold but in such small quantity that although the price of the orpiment was only four denarii a pound, he found that he had lost by the experiment which was inspired by greed alone, the attempt has not been repeated." No doubt the first batch which the emperor tested was a "salted" consignment!

Massicot or yellow lead oxide was used in Egypt from Predynastic times onwards and it was found on a painter's palette of 400 B.C. Massicot or litharge, the yellow monoxide of lead was of course quite common in classical times, being from very early times a pigment that was recovered as a fairly pure by-product of silver refining. It was sometimes made from white lead it seems if we read what PLINY has to say (43):

"*Burnt ceruse* (usta, here clearly litharge) was accidentally discovered when the flames reached the ceruse-pots, during the burning of the

TABLE XXII

Green pigments

	Prepared from	Egyptian	Sumerian	Accadian	Hebrew	Greek	Latin
Malachite (chrysocolla)	basic copper carbonate	w3ḏ (I.267.15)	[a]NINI-MUS GIR	[a]mušgarru	?	chrysocolla	chrysocolla
Green frit	artificial ground glaze		ŠE-ZA-GÌN-DUR$_5$	?	?	—	—
Verdigris / Vert de Grèce	basic copper acetate	—	URUDU-SUN	šuḥtu	?	ios xustos / chalkon anthos	aeruca
Green earth (terre verte)	natural caledonite	ḥb (III.61.2)? —	—	—	?	theodotaion	creta viridis

TABLE XXIII

Black pigments

	Prepared from	Egyptian	Sumerian	Accadian	Hebrew	Greek	Latin
Carbon black, soot	bones or wood	wbd (1.297.9) ḏ'b.t (V.537.1)	IM-GÍG	—	ḥéret	aithale / asbolos	fuligo / atramentum
Charcoal	—	ḏ'b.t (V.537.1)	—	pentû	—	—	—
Bitumen	—	—	ESIR	iddû, kupru	hemār	asphaltos	bitumen
Iron oxide	black haematite	sš.w (III.481.II/12)	[a]KA-GIG	šadanu	—	—	—
Stibnite	antimony sulphide	mśdm.t (II.153.8)	ŠEM-BI-ZI(-DA)	guḫlu	kahâl	stimmi	stibium
Chinese ink	—	—	—	—	—	melan indikon	indicum

Piraeus. The first painter to employ it was Nicias, whose work has already been described. The Asiatic brand, known as purpurea is now considered the best and costs six denarii a pound. The pigment is manufactured also at Rome by burning hard lumps of sil and pouring vinegar on them while hot. It is indispensible for shadow-effects."

to which information DIOSCORIDES has the following to add (44): "The Attical is the best, the next to this is the Spanish, after these that from Puteoli in Campania and in Sicilia for much is made in these and those places where silver and lead are refined. The yellow and glittering is called Chrysitis which is the best, but that in Sicilia Argyritis and that of silver Lauritis." The preparation of litharge was a complicated process. The lead ore, galena, which was to yield silver, was heated in an elevated cauldron and the layer of molten litharge was run off continuously in a lower vessel. Its purification was a complex process including boiling with wheat, barley and beans, apparently absorbing some of the impurities. Then the litharge was ground in mortars together with salt or soda in order to obtain lighter hues (by the formation of basic chlorides and lead carbonates). These recipes of which DIOSCORIDES gives the clearest version give excellent results as BAILEY proved by his experiments (46), he obtained a series of colours ranging from orange to the palest yellow.

Finally there was Napels yellow, lead antimoniate or a compound of lead and antimony oxides, which was an important pigment in Babylonian glazes. A cake of this pigment was found in the palace of Sargon II at Chorsabad, but it was never found in Egypt, though possibly occuring in a XIXth dynasty glass.

Brown colours were produced in Egypt from natural ochres such as occur in Dakla Oasis. Sometimes red over black pigments were used and the brown paint on a XVIIIth dynasty box is a mixture of ochre and gypsum. Other combinations are haematite over black or yellow over haematite.

In Egypt *orange pigments* were obtained by mixing red and yellow ochres, but this colour is not frequently used.

The classical painters used similar combinations of pigments. Thus the orange on a piece of stucco found in the ruins near the monument of Caius Cestus at Rome consisted of a mixture of massicot and minium (46).

The choice of *green pigments* was rather limited. The ancients started to use powdered malachite or chrysocolla both in Egypt and the Near East. In Egypt and Mesopotamia artificial frit was then developed by smelting sand, alkali and copper minerals, which when powdered could be used as pigment. This green artificial frit occurs in Egypt from the VIth dynasty onwards (47). Sometimes mixes of the artificial blue frit and yellow ochre were used (in tombs at El-Bersheh and Kahun of the XIIth and XVIIIth dynasties). The manufacture and use of verdrigis in ancient Mesopotamia is well-attested but it was unknown to the ancient Egyptians. Both malachite (or chrysocolla) and green frit were used in Mesopotamia.

The green frit was not used by classical painters, but they did know malachite, terre verte and verdigris. Malachite is usually called chrysocolla by the ancients. This is the cause of some confusion as at present the term chrysocolla denotes the natural copper silicate, which was indeed used in some XIIth dynasty tombs of Kahun and El-Bersheh (Egypt). The pigment commonly denoted by "chrysocolla" was the natural basic copper carbonate which we now call mountain green or malachite and which was not only used in Egypt since predynastic times as a pigment and as an eyepaint, but which was also found in early Chinese paintings. This natural pigment was often dyed with the yellow dye-wood or dyer's weld, using alum as a mordant, in order to obtain the correct shade. This will be clear from the long passage which Pliny devotes to chrysocolla (48):

"Chrysocolla ("gold-solder") is an exudation found in the shafts (in gold mines) which we have already mentioned. It oozes down the vein of gold, and its muddy substance is congealed under the influence of the winter cold till it is as hard as pumice. It is well established that the best quality forms in copper mines and the next best in silver mines. It occurs in lead mines also, but this kind is inferior to that found in gold mines. In all these mines, however, it is also prepared artificially (though its worth is far below that of the natural product) by leading a gentle stream of water into the vein all through the winter till the month of June, and evaporating the extract in June and July. It is therefore perfectly clear that chrysocolla is none than a decomposition product of a vein of metal. Natural chrysocolla which is called uva differs from the artificial mainly in hardness, and yet it also is dyed with the herb called lutum (weld). It resembles flax and wool in its property of absorbing vegetable dyes. It is ground in a mortar, sifted through a fine sieve, ground again and sifted more finely. Whatever does not pass through is put back into the mortar and ground once more. The powder from each sifting is distributed into vessels and digested with vinegar to break up all the hard particles. It is then ground once more, washed, and dried in shell-shaped vessels. Finally it is dyed with fissile alum and the herb mentioned above, being itself painted before it is used as a paint. It is essential that it should possess the property of obedient adsorption. If it fails to take up the dye, those mordants which are known as scytanum and turbistum are added.

The dyed product is called orabitis by painters who distinguish two species, the eluta (washed) which is kept for making lomentum and the liquida, in which the small lumps are blended to a paste with liquid. Both these kinds are found in Cyprus, but the best quality comes from Armenia and the next best from Macedonia. Spain provides the greatest yield. The most esteemed variety closely resembles in colour the joyous verdure of the blade of corn. Ere now we have seen the arena of the circus strewn with chrysocolla at the spectacles given by the Emperor Nero, when he himself was to appear as a charioteer, dressed in a robe of the same colour. Ignorant workmen in general distinguish three varieties, the "rough" valued at seven denarii to the lb., the "medium", valued at five and the "powdered", also called "grass-green" valued at three. But before they put on the sandy kind, they lay a foundation with atramentum (carbon black) and paraetonium (chalk). These hold chrysocolla and soften its hue. The paraetonium being naturally very unctuous and adhesive by reason of its smoothness. is covered thinly with atramentum, lest the glossy whiteness of the paraetonium should make the chrysocolla too pale. The name lutea is said to be derived from the herb lutum which is itself ground up with caeruleum and put on as a substitute for chrysocolla, "a most inferior adulteration".

"Armenia exports the substance which bears its name. It is a mineral (mixture of malachite and azurite?) which is dyed like chrysocolla, and the best quality is that which approaches most closely to chrysocolla, but with a tinge of the blue colour of caeruleum.

It used to be valued at thirty sesterces a pound. Then a sandy material was found in Spain, which admits of a similar preparation and the price fell to six denarii a pound. It differs from caeruleum in that it has a certain pallor which enables the pigment to produce more delicate effects...."

Similar data are given by other classical authors (49). Bailey found the dyeing process described by Pliny to work well (50). The description of chrysocolla manufacture quoted above includes that of verdigris (vert de Grèce), a dibasic copper acetate, which many classical authors describe. Dioscorides (51) informed us that it was sometimes adulterated with pumice stone (which gave it a gritty taste) and with chalcanthum which would produce a red colour on heating.

Finally there was terre verte or green celadonite earth which is found in certain restricted areas such as Monte Baldo near Verona (terre de Vérone), Germany, France, Cyprus and Cornwall. It was found in wall paintings of Pompeii and Dura Europos and has been used since. PLINY (52) informs us that "one of these new-fangled colours of the cheapest sort was called Appian green, an imitation of chrysocolla, as if there were not enough counterfeits of it already. It is made from green earth and costs one sesterce a pound". VITRUVIUS (53) adds that "green chalk is found in many places but the best is from Smyrna, which the Greeks call theodoteion, because Theodotus was the name of the man on whose land it was found first."

A variety of *black pigments* were available. Though galena and stibnite (stibium, eyepaint) were available at an early date they were used for a short period only. The use of pyrolusite is very doubtful. Most of the pigments analysed upto the present contain carbon in some form, mostly a finely divided soot (lamp black, bone black) and in some cases powdered charcoal. The use of bitumen as a paint was restricted to Mesopotamia. In some cases a black iron oxide may have been used.

The greys were obtained in Egypt by mixing gypsum and charcoal or a pale yellowish earth (ochre?) with lamp black.

DIOSCORIDES informs us that the best "atramentum", soot or carbon black (54) is obtained from glass furnaces, but PLINY prefers wine-lees (55):

"Some make atramentum by drying and igniting wine-lees, and assert confidently that, if the lees come from good wine, the atramentum produced resembles Indicum (indigo). Polygnotus and Micon the celebrated Athenian painters made their black from grapeskins and called it tryginon. Apelles had the idea of making it by burning ivory and the product was called elephant black."

VITRUVIUS gives many more details on the manufacture of carbon black (56):

"I will now proceed to those materials which by special processes, are changed substantially and acquire the properties of colour. And first I will deal with black. The use of this in buildings is often necessary, so that we must know the tempering of materials for the purpose is carried out by special craftsmanship.

A vaulted apartment is built like a sweating chamber, and is covered carefully with a marble facing and smoothed down. In front of it a small furnace is built with outlets into the chamber, and the mouth of the furnace is carefully enclosed, so that the flame does not escape. Resin is placed in the furnace. Now the fiery potency burns it and compels it to emit soot through the outlets into the chamber. The soot clings round the walls and vaulting of the chamber. It is then collected and in part compounded with gum and worked up for the use of writing ink; the rest is mixed with size and used by fresco-painters in colouring walls.

But if this cannot be obtained, we must satisfy our requirements without holding back the works by the delay involved. Brushwood or pine-chips must be burned, and when they are charred they are to be pounded in a mortar with size. Thus the fresco-painters will have a not unpleasant black colour.

Again, a black colour even more pleasant than this is produced if the dregs of wine are dried and burnt in a furnace, and applied to the wall after being ground with size. The use of finer wines will allow us to imitate not only black but indigo."

The manufacture of inks and shoemaker's black, the copper compounds used to dye leather will be dealt with later on.

White Egyptian pigments used from pre-dynastic times onwards are either some form of calcium carbonate (whiting, chalk) or gypsum. Both occur in many places in that country. The Sumerians prepared their gypsum (pigment and plaster) by calcining the calcareous gypsum so plentiful in their country with cow-dung and crushed the mass thus obtained in mortars. They also disposed of white lead which they prepared by the action of vinegar on lead as described later by THEOPHRASTUS and PLINY. It is aptly called "the acetated thing". Again they used terra melia in certain cases. In Assyrian glazes tin oxyde is used, but it has not been spotted as a pigment in the few traces of wall-paintings that survived in Mesopotamia. Mercury, aptly termed "sublimate of cinnabar" was used in a few cases to colour the surface of little metal figurines.

The Greeks and Romans continued to use lime, gypsum, whiting (chalk) and china clay and they produced white lead too. The gypsum or terra alba was seldom used in unburnt form, in fact the Greek "gypsos" means burnt gypsum. It was not only used in cements and plasters but also as a basis for lake pigments, sometimes competing with the pigments which we have discussed. Amongst the limestones and carbonates of lime there was one which was preferred as a white

TABLE XXIV

White pigments

	Prepared from	Egyptian	Sumerian	Accadian	Greek	Latin
Limestone, chalk	calcium carbonate	inr ḥḏ (I.97.12)	—	[a]kak-ku-us	creta	creta paraetonium
Lime	calcium oxide	—	[a]ZALÁG (BIR)	namru, namrûtu	titanos	calx
Gypsum	calcium sulphate	ḳd (V.82.8)	IM.PAR	gassu	gypsos	gypsum
Ceruse, white lead	bas. lead acetate	dḥtj hḏ (?)	[a]ZA-TU, [a]NINI	ni-ir, ḫulâlu	psimithium anulare	cerussa
Terra Melia	"white haematite, ochre"	—	[a]KA-PAR	?	ge melia	melinum

pigment. This was a limestone called "paraetonium", which PLINY (57) describes thus:

"*Paraetonium* is called from the place of the same name in Egypt. The discovery in it of tiny shells gives rise to the opinion that it is compacted of sea foam and slime. It is prepared also in the island of Crete and at Cyrenae. At Rome it is sophisticated by boiling it down to a thick paste with Cimolian earth. The best kind costs fifty denarii for six pounds. It is the most unctuous of all white pigments, and, by reason of its impalpable fineness, the one which adheres most firmly to a plaster surface."

Then there were several natural earths of the China clay type, the most famous of which were Melian earth (58), Eretrian earth (59) and Samian earth (60). Melian earth is described in detail by PLINY:

"Melinum, the best variety of which comes from the island of Melos, is another white earth. It occurs in Samos also but painters find the latter kind too unctuous to be useful. It has to be mined there by men lying at full length, picking out the vein of earth from among the rocks.... It costs one sesterce a pound."

The other two are characterised by DIOSCORIDES in this way:

"Eretrian earth (eretrias) is exceedingly white in some cases and some is of ashy colour, but the best is that which resembles ashes in colour and is very soft and being drawn along brass-works yield out a violet-like lineament.

But of the Samian earth (samia) that is preferred which is very white and which is light and in touching the tongue holds fast like glue and with all full of juice and soft, and brittle such as that which some call Collyrium."

White lead or sugar of lead was a very important synthetic white the manufacture of which is described in detail by PLINY and several other authors (61). This artificial basic carbonate of lead was identified on a Fayum portrait and used widely in classical times. PLINY gives a good description of its manufacture:

"Psimithium also, that is cerusa or lead acetate (sugar of lead) is produced at lead works. The most highly spoken of is in Rhodes. It is made from very fine shavings of lead placed over a vessel of very sour vinegar and so made to drip down. What falls from the lead into the actual vinegar is dried and then ground and sifted, and then again mixed with vinegar and divided into tablets and dried in the sun in summertime.

There is also another way of making it, by putting the lead into jars of vinegar kept sealed up for ten days and then scraping off the sort of decayed metal on it and putting it back in the vinegar, till the whole of it is used. The stuff scraped off is ground up and sifted and heated in shallow vessels and stirred with small rods till it turns red and becomes like sandarache (realgar). Then it is washed with fresh water till all the cloudy impurities have been removed. Afterwards it is dried in a similar way and divided into tablets. Its properties are the same as those of the substances mentioned above, only it is the mildest of all of them and besides, that it is useful for giving women a fair complexion; but like scum of silver, it is deadly poison. The lead acetate itself if afterwards melted becomes red."

"A third white pigment is *ceruse*, the manufacture of which is described in the section on the ores of lead. Originally it was found as a natural earth on the land of Theodotus at Smyrna and was used by the early masters in painting ships. At present, all ceruse is made from lead and vinegar, in the way already described."

The natural cerusa mentioned by PLINY is of course not sugar of lead but lead carbonate (cerussite). White lead was produced in Rhodes, Corinth and Lacedaemonia and later at Puteoli too. It was not only an important pigment but it was an important cosmetic powder too (62), found in covered bowls called pyxis in women's graves of Greece since the fifth century B.C.

INKS

The inks used in Antiquity consisted of a black pigment suspended in a solution of gum or glue and they were generally of the Chinese ink type using soot as a pigment.

Though in Mesopotamia most of the perishable writing materials have disappeared we know that in Egypt bone, clay, ivory, leather, linen, metal, papyrus, parchement, vellum, pottery, reed, stone, wax and wood were used to write upon. The pens were made from rushes (Juncus maritimus). From Graeco-Roman times onwards reed (Phragmites comm.) pens were used. The grinders were small rectangular pieces of stone with a slight depression in the middle and a raised edge all around. Small pestles or stone spatulas are used to ground the pigment mixed with gum-water and this is then dried into cakes.

The scribes and painters and even noblemen had beautiful palettes made of ivory, wood, alabaster, sandstone, schist or serpentine. Still scribes usually stuck to a wooden palette with a sliding lid, oval or circular hollows for the cakes of ink and grooves for pens. Their pens were originally frayed out into a kind of brush but in Hellenistic days they were cut like quill pens. Though they disposed of many pigments, papyrus scrolls demanded black ink only, red being frequently used for initials or titles. The scribe, often depicted with his brushes behind his ear, dipped them into a water-pot and then rubbed them on the cake of ink like a modern water-colour artist (63).

Sometimes a sponge is attached to the low table on which the papyrus is spread out. In a few cases wooden tablets covered with stucco were found (Lahun, XIIth dynasty) prepared for writing. Vellum and parchement may have been used from 1500 B.C. onwards.

The common black ink was prepared from carbon black and gum-water. Various kinds of carbon-black are mentioned in medical papyri. It was certainly invented in Egypt but may be independently outside Egypt too. Iron-gall ink comes very late, so does an ink prepared from green vitriol and oak-bark (400 B.C.). Marking inks used on linen, etc. are usually iron-oxide inks, in one case an organic dye, may be bistre was used (64).

In classical times a mixture of one part of gum and three parts of carbon black was used (65). Apart from this "Chinese ink" a mixture of two parts of soot, twelve parts of gum, one part of glue and one part of "chalkantos" was used, but as here the copper and iron compounds do not form a pigment with the rest of the components this was still a Chinese ink. Red dye solutions were also in use and Plutarch mentions a "chrysographia" or a suspension of gold powder for use in manuscripts.

Modern black inks are essentially extracts of galls or other sources of tannin, a salt of iron (usually ferrous sulphate or green vitriol) and a gummy substance to keep the insoluble tinctorial matter of the ink in suspension. The blue-black ferrosoferric gallate formed by oxidation in the air is precipated onto the fibres of the paper and by further oxidation of the ink is so mordanted into the fibre.

The ancients had some inkling of this process. Theophrastus (66) mentions that kekides (oak-galls) were used as mordants for woollens. Philo of Byzantium talks of a type of secret writing with the help of extract of oak-galls which becomes legible by sprinkling the paper with a solution of chalkanthos. The reaction of this chalkantos or iron vitriol was used in Roman times to blacken shoes. Hence we find both "sory" (decomposed copper sulphate) (67) and "chalcanthos" or "atramentum sutorium", green vitriol or ferrous sulphate prepared by dissolving pyrites and inspissating the green solution (68) used as shoemaker's black. This is what PLINY has to say on chalcanthos:

"The Greeks indicated the relationship of copper to shoemaker's black, also, by their name for the latter substance which they call chalcanthos (flower of copper). This substance is so strange as to be unique. It occurs in Spain in wells or pools the water of which holds it in solution. This solution is mixed with an equal volume of fresh water, concentrated by heat and poured into wooden tanks. From beams fixed permanently over these tanks hang ropes kept taut by

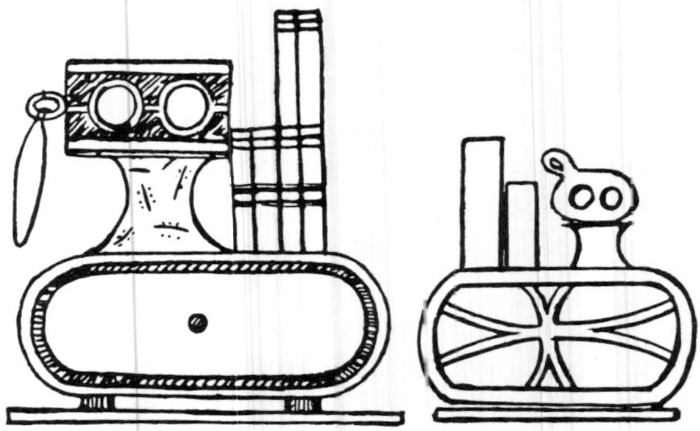

Fig. 41. Inkstands of the Egyptian scribes. (After LEPSIUS)

stones, and on these the slime deposits in glassy berries not unlike grapes. This material is taken out and dried for thirty days. It is blue with a very notable brilliance and may be mistaken for glass. A solution of it is used as a dye for staining leather black.

It can be made in several other ways. For example, if pits are sunk into the right kind of soil, stalacites form in the drippings from the sides during the frost of winter, and this kind, called stalagmias, is the purest known, but one variety of it whose violet colour is decidedly lighter in shade is called lonchoton (lanceshaped). Again it forms in holes in the rocks where the material which has been accumulated thereby the rain-water freezes. It is made also, after the fashion of salt, by using fresh water as a solvent and evaporating the solution by the burning heat of the sun. So a double distinction is sometimes made between the natural and the artificial substance, the latter being paler, and as inferior to the former in quality as it is in colour."

which should be read in conjunction with another passage of PLINY's (69):

"*Atramentum* (shoemaker's black), too must be considered an artificial pigment, although the earth also provides it, and in two different ways. For in some places it oozes from the ground like brine, in others the earth itself is sulphur-coloured and proves suitable for the purpose.

Painters have been found who are prepared to dig up charred material from the tombs in which it was interred. All such methods are indecent and new-fangled for atramentum is already prepared from soot in various ways, but burning turpentine, resin or pitch, and special buildings, without exit for the smoke, are constructed for the purpose. The finest kind of atramentum is thus made from the wood of the pitch-pine. It is sophisticated with the soot from furnaces and bath-houses, wihch is used as ink for writing books."

The modern type of gall-iron ink is mentioned for the first time by ISODORE of Seville in the seventh century. A.D. and Lucas found that it was used in vellum manuscript of the seventh to twelfth centuries in Egypt. Hence in general Antiquity has used inks of the Chinese ink type only except in very special cases when inks of the gallate type were applied or the basic reaction of these inks used to convey secret messages.

PAINTS, MEDIA, VARNISHES, GROUNDS AND PAINTING

Painting which plays such a large part in the life of the ancients certainly began with the decoration of pottery (and the body) as we can prove from the analysis of the words used in this trade (70). The colours, the scala of which was taken from nature (71), had religious and magical meaning, the symbolism of which we will not discuss here. Nevertheless we must always be aware of the fact that the colours had an highly important meaning for the ancients and that painting in the proper colour, dyeing and staining were not simply technical operations but carried something of the creative act in them as did all arts and crafts.

Early in this century much time has been devoted to the discussion of the sensitivity to colours of the ancients. It was argued (72) that the colour sense developed but slowly in mankind and that even the Greeks and Romans were incapable of distinguishing between blues and violets seeing them as a dull hue only, whereas their sensitivity to red, orange and yellow colours was already fully developed. It is true that the Pythagoreans like the earliest Greek painters used but four primary colours; white, black, red and yellow but there is no doubt that as they acquired more dyes and pigments the new colours were properly distinguished and used specifically with great taste (73). We have already noticed that good blue and green pigments were fairly scarce (74) and this may be one of the reasons why they were not reckoned amongst the primary colours. It is true that in classical literature many objects which do not, as we should think, vary much in colour in their different manifestations receive many different colour epithets but then many of these epithets have meanings which are not visual at all. What seems to have arrested their eye is not so much the qualitative as the quantitative difference between colours. The Greeks seem to have felt little interest in the qualitative differences of decomposed and partially absorbed light (75).

The less refracted reds and oranges or yellows were called "warm" colours in contrast to the "cold" blues and violets. The Greeks show little discrimination among the various shadings and gradations of brown, purple, grey, black and white and have but few terms in the green and blue range. In Hellenistic times a few colours were added by the acquisition of artificially produced or newly found natural pigments, except in respect to green and blue. In Roman times a few more terms were added but not in blue and green (76). It would be dangerous to conclude that they had an underdeveloped colour sense from this evidence only. Neither of these ancient peoples can compare in abundance of colour terms with us, but this is to be expected since we find it possible to create artificially not only all colours that already exist but many more new ones every year.

When PLATO defined colour (77), he called it "an effluence of form commensurate with sight and palpable to sense" (*Meno*, 76 d) using terms which belong both to physics and to the stage where colour was so important. Since NEWTON's *Opticks* and his experiments on the spectral colours we have gone far into the relationship between colours. We now define colour as "that aspect of the appearance of objects and lights which depends upon the spectral composition of the radiant energy reaching the retina of the eye and upon its temporal and spatial distribution thereon" (78). We can define them by three independent attributes indicated by the terms: hue, lightness and saturation, or we can measure them more scientifically by tristimulus colorimetry. Still even now our practical terminology of colours is often still confused and vague and we need not wonder that this was the case in Antiquity with its limited scale of pigments, the more so as these terms are often poetical rather than scientific efforts.

Another recurrent story is that of the "good old pigments" the secret of which is now lost (79). We forget that the vivid paintings we still admire are tomb or cave paintings which never saw daylight for 6000 years or more and hence they stand a very good chance that their colours are still fresh though even this is just a fancy story in many cases. In many cases and notably on the exterior of monuments the frescoes and paint on walls and pillars have vanished with the supporting lime plaster, their medium (glue) has suffered oxidation and darkening or humidity has detached them. Indigo and cinnabar were fairly strong colours but not everlasting, verdigris and orpiment are dangerous pigments if mixed with others. Malachite and Egyptian blue have long been abandoned by oil painters. Ultramarine is now artificially produced in a more concentrated and more stable form and so are the dyestuffs of madder, Tyrian purple and kermes. Only the good pigments like ochres and certain earths have staid. Even with our better quality ingredients no paintings could be garantueed to last indefinitely for pigments, media, varnishes and grounds are all susceptible to gradual corrosion by air and humidity aided by the active radiation of sunlight.

We have hardly any information of the painter's craft from Mesopotamia. In Egypt most of the craftsmen seem to have done their own painting for centuries. We find the sculptor painting or gilding his statues and the carpenter or leatherworker attending to this part of his work. Yet we have traces of individual painters and even of easel-painting and its products (80) as far back as 2600 B.C. We know that they made decorated screens and by 1500 B.C. painters emerged as fully independent craftsmen. Names of individual artists like Nebre, Heje, Mery-re and Juti crop up and the possessors of graves are depicted making the plans and designs for their own graves. Reliefs also show the painting of pillars, woodwork and other objects but we never find any picture of the painting of reliefs or tomb walls, probably on account of religious taboos. Sketches have also been found and a picture of an artist's workshop dates of the Amarna period.

We now have ample evidence to prove that their palette increased considerably during Egyptian history. Early wall paintings at Hierakonpolis show the use of yellow, red, green, white and black. In Meydum and other Old Kingdom mastabas this palette is completed with brown (mixing haematite and soot), grey (mixing gypsum and soot) and two blues (chessylite and blue frit). During the Twelfth Dynasty new green, red and black colours are introduced but only one blue (Egyptian blue) is now used. From the Eighteenth Dynasty onwards yellow orpiment is introduced as well as more ochres and frits. A pink gypsum stained with madder is an acquisition of Roman Egypt.

The painting grounds of the ancients were pottery, plaster, stone, wood, canvas, papyrus, ivory and semi-precious stones or metals. As the style and method of painting is closely related to the support on

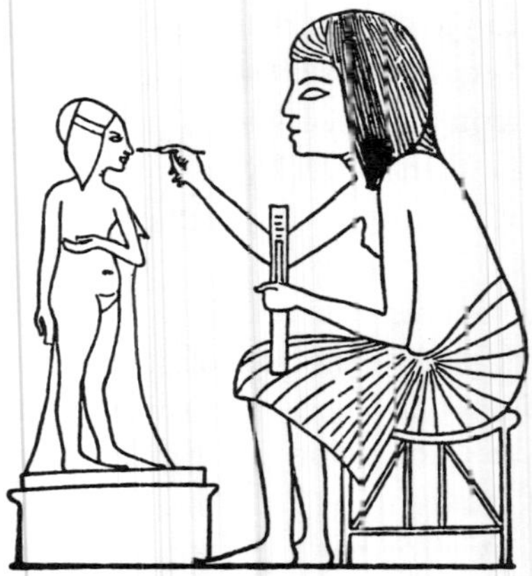

Fig. 42. The Egyptian chief sculptor Auta painting a statue

which they painted (apart from the painting materials and their own aims) we must need discuss them first. From prehistoric times onwards pottery was decorated. In Egypt a white slip was applied or red ochre, blue frit, black iron oxide or carbon paints were used. In Mesopotamia black, white or red lines were used to fill incised lines or glazes were made using bone ash, black manganese oxide, blue and green copper oxides or yellow lead antimoniate as pigments.

Plastering walls started very early in the history of architecture. Materials such as clay, lime, gypsum or pozzolano were mixed with water and left to set on the wall by drying, carbonation or evaporation. Sometimes inert material like sand, crushed bricks and stone or binders like hair, straw and jute are added.

In Egypt clay plaster occurs since Predynastic times but it went out of fashion for more important buildings except for the brief Amarna period. It consisted of the ordinary Nile alluvium mixed with straw. Better quality plaster was obtained by adding a finishing coat of somewhat finer clay. The clay best suited for this purpose is the natural mixture of clay and limestone found in hollows and pockets at the foot of the hills and still called "hib" by the Egyptians. In Mesopotamia clay plaster with chopped reeds or straw was also very common. This ground was not very suitable for painting.

Mural paintings were usually drawn on gypsum plaster. In Egypt this was applied since pre-dynastic times (Maadi) and prepared by burning crude gypsum at 130° C, powdering and slaking the burnt product. The very pure gypsum employed in the tombs of Gizeh and Saqqarah was taken from quarries in the Fayum. In the early period great care was taken to select good quality gypsum and often a second layer of gypsum and powdered limestone (upto 85%) was applied to obtain a smooth painting ground.

In Mesopotamia gypsum plaster was also applied but it was more usual to prepare a lime mortar. The knowledge of burning lime was very old in that country but not in Egypt where it was introduced only in Graeco-Roman times. At Chafadje a lime-kiln was discovered which dated back to at least 2500 B.C. The white lime mortar was sometimes mixed with ashes and applied in layers about 4 mm thick. In later period there was a tendency to add coarse powdered brick to the lime mortar.

The same coarsening of the quality of plaster is observed in Egypt. When applied on brick walls it first was a thin coat of about 1/16" to 1/10". It became more and more coarse until in Ptolemaic times it was a mere daub of plaster. The finishing coat was a priming coat to which glue had been added and hence we can call it gesso, a word derived from gypsum but denoting any aqueous white priming coat.

When painting on stone such a gypsum or lime plaster was first applied in many cases. But often this layer of whitewash is missing and both in Egypt and Mesopotamia we find traces of paint directly applied to the stone surface of statues (red, yellow, blue and black pigments!). In Mesopotamia where brick architecture is more prominent brick walls are sometimes painted directly (white, black, blue and orange) and in a few cases even silvered or gilded. It was, however, more common to paint on stuccoed brick walls.

Painting on wood directly was avoided in ancient Egypt. Even the wooden panels of the easel painters were primed with a layer of gypsum or whiting as were coffins, boxes and stelae, unless a single colour was used.

Too little remains of the Assyrian mural paintings to inform us on the medium used there. But the Egyptian woman Aholah saw "men portrayed upon the wall, the images of the Chaldeans portrayed with vermilion" (82).

Neither in Mesopotamia nor in Egypt were oil paints known. Linseed oil as well as other drying oils were probably known at an early date but they were used for medicinal, culinary or cosmetic purposes only. Again such thinners as oil of turpentine were not known until the days of early Greece but even then they were not employed in painting. All Egyptian paintings were executed in tempera colours that is some adhesive was used in their production, such as size (gelatine, glue), gum or albumen (white of egg). This conclusion from analyses agrees with PLINY's statements on Egyptian painting.

Casein prepared from curd or milk forms a strong glue used for centuries in woodwork in Egypt. Hebrew texts also speak of the use of curd for house painting and decoration. Gum arabic (83) was imported in Egypt from Punt and southern Arabia, it was also known in Mesopotamia. Starch prepared from grain was used in Egypt, gelatine, tragacanth from various species of Astralagus and the gum from species of Accacia were available. Shellac, the resin prepared in India from the Tacchardia lacca insect living mostly on Butea frondosa Rexb., is not mentioned before 250 A.D. (Aelian). Nor does it seem plausible that Chios mastix was available, a resin produced from Pistacia Lentuscus since the days of DIOSCORIDES. We know however, that white of egg was probably used in a few instances. Though fowl play no part in the earlier history of Egypt geese and ducks of many varieties were used and kept. We also know that sometimes honey was added to such water-soluble media as gum arabic or size, as it retained some water and thus prevented the gum from becoming too brittle.

We have many mortars, pestles and palettes to show us that paints were ready-mixed before use (84). The pigments were made into cakes or kept in small bags. The crude mineral colours were finely ground with a stone grinder upon a small slab of stone or slate. This done, they were mixed with some kind of gum medium to make them adhere, and with water to make them flow easily. The cakes found on palettes are often made by drying the mixture of pigments and gum-water. An eighteenth dynasty palette contained no less than 3 yellows, 3 browns, 2 reds, 2 blues, 2 greens, and one cake each of white and black. A case in the Cairo Museum exhibits the various articles required for painting. Among them is a block of wood measuring 19.5 × 6.5. × 2.5

cm the top of which is divided into six oval pans some 7 mm deep hollowed out to receive the paints; these pans are all nearly full of solid and partly disintegrated colours (red, dark, yellow, light green, blue, and white). The same case also contains a bunch of different-sized brushes still tied together with the string dipped in red which was used for setting out the design. One of these brushes is short an stumpy, rather like a stencil brush; it is apparently made of grass fibres

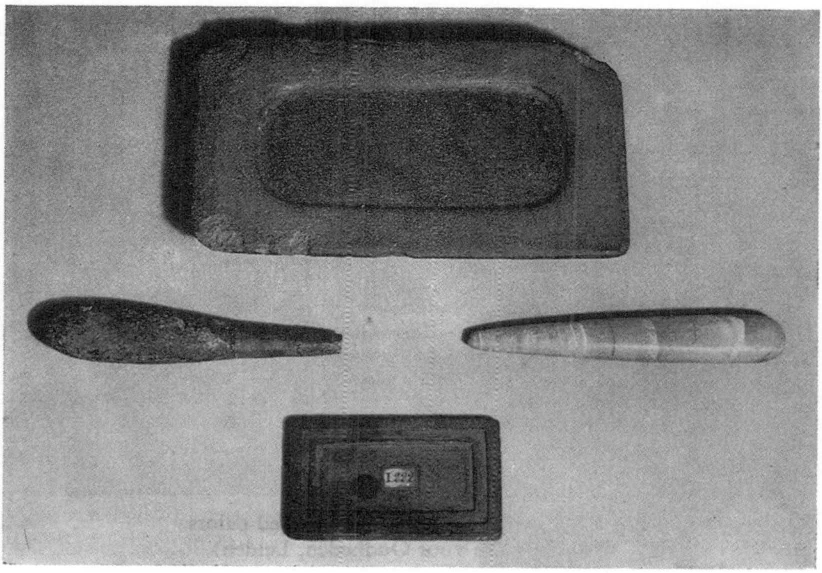

Fig. 43. Egyptian pestles and mortars for grinding pigments. (Rijksmuseum voor Oudheden, Leiden)

doubled over and bound back. The rest are sticks of a fibrous wood about 5.5 cm long, one end of which has been soaked in water, frayed out and cut either round or into the shape of a wedge. On these frayed ends are traces of red, green, yellow, black, and white, each brush being evidently kept for its own particular colour. The traces on the other ends of the brush show that they have been used to stir the paint in its pan. For outlining pens or brushes made from the rush called Juncus maritimus were used, the same pens or brushes as are found attached to the long scribe's palettes so often depicted (85). Animal hairs were used in a few brushes only.

As to the methods by which the ancient Egyptians decorated their walls we can quote with profit the opinion of one who has studied them for many years (86):

"Mural paintings as practised in Ancient Egypt may be defined as distemper or gouache methods of applying powdered colours mixed with gum or size to a surface of dry plaster, or less commonly to one of stone. To speak of Egyptian wall paintings as "frescoes" is a misnomer, since true fresco-painting consists of applying colours mixed

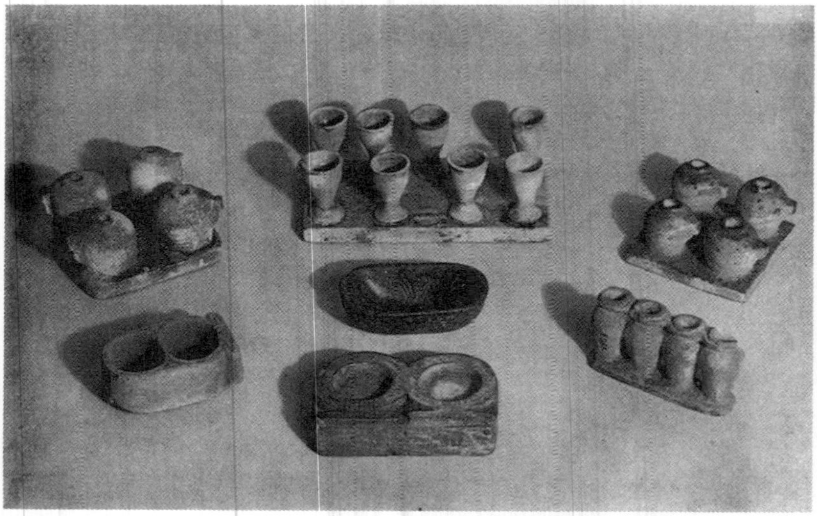

Fig. 44. Egyptian sets for ready-mixed paints.
(Rijksmuseum voor Oudheden, Leiden)

with lime and water to a surface of damp plaster with which they become incorporated; thus only the amount of wall space that could be kept damp during the day's work was coloured at one time, and when fresh plaster was added a join may be seen.

Once the colours have been prepared and mixed with gum, they will last for any length of time and when hardened need only softening with water to become ready for use. One opaque colour can be painted over another when the latter has dried and then completely hides it.

We have no certain trace in Egypt of the use of egg medium such as common amongst the medieval Italian painters. It is evident from Pompeii and elsewhere that first the Greek and Roman artists, and later the Italians inherited their tempera technique from ancient Egypt where it had been perfected already in the Fourth Dynasty (2500 B.C.)"

In these tombs the inequality of the limestone surface was compensated by a layer of mud or clay plaster mixed with straw. On top of it a layer of fine plaster (often buff) was applied, perfectly smooth to receive the painting. Squares of various sizes made by lines snapped across the wall by means of a string dipped in red paint served to sketch the design in roughly. On some places a thin wash of light blue-grey was applied. White masses or places intended to become a bright red or yellow patch were painted dazzling white. Deep pinks were achieved by mixing reds and whites, bright yellows by glazing a thin transparent film of yellow over a brilliant white underlay. Bright vermilion reds were obtained by stippling red over white. The blue powdered frit is applied rather thickly. In general the brushwork is astonishingly fine.

The Egyptian artists were more concerned at obtaining a brilliant colour scheme than with the approximation of their tints to those of nature, though they were excellent imitators of materials. The love of diversity and the desire to keep adjacent objects of like colour distinct from one other predominate. Sometimes a combination of relief and painting was used, modelling on plaster or even relief "en creux".

In many cases these wall paintings were varnished either with wax or with a true varnish.

In the reigns of Amenophis I & II beeswax was used as a fixative or as varnish in tombs. Its application seems to improve the brilliance of red, blue and green pigments (87). As suitable solvents were still unknown it must have been applied hot. Sometimes the varnish is applied to the whole surface sometimes to some specific colour only. In the later case we have no reason to suspect that it was intimately mixed with the pigment and that we have here the first experiments in "encaustic painting" so dear to the Egyptians of the Roman era. The earlier experiments with beeswax were soon discontinued.

The composition of the varnish applied to other Egyptian mural paintings is still a mystery. Like the varnish on wooden objects it is now often brown, red or yellow, but originally it must have been colourless. A varnish made of accacia gum was applied after 1000 B.C. only. The earlier varnishes must have been natural semi-liquid oleo-resins applied hot with a brush as solvents for resins were unknown then. The gum arabic from the Red Sea coasts was sufficient for varnishing wood and making "papier maché" (gummed layers of linen) for mummy cases. The gum produced from Accacia Nilotica (88) was used in making sheets of papyrus. But neither had the qualities needed for the paint-varnish. The unknown varnish has certain qualities in common with shellac. It disappears in Ptolemaic and Roman times as if supplies were cut off by war. Its source may have been Persia from which country the inhabitants of Mesopotamia also imported a varnish of unknown composition (89), though its name seems related to the gum produced from the Accacia Nilotica in Egypt and exported in large quantities.

The Egyptians used a naturally black varnish from about 1500 B.C. onwards which forms a black lustrous surface lacquer. It may be related to or identical with the black dammar resin produced from Canarium strictum in western and southern India. However, the whole subject of the Egyptian varnishes is still unsettled.

From direct information on potsherds these paintings were made with the light of small oil lamps. The modern use oil large mirrors or sheets of paper would have failed the ancients who had only small hand mirrors. The artists and craftsmen of Pharaonic times belonged to a large fraternity which must have comprised many grades. It is likely that different artists outlined the picture and carried it to a finish. We have, however, no precise information on such division of labour.

Many tombs were subjected to the action of fire and smoke in the course of their history but in general this added but a film-like coating which can often be removed. The red and yellow pigments have proved most durable, blue being the next best, but the greens and blacks were most prone to disappear or to suffer change. In some cases the yellow ochres were burnt to red, blue became dark green and the greens darkened. In general it may be said that all the colours of a painting are seldom preserved with their original values.

In Egypt canvas or cloth paintings were found dating back to about 1500 B.C. In Graeco-Roman times painting on linen shrouds and portrait painting on linen or wood had become quite common. Both in Egypt and in Mesopotamia leather was dyed white, green, yellow, black and red since Predynastic times but we have no details on the methods used. Nor do we know how ivory was coloured but some of our museum pieces show traces of blue and red paints or dyes.

We should mention the artificial staining of metals practised in ancient times for coloured metals were highly valued in art work. The variety of colours of the native alloys was increased both by preparing artificial alloys or by painting metal surface. Thus the Egyptians coloured gold surfaces pink by dipping the gold in a solution of iron salts and then heating it. This art and that of staining semi-precious stones both contributed to the rise of chemistry.

Mesopotamia seems the country where the art of colouring semi-precious stones (90) was discovered. Not only were small blackened shells discovered at Niniveh which may represent PLINY's "cochlides of Arabia" (91) but texts inform us of artificially stained stones (92). A seal stone is dyed with iron vitriol. Other examples remind us of Pliny's artificially stained Indian beryls (93).

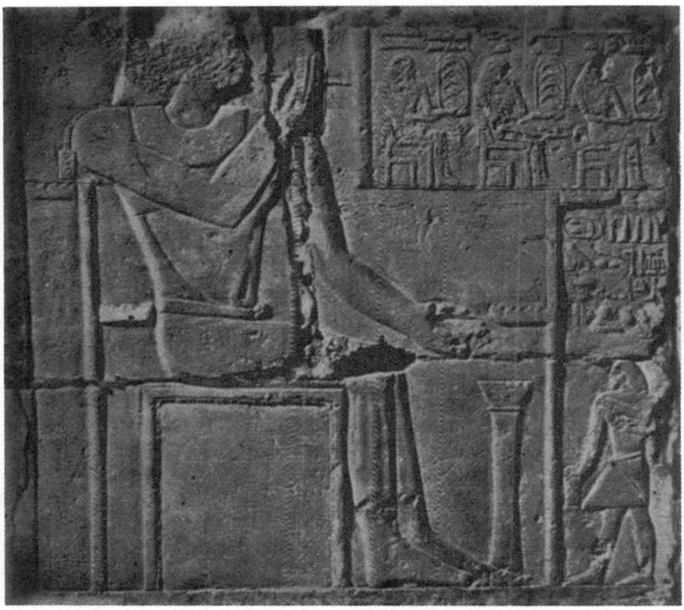

Fig. 45. Egyptian artist in front of his easel

The Egyptians never practised fresco painting, that is they never painted on a wet surface made caustic with lime. Nor did the inhabitants of ancient Mesopotamia know this art as far as we can conclude from the few fragments of mural paintings in that country. More will certainly be revealed on this problem when the recently discovered mural decorations of Mari, Chorsabad, Tell Aḫmar, and Dura Europos have been examined and analysed by experts (93a). The home-country of the real "buon fresco" paintings was ancient Crete, where mural paintings were executed on wet pure lime plaster since 2500 B.C. In later periods this lime plaster coat became thinner and overlay a thicker gypsum backing. Red, white, black, yellow, deep red, orange, green and blue (frit imported from Egypt) colours were here applied directly to wet lime coatings the contours having been incised.

During the second millenium B.C. paintings were laid on two layers of plaster, the top one of which was finer and often coloured by a slight addition of red. Gradually the burning of lime became more common. The total thickness of the ground is generally 6—8 cms (94). HEATON's conclusion that some of the Aegean wall paintings were done in true "buon fresco" after the manner of the Italian painters, was challenged by later researches by DUELL and GETTENS. They concluded that the lack of proper evidence for true fresco techniques rather points to some sort of tempera as common in the Ancient Near East and Egypt.

The Cretan-Mycenean group of wall-paintings are certainly primarily fresco paintings, but apart from the true fresco techniques other techniques have been applied. Thus "fresco secco", e.g. mixing the colours with lime water has certainly been applied as a supplementary device, and in certain cases we suspect the use of techniques of putting on colours with lime or gypsum in a lime-gypsum technique or even the use of a lime and milk process. As to the latter medium we should be very wary for Laurie has correctly pointed out that the presence of organic material in the remains of ancient frescos may be quite accidental and does not definitely point to an original organic binding medium.

Greek and Roman painting methods have been the subject of many publications and even experiments (95), several of the outstanding problems, however, remain unsolved. Painting as a fine art existed no doubt, the words "pictor" and "pingo" are always used in this sense. The painter may have been a subject of wisecracks by the comic poets, his trade is mentioned very often (96) and we have a fair knowledge of the tools of his trade (97). We know that the Greek painters preferred boxwood to paint on (98). Unfortunately no original Greek easel paintings have survived, but the usual process employed seems to have been tempera. The details of these methods may have differed from those of the medieval painters, but they certainly never used oil as a medium but were limited to the use of size (mainly of animal origin) (99), gum arabic or glue (100), white of egg, milk or the like (101) some of which may have acted as a kind of varnish when used on the plaster background of a wall. There is no doubt that white of egg and glue were the favourite binding media, the pigments being often mixed with powdered pumice stone to disperse them properly. Some of the Roman wall paintings have a shining coat above the coloured layers which contains no lime and which was not applied by any fresco method and hence was equivalent to the modern varnish. Often this was wax applied according to PLINY's "ganosis"-method. The easel paintings, however, seem to have been painted in pure tempera for we have several allusions to the fact that these colours faded (102) and also that they could be wiped off with a sponge (103) in the same way as PLATO used a sponge to erase the name of a disciple from a slate.

We possess much more information on mural paintings. The external decoration of houses seems to have been rarely practised but it certainly occurs in Pompeii and Rome. It was as intelligible to the public of Plautus as was easel painting. Actual traces of red, blue, black, green and white pigments on archaic Attic gravestones show us that this practice was no Roman innovation (104). The ancients used fresco, tempera and encaustic techniques, but the latter was unsuitable for wall-paintings as PLINY already explained. Hence wall-paintings were executed on wet lime or on dry ground (105) according to VITRUVIUS and PAUSANIAS suggests (106) that Polygnotus was the first Greek painter to take up fresco painting again after Mycenean times.

Two methods of fresco painting were used in classical times: the true fresco technique of painting on wet lime plaster and the "fresco secco" technique of applying colours mixed with lime water on dry plaster. In both cases the ground had to be carefully prepared and the ancients were quite aware of this (107). In classical times lime plaster was favoured. We have considerable information on the ground of ancient wall paintings from Italian excavations. CATO lays down the rules for burning lime and bares witness to its usefullness in building (108). It was occasionally used in pure form to conceal the joints but not as a mortar unless mixed with sand and the like. With water it is used as a whitewash or coating of tiles in preparation for "opus signium" masonry; combined with oil it is a valuable sealing material for the joints between earthenware water pipes. Greece passed on the knowledge to Italy that sand mixed with lime makes a stronger mortar than pure lime. Still there a mortar was only used for water conduits (as early as the seventh century water tunnel at Olympia and in the fountain of Glauce at Corinth which in all probability was built not so very much later). In any case, the Latin word calx, meaning small stone is manifestly derived from the Greek chalix, small stone, pebble. The Romans however also came to apply it to lime, a usage which apparently did not obtain in Greece proper. The inference is strong that they learned the word and the process of making lime at one and the same time (the third cy. B.C.?) (109).

Plastering of some sort goes back to times immemorial. But it is impossible to tell when a plaster of lime and either sand or pozzolana or a stucco of lime and marble dust followed the earlier simple white-wash. The former would be employed primarily to protect the outer surface; the latter, though affording some protection, would serve to conceal an inferior material. Both are so perishable and often renewed and their origin hard to trace in old buildings. The Romans based their earlier temples on Etruscan models rather than on Greek ones.

Tomb paintings in Egypt and Minoan wall paintings prove the art of plastering was well known. The Etruscans brought to their tombs their own technique, painting either directly on the stone or on a very thin coat of sand and lime. The Oscans of the V & IVth centuries B.C., on the other hand, before applying their frescoes covered the walls of their tombs with plaster, sometimes as thick as 4 cm. The Hellenistic paintings at Pompeii conceal a plaster sometimes 7—8 cm thick, made up of several layers.

The oldest stucco in Rome is believed to go back to the fourth century B.C. LIVY refers to a stuccoing of the Temple of Jupiter Capitolinus in 179 B.C. (110) and stucco on the facade of the Tomb of the Scipios goes back to last decade of the second century B.C. We may therefore assume that by the middle of the fourth century B.C. stucco was used to conceal the ugly building materials which were all that were readily available to the Roman builders. The preparation of the plaster itself calls forth from Vitruvius few directions which are not implicit in the process of making mortar of any kind (111). He who followed VITRUVIUS (112) must use a rendering coat, three layers of harenato (sand mortar) and three layers of marmorato (creta aut marmor) before his walls were ready for decoration. As soon as the last coat was on, while it was still damp, colour could be applied. The surface was then polished with a tool known as a liaculum (113). Sufficient samples of the seven layers have come to light in Rome to convince us that the instructions of Vitruvius were generally followed except in the humbler rooms. The Roman builders of the Augustean period were likely to content themselves with 2 or 3 coats, the rough-cast and the stucco, with possibly an intermediate layer of sand and lime, before applying the painting. Special preparation must be made before plastering walls in damp places, a special roughcast made with powdered terracotta instead of sand being favoured to protect the plaster (114). Before painting the plaster had been treated by beating, rubbing with planes and polishing and modern experiments have shown that this will yield a perfectly smooth surface. Thin coats of plaster were also applied to statues when they had to be painted.

However such elaborate grounds were not used in earlier times, and even the Etruscans, like the cave painters of prehistoric France, Spain, sometimes painted on the bare rock of their tombs, without even smoothing the surface. In such cases it is extremely difficult to detect any binding medium like animal fat, plant saps, balsams, milk or blood, the last traces of which have long disappeared. As the rock

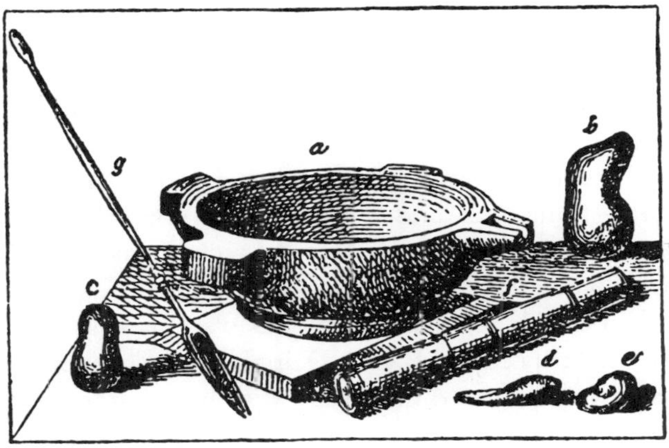

Fig. 46. Materials of a Roman artist.
a. Alabaster mortar; b. & c. Pestles; d. & e. Lumps of pigments; f. Basalt plaque; g. Bronze cauterium of wax-painter

is often composed of limestone it has been suggested that true fresco painting in its most primitive stage goes back to prehistoric cave paintings.

Applying pigments mixed with water to fresh lime plaster has been called "*al fresco*" painting since the fourteenth century but classical authors like PLINY speak of "illinere udo". The surviving later PLINY manuscripts have caused much confusion by speaking of "*nudo*" (bare) instead of "*udo*" (damp). The thick Roman ground must have held moisture for a considerable time and it could be kept damp by sprinkling water or covering it up with wet cloths. In Egypt this plaster (made of gypsum in that country) would have dried much too quickly, and hence the ancient Egyptians had to apply tempera painting. In fresco painting only such pigments can be used as are compatible with lime, as are most earth colours, for the plaster has to fix the pigments after drying. This the classical authors evidently knew (115).

VITRUVIUS' description:

"For colours when carefully laid on *damp* (udo) plaster do not get loose, but are for ever permanent. For his reason that the lime, losing all its moisture in the kiln, is so dry and porous that it readily imbibes whatever chances to touch it and soldification taking place from the mixtures of the various potentialities whose elements or first principles are brought together, the resulting substance, of whatever it is composed, when it becomes dry, is such that it seems to have special qualities peculiar to itself", records the action of carbonic acid on the lime most completely for one who knew nothing about the chemical background.

Such incompatible colours could be applied only on some type of underpainting as was discovered at Pompeii and which describes PLINY when he discusses the ways of obtaining different shades of red and purple (116). Pompeiian and indeed many other classical paintings therefore combine fresco and tempera techniques, but true fresco techniques dominate.

For certain details tempera techniques were used as in the case of remains of the fifth century B.C. at Delphi (the Lesche) but more often these details were executed in colours with lime water applied on dry plaster, e.g. "fresco secco" technique, as in Pompeii. In this case the ground must be very smooth to ensure proper succes.

The Etruscan wall paintings (117) herald this more elaborate technique. They are painted either directly on the bare limestone rock, on a lime mortar, a lime mortar finished with a lime wash or on a series of layers of the stucco type. The pigments used were mostly earth colours obtained locally, and we have reason to believe that in certain instances glue was used as a medium. During the third and last period of Etruscan mural art real fresco painting was applied and new pigments like cinnabar, azurite and malachite are applied over other colours like Pliny's "colores floridi". Here as well as in the classical period one should not assume too readily the use of sophisticated recipes which we now use. LAURIE has rightly pointed out that high skill of the ancient craftsmen could very well overcome difficulties arising from the simplicity of the materials available to him.

During the later Empire a poor stucco with little admixture of marble and more like our sand mortar such as could be found in less prominent places at Pompeii and Rome at earlier periods became quite common. One volume of lime was mixed with 1.5 volume of quartz, powdered bricks and volcanic ash and layers of plaster from 25—30 form the ground of the paintings. The next layer consisted of equal volumes of lime and limestone powder, which layer of 15—25 mm was smoothed with a finish of powdered marble, 1—2 mm thick. But this held only for the most important buildings, in other cases the quality of the stucco becomes much less. Incompatible pigments are applied in paste form and as only patches representing a day's work can be finished properly, the separating lines of such patches can be easily detected.

In the early Christian churches, notable those of the tenth century and later the stucco was no longer built up with so much care. A mixture of 30% of lime and 70% of sand is the general rule (119). There is no addition of new pigments, earth colours and local pigments being used. Organic dyes, lazurite, orpiment, red lead or white lead occur only rarely. Both fresco techniques and tempera using white of egg medium were used. Both ingredients and techniques show a marked resemblance to the prescriptions given by THEOPHILUS Presbyter in his Diversarium Artium Schedula.

The same changes in ingredients and techniques can be observed in other domains of art. Whereas Byzantine illuminated manuscripts use beautiful and very pure qualities of cinnabar, orpiment, ultramarine and crimson lakes obtained from Murex purple, the Scoto-Irish monasteries of the West are shut off from the sources of such costly pigments by the fall of the Roman Empire and use red lead instead of cinnabar and pigment obtained from the local Purpura capillus instead of real Tyrian purple or crimson lakes made from kermes.

The Greeks gave a new form of painting to the world, "encaustic painting", Polygnotus (fifth century B.C.) being mentioned as one of the earliest to have worked in it. The masterpieces of the Hellenistic and Roman periods of Egypt became known by the publication of the excavations of Hawara (120). Our knowledge of the technical process of encaustic painting rests on two passages in PLINY (121) as we have only one other more detailed reference in Roman literature (122). This is what PLINY has to tell:

"The pigments which require a dry cretaceous surface and cannot be applied to fresh plaster, are purpurissum, indigo, caeruleum, melinum, orpiment, Appian green and ceruse. The same pigments may be incorporated in wax for encaustic painting, a process unsuitable for mural decoration but usual for ships of war, and applied now even to merchant vessels. This decoration of ships, the use of which is fraught with so much peril should prevent anyone from feeling surprise at the painting of funeral pyres. It is even our pleasure that gladiators should be borne in state, to slay or to be slain."

"In early days there were two kinds of encaustic painting, with wax and on ivory with a graver or cestrum but later the custom came in of decorated battleships. This added a third method, that of employing a brush, when the wax had been melted by fire. This process of painting ships is not spoilt by the action of the sun nor salt water or winds."

It is believed that the wax process arose in Egypt, where handling the medium was easier than in Greece. The first Greek artist to specialize in this art was Pausias (123). The colours were blended in powder form with wax and kept fused by the heat of the sun or on a hot plate. The panel of wood on which these colours were applied recieved a) a priming of distemper, b) a grounding varying in tint with the object to be portrayed and on top of these the wax-colours were applied. It seems that three methods were employed: 1) painting on wooden panels with the aid of a brush and using a bronze spatula called cauterium for spreading the wax; 2) painting on wood, linen and marble with a brush and 3) painting on ivory and marble after having incised the design with a pointed cestrum or burin and then laying on the colours mixed with wax.

In the Fayum pictures we find that backgrounds and garments were often executed with a brush dipped in the fluid wax colours, and that facial details were executed by means of the cauterium, which "modeled" the colours from the sticks of coloured wax on the panel in low relief. In certain cases we suspect that the panel or wall were heated before applying the colours. The result is very much like a true oil painting and by the time of Apelles a very adequate palette had been acquired with which paintings could be made which surpassed frescoes and tempera paintings in depth and richness of colour. Wax was of course well-known in Antiquity (124) and apart from encaustic painting we have discussed its use as a varnish, by a process called "ganosis" by Pliny.

This was not true oil painting which makes use of the drying properties of certain oils. Such oils were of course known in Antiquity, e.g. linseed oil and poppy oil (125) but not before the sixth century A.D. is the drying property of these oils described. Hence oil painting was unknown to the ancients.

Bibliography and notes

(For additional information see the author's Bibliographia Antiqua (Leiden, 1950), Suppl. I (1952), Suppl. II (1963) and the I.I.C. Abstracts (London))

(1) Wunderlich, E., *Die Bedeutung der roten Farbe im Kultus der Griechen und Römer* (Leipzig 1925)
Kühn, H., *Färben und Farbe in der Malerei* (*CIBA Rundschau* 1963/1, 2—36)
Wehlte, K., *Ein Beitrag zur Werkstoffgeschichte* (*Maltechnik* 62, 1956, 45—51)

(2) Pliny, *Nat. Hist.* XXXV.15
The Elder Pliny's *Chapters on the History of Art* (edit. Blake and Sellers, London 1896)

(3) Gehant, John C., *Tracing our Industry through the centuries* (*Paint, Oil Chem. Review*, Vol. 102, December 1940, pags. 9—11)

(4) Obermaier, H., *Die Uranfänge der Malerei beim Eiszeitmenschen* (*Forsch. und Fortschr.*, Vol. XVII, 1941, No. 19/20, pags. 216—218)
A Paint mine from the Early Upper Palaeolithic Age near Lovas (*Hungary*) (*Acta Archaeologica Acad. Sci. Hung.* vol. V, 1954, 1/2, pags. 1—32)

(5) The Egyptian terms for pigments (drwj, V.601.5; wtrj, I.381.5) point to the use of granular substances
The Sumerian terms for pigments are often compounds of "IM, ṭiṭṭu", clay

(6) Windels, F., *The Lascaux Cave Paintings* (Faber, London 1949)
Riddel, W. H., *Altamira* (London 1938)
Bryson, H. Courtney, *The earliest known paints* (*Paint Manufacturing*, 22, 1952, 243—246)
Pietsch, E., *Altamira* (*Abh. Ber. Dtsch. Museum* 31, 1963, Heft 1)

(7) Obermaier, H., *Probleme des paläolithischen Malerei Ostspaniens* (*Quartär*, Vol. I, 1938, pags. 111—119)

(7a) Ur Excav. IV, 58, 67

(8) Pliny, *Nat. Hist.* XXXV. 50

(9) Pliny, *Nat. Hist.* XXXV, 30

(10) Rokuro Uyemura, *Studies on the ancient pigments of Japan* (*Eastern Art*, Vol. III, 1931, pags. 47—60)
Yamasaki Kazuo, *Chemical Studies on ancient pigments in Japan* (*J. Chem. Soc. Japan, Pure Chem.* Sect. 711, 1950, 411—412) (*Sci. Papers Japan. Antiques* no. 1, 1951, 27—30; no. 2, 1951, 8—14)
Schafer, E. H., *Orpiment and realgar in Chinese technology and tradition* (*JAOS* 57, 1955, 73—89)

(11) Dioscorides, V.112; Vitruvius, VII.7.2

(12) Pliny, *Nat. Hist.* XXXV, 31—35. See also Theophrastus, *De Lap.*

93 & 94; VITRUVIUS, 7.7.2; ISIDORE, 19.17.3; DIOSCOXIDES, V. 110—112; STRABO,X II.2.10. cap. 540

(13) PLINY, *Nat. Hist.* 33.118; DIOSCORIDES, V.96, PLUTARCH, *Def. Orac.* 47.436; VEG., *Mulom.* 11.16

(14) BING, H., *Zur Farbgeschichte der Sinopia, vom Bolus und vom Poliment* (*Farbe und Lack*, 1925, pags. 471—472, 482, 496—497)

(15) TOCH, M., *The Pigments of the Tomb of Perneb* (*J. Ind. Eng. Chem.*, Vol. X, 1918, 118—119)

DIOSCORIDES, V.144—145

(16) BENEDETTI-PICHLER, A. A., *Microchemical Analysis of Pigments use in the fossae of the incisions of Chinese oracle bones* (*Ind. Chem. Eng. Anal. Ed.*, Vol. IX, 1937, pags. 149—152)

(17) PLINY, *Nat. Hist.* XXXIII, 111—122

(18) BAILEY, K. C., *The Elder Pliny's Chapters on Chemical Subjects* (2 vols. London 1929/1932)

BAILEY, K. C., *The pigments of the ancient Romans as described in the Natural History of Pliny the Elder* (*Chem. & Ind.* 1925, pags. 1135—1137)

RABATÉ, H., *Red pigments of antiquity* (*Peintures, pigments, vernis* 23, 1947, 69)

RABATÉ, H., *Ancient yellow, white and black pigments* (*Peintures, pigments, vernis* 23, 1947, 358—359; 24, 1948, 40—41, 104—105)

PLENDERLEITH, H. J., *History of artists' pigments* (*Science Progress* no. 150, 1950, 246—256)

MARGIVAL, F., *Colors and coatings in antiquity* (*Peintures, pigments, vernis* 26, 1950, 467—474)

(19) VITRUVIUS, 7.8.1—2; 7.9.1—5

(20) STEPHANIDES, M., *Petites contributions a l'histoire des sciences* (*Rev. Etud. Grec.*, Vol. 31, 1918, pags. 197—198)

SCHRAMM, A., *Zur Prüfung der Zinnobers auf seine Verfalschung mit Kalk nach Vitruvius* 8.7.5; (*Philol. Wochenschr.* 1930, pags. 94—96)

LIBERTY, S., *Ricerche sulle alterazione del cinabro* (*Boll. Inst. Centr. Restauro* II, 1951, pags. 59—60)

(21) *A.J.A.*, Vol. 31, 1927, page 30; *Klio*, Vol. 22, 1928, page 375

(22) THEOPHRASTUS, *De Lapid.* 58; DIOSCORIDES, V. 109; FLORUS, 2.33.60; SUETONIUS, *Calig.* 18; PETRONIUS, *Cena* 68

(23) *Jeremiah*, 22.14; Ezek. 23.14

(24) VITRUVIUS, 1.12.1. See also DIOSCORIDES, V.103; AETIUS, 1.2.82

(25) PLINY, *Nat. Hist.* XXXV. 39—40. See also ISIDORE, 19.17, 5—6 & 11

(26) PLINY, *Nat. Hist.* XXXIV. 177

(27) STRABO, XII.3.40, cap. 562; DIOSCORIDES, V. 122, VITRUVIUS, 7.7.5; ARRIAN, *Periplous* 13

(28) VITRUVIUS, 7.7.5; THEOPHRASTUS, *De Lapid.* 89

(29) RÖHRIG, H., *Dreitausend Jahre Ultramarin* (*Naturwiss.* 1935, page 312);

GETTENS, R. J., *Lapis lazuli and ultramarine in ancient times* (*Alumni* 19, 1950, 342—357)

KUMINS, CH. A., *Ultramarine blue* (*Amer. Ink Maker*, 32, 1954, 47—49, 51—55, 113)

(30) "armenium, armenion". DIOSCORIDES, V. 105
(31) This pestle is called "duktu"
(32) LAURIE, A. P., *Pigments, Mediums and Technical Methods of Classical and Medieval Painters* (*J. Chem. Soc.* 1937, pags. 163—169)
JOPE, E. M. and HUSE, G., *Examination of Egyptian blue by X-Ray Powder Photography* (*Nature*, Vol. 146, 1940, page 26)
(33) HODGSON, L., *Egyptian blue frit* (*Papers Soc. Mural Decorators and Painters in Tempera*, Vol. III, 1925/35, pags. 36—38)
(34) PLINY, *Nat. Hist.* XXXIII, 57—58
(35) VITRUVIUS, 7.11.1
(36) DIOSCORIDES, V. 106; THEOPHRASTUS, *De Lapid.* 70, 98—100
(37) VITRUVIUS, 7.11.2
(38) PLINY, *Nat. Hist.* XXXIII. 158—163
(39) VITRUVIUS, 7.7.1; see also DIOSCORIDES, V. 108; THEOPHRASTUS, *De Lapid.* 52; GALEN, 19.736 k
(40) PLINY, *Nat. Hist.* XXXV. 36
(41) VITRUVIUS, 7.7.5; DIOSCORIDES, V.121; ISID., 19.17.2
(42) PLINY, *Nat. Hist.* XXXIV. 178
(43) PLINY, *Nat. Hist.* XXXV. 38
(44) DIOSCORIDES, V. 102; V. 96 (throughout this essay we quote from R.T. GUNTHER's edition of DIOSCORIDES (Oxford, 1934)
(45) PLINY, *Nat. Hist.* XXXIII. 79
(46) BAILEY, K., C. *The pigments of the ancient Romans as described in the Natural History of Pliny the Elder* (*Chem. & Ind.*, 1925, pags. 1135—1137)
FARNSWORTH, M., *Ancient Pigments* (*J. Chem. Educ.* 28, 1951, 72—76)
CALEY, EARLE R., *Ancient Greek Pigments* (*J. Chem. Educ.* 23, 1946, 314—316)
AUGUSTI, S., *Imitazioni e falsificazioni dei colori presso gli antichi* (*Ind. Vernice* 25, 1949)
(47) The term ḥb denoting the artificial green frit is sometimes loosely used for malachite too
(48) PLINY, *Nat. Hist.* XXXIII, 86—91; XXXV. 47
(49) DIOSCORIDES, V. 104; VITRUVIUS, 7.7.6; FLORUS, 2.33.60; SUETONIUS, *Caligula* 18
(50) Note in *Nature* 1925, page 764; AUGUSTI, S., *Sui colori degli antichi, la chrysocolla* (*Rend. Acad. Arch.* Napoli XXXIV 1959, 7—13)
(51) DIOSCORIDES, V. 91
(52) PLINY, *Nat. Hist.* XXXV, 48
(53) VITRUVIUS, 7.7.4
(54) DIOSCORIDES, V. 182
(55) PLINY, *Nat. Hist.* XXXV, 42
(56) VITRUVIUS, 7.10 1—4
(57) PLINY, *Nat. Hist.* XXXV. 36; see also VITRUVIUS, 7.7.3
(58) PLINY, *Nat. Hist.* XXXV. 37; THEOPHRASTUS, *De Lapid.* 107—108, DIOSCORIDES, V. 180
(59) DIOSCORIDES, V. 171; PLINY, *Nat. Hist.* XXXV. 192
(60) DIOSCORIDES, V. 172; VITRUVIUS, 7.7.3; PLINY, *Nat. Hist.* XXXV, 191

(61) PLINY, *Nat. Hist.* XXXIV. 175—177; XXXV. 36; VITRUVIUS, 7.12.1; DIOSCORIDES, V. 103
(62) LESLIE SHEAR, *Psimythion* (*Classical Studies presented to* E. CAPPS, Princeton 1936, pags. 314—317)
(63) Cake of ink, pigment = "rj.t" (II.399.9)
Waterbowl of the scribe = "p3ś" (I.499.5)
Palette of the scribe = "gs.tj" (V. 207.11)
(64) LUCAS, A., *The Inks of Ancient and Modern Egypt* (*The Analyst*, Vol. XLVII, 1922, pags. 9—15)
AINSWORTH MITCHELL, C., *An Ancient Egyptian Marking Ink* (*The Analyst* 1940 ,pags. 100—101)
POSENER, G., *Sur l'emploi de l'encre rouge dans les mss égyptiens* (*JEA* 37, 1951, 75—80)
KOBERT, R., *Ueber antike Tinte* (*Arch. Naturwiss. u. Technik* 1908, pags. 103—112)
LEVEY, M., *Some black inks in early medieval Jewish literature* (Chymia 9, 1964, 27—31)
SJÖQVIST, E., *Hellenic Inkstands* (*AJA* 63, 1959, 3, 275—276)
(65) DIOSCORIDES, V. 183
(66) THEOPHRASTUS, *Hist. Plant.* 3.8.6
(67) PLINY, *Nat. Hist.* XXXIV, 120; DIOSCORIDES, V. 119
(68) PLINY, *Nat. Hist.* XXXIV. 123—125; see also XX.123, XXXIV.112; DIOSCORIDES, V. 118; CELSUS, 5.8; SCRIBONIUS LARGUS 208 & 248
(69) PLINY, *Nat. Hist.* XXXV. 41
(70) The verb "ḳd" (V.73.24) means "to form pottery, to create (in general) to build, to make". From this verb the word "ḳdwt" (V.81.2) is derived which originally means "contours" and hence the "sš ḳdwt" (V.81.4) is the "painter, engraver, draughtsman" and the "sš ḳdy" (III, 480.11) is the "scribe of contours, draughtsman". But the "ḳd(y)" (V.52.8) is the "provider of gypsum" and the "irt ḳd" the "preparer of gypsum, plasterer".
This same intimate connection between building and decorating is found in the derivates frow the verb "sš" (III.475.6) which not only means "to write, to paint" but also "to draw" (III.476.7), "to paint on a wall" (III.476.8), "to paint in colours" (III.476.15). Therefore the "ḳsš dwt" (III.480.11) is both painter and draughtsmen working on a wall or any other prepared ground.
Two more terms are clearly connected with painting. The verb "śpẖr" (IV.106.11) also combines the idea of writing, drawing and painting and is used for the painting of texts and scenes on walls. The verb "sšr" (IV.294.9) means "to stroke, coat or smear" and it refers particularly to the plastering or white-washing of walls.
Similar combinations of ideas are found in Sumerian and Accadian.
(71) If we confine ourselves to the Egyptian language only we find that "iwn" (I.52.10), colours refer to natural objects. Black is either ḏ'b.t (V.536.8), charcoal or more often "km" (V.123.1), the colour of the black fertile soil of the Nile valley. "mfk3t" (I.65.13) describes the "turquoise green of herbs", "w3ḏ" the green of papyrusreed

and young plants. The word olive-oil "b3ḳ" (I.424.17) is used for light coloured, "mkrr" (II.163.5) for the colour of timber "between black and white". Golden and silver are named after the metals (nb, II.239.12; hḏ, III.210.20) but the earlier "golden" (ḏ'm, V. 539.5) refers to electron. Blue is the colour of lapis lazuli (hsbḏ, III. 334.15), pale red that of myrrh (mrš, II.113.1). We also find "blood red" (dšr V.488.1; ins, I.100.5).

Colours are used both as a mark and value of things. Blue is weapons stands for steel, in persons for certain ranks. Men are usually painted, red, women white. Iron is either brown or black.

(72) Magnus, H., *Histoire de l'évolution du sens des coleurs* (Paris 1878)

(73) Benaky, N. P., *Des termes qui désignent le violet dans l'antiquité et de la signification des épithètes composées de "ion"* (*Rev. Etud. Grec.*, Vol. XXVIII, 1915, pags. 16—38)

(74) Wolff, Th., *Von Antiken Farben und Farbenfabrikation* (*Farbe und Lack*, 1928, pags. 190—191; 203—204; 231—232; 240)

(75) Platnauer, M., *Greek colour-perception* (*Class. Quart.*, Vol. XV, 1921, pags. 153—162)

(76) Kober, A. E., *The uses of colour terms in the Greek poets* (New York, 1932)

André, J., *Etudes sur les termes de couleur dans la langue latine* (Paris 1949)

Gradweh, R., *Die Farben des Alten Testaments*, 1963

Thorndike, L., *Some medieval texts on colours* (Ambix (GB) 7, 1959, no. 1, 1—24)

Till, Walter C., *Die Farbenbezeichungen im Koptischen* (Roma, 1959) (*Analecta Biblica* no. 11, 1959, 331—342)

Vels, Heyn, *Kleurnamen en kleurbegrippen bij de Romeinen* (Utrecht, 1951)

(77) Wright, F. A., *A note on Plato's definition of colour* (*Class. Rev.*, Vol. 33/34, 1919, pags. 31—32)

(78) Standard Definitions of Terms Relating to Paint, Varnish, Lacquer and Related Products (ASTM Designation D 16—47, ASTM Standards Part II, Suppl. 1947, page 187)

(79) Norblin, *Les bonnes couleurs d'autrefois* (*Recherches et Inventions* 1935, pags. 351—354)

(80) Duell, P., *Evidence for Easel Painting in Ancient Egypt* (*Tech. Studies Field of Fine Arts*, Vol. VIII, 1939/1940, 175—191)

Junker, H., *Der Maler 'Ity* (*Oesterr. Akad. Wiss. Phil. hist. Kl., Anzeiger* vol. 93, 1957, 59—79)

(81) Glanville, S. R. K., *Materials and Technique of Egyptian Painting* (*Papers Soc. Mural Decorators and Painters in Tempera*, Vol. III, 1925/35, pags. 13—35)

Lucas, A., *Ancient Egyptian Materials and Industries* (London 1962)

Iversen, E., *Some ancient Egyptian paints and pigments* (*Dansk. Hist. Filol. Medd.* 34, 1955, no. 4)

Harris, J. R., *Lexicographical Studies in Ancient Egyptian Materials* (Berlin, 1961)

Wagenaar, M., *Microscopisch en Microchemisch onderzoek van enige Egyptische kleurstoffen* (*Pharm. Weekblad* 1933, pags. 894—901)

Wulkan, H. E., *Wat weten wij van de verven der oude Egyptenaren* (*Verfkroniek* 1950, pags. 41—46)

BAUD, M., *La peinture en bâtiment en Egypte ancienne* (*Recherches et Inventions*, 1935, pags. 355—358)

BAUD, M., *La décoration intérieure en Egypte Ancienne* (*Ann. Instit. du Bâtiment*, sept. 1936, pags. 62—65

SCHOLZ, H. A., *History of water-thinned paints* (*Ind. Eng. Chem.* 45, 1953, 710—711)

STOPPELAERE, A., *Introduction à la peinture thébaine* (*Valeurs* 7/8, 1947, 3—13)

(82) Ezech. 32.14

(83) Gum water = "ḳmjt" (II. 51.3); ḫil, [is]Ú-GIR = gum of thorn = ašagi, dardanu

(84) Rubbing stone = "s3.ś (III.422.6)
Mortar = "šd" (IV.566.11)
Triturate pigment in medium = "s n" (III.426.6)

(85) GARIS DAVIES, N. DE, *Five Theban Tombs* (London 1913, page 5, plate XVII)

(86) GARIS DAVIES, N. DE, *Ancient Egyptian Paintings* (Vol. III, 1936, pags. xxi—xlvi)

(87) MACKAY, E., *On the use of beeswax and resin as varnishes in Theban tombs* (*Ancient Egypt*, 1920, 35—38)

MARGIVAL, F., *Colour and coatings in Antiquity* (*Peintures, pigment, vernis* 26, 1950, 467—474)

MERCIER, M., *La propolis* (*BSAF* 1952, 127—160)

(88) The "akanthos" of Herodotus II.96

(89) ŠE-DÚN, šindu = varnish compare "šnḏ.t" (sunt) = Accacia Nilotica

(90) Dyeing of a stone = [a]SIM-SIG$_7$ = ṣurrupu ša abni

(91) PLINY, *Nat. Hist.* XXXVII. 74

(92) HARPER, R. F., *Assyrian and Babylonian Letters*, No. 570

(93) PLINY, *Nat. Hist.* XXXVII. 20

(93[a]) SNEYERS, R. & THISSEN, J., *La technique des lames minces appliquée à l'examen d'un relief assyrien en gypse* (*Bull. Inst. R. Patrim. Artist.* I, 1958, 94—96)

(94) BESQUES, S., *La peinture murale de l'époque préhellénique en Crète* (*Recherches et Inventions* 1935, pags. 359—361)

NOEL HEATON, *The decorator of ancient times* (*Proc. and Varnish Soc.* 1910/11, 1911, no. vi, pags 93—114)

DUELL, P. and GETTENS, R. J., *A Review of the problem of Aegean wall painting* (*Techn. Studies Field Fine Arts*, Vol. X, 1941, pags. 179—223)

(95) RAEHLMANN, E., *Ueber die Maltechnik der Alten* (Berlin 1910)

BERGER, E., *Beiträge zur Entwicklungsgeschichte der Maltechnik* (München 1904)

SCHMID, H., *Enkaustik und Fresko auf antiker Grundlage* (München 1926)

BORELLI, L., *Sulla tecnica della pittura greca* (*Boll. Ist. Centr. Restauro* I, 1950, 55—57)

HOFMANN, U., *Die chemischen Grundlagen der griechischen Vasenmalerei* (*Angew. Chemie*, 74, 1960, 397—406)

KRONSTEIN, M., *Ancient surface technology* (*Amer. Paint J.* 32, no. 8, 39,

42—43, 46, 48, 51—52; no. 10, 16, 18, 22, 24, 26—27; no. 17, 68, 70, 72)
BERGER, E., *Die Wachsmalerei des Apelles und seiner Zeit* (München 1917)
HERBERTS, K., 10.000 *Jahre Malerei und ihre Werkstoffe* (Wuppertal 1939)
LAURIE, A. P., *The Technique of the Great Painters* (London, 1949)
ALETTI, E., *La tecnica della pittura all' encausto* (Roma 1951)
COCHE DE LA FERTÉ, E., *Les portraits Romano-Egyptiens du Louvre* (Paris, 1952)
AUGUSTI, S., *La tecnica dell'antica pittura parietale Pompeiana* (Napoli, 1950)
LÜDECKE, C., *Die Wachsmalerei der Alten* (*Fette, Seifen, Anstrichmittel*, 63, 1961, 38—41)
COCHE DE LA FERTÉ, E., *Imagines majorum ou portraits de momies* (*Revue des Arts* 34, 1953, I, 54—55)
PLENDERLEITH, H. J., *The history of artist's pigments* (*Science Progress* no. 150, 1950, 246—256)

(96) MILLER, W., *Daedalus and Thespis* (*Univ. of Minnesota Studies*, Vol. VII, 1932, pags. 609—612)
KNAPP, CH., *References to Painting in Plautus and Terence* (*Class. Philol.*, Vol. 12, 1917, pags. 143—157)

(97) LOUMYER, G., *L'outillage et le matériel du peintre de l'Antiquité grecque et romaine* (Van Oest, Bruxelles, 1922)

(98) ANAXANDR., Ζωγ, Frag. 13 K

(99) PLINY, *Nat. Hist.* 28, 71; 25, 26; 36, 55

(100) PLINY, *Nat. Hist.* 13.20; VITRUVIUS, 7.10; DIOSCORIDES, III.83.84

(101) ARZENS, R., *L'évolution de la technique du vernis* (*Ing. Chimiste*, Vol. 22, 1938, pags. 77—83)
CRIVELLI, E., *The origins of pigment and varnish techniques* (*Ind. Vernice*, V, 1951, 134—138)
HOWES, F. N., *Age-old resins of the Mediterranean region and their uses* (*Econ. Botany* 4, 1950, 307)
BRANDI, C., *Some factual observations about varnishes and glazes* (*Boll. ist. centrale restauro* 3/4, 1950, 9—29)
MACLAREN, N. and WERNER, A. E., *Some factual observances about varnishes and glazes* (Burlington Mag. 92, 1950, 189—192)
GREBER, J. M., LEHMANN, H. & WERTH, A. VAN DER, *Die Tierischen Leime* (Heidelberg, 1950)
WILLETS, W., *China* (London, 1958, I, 188—197) (on lac)

(102) ANTIPHON, *Eup. Frag.* 98 K; ANTIPHON, *Inc. Frag.* 232, 1—4 K; EURIPIDES, *Helen.* 262—263; EURIPIDES, *Peleus Frag.* 618 N

(103) AESCHYLUS, *Ag.* 1327—1329; PLATO, *Theat.* 187 B; PLINY, *Nat. Hist.* XXXV. 101

(104) HALL, L. F., *Notes on the colours preserved on the archaic Attic gravestones in the Metropolitan Museum* (*Amer. J. Archaeol.* 1944, pags. 334—336)

(105) VITRUVIUS, 7.3.5

(106) PAUSANIAS, IX. 4.2

(107) AFRANIUS, *Augur* V (1) 14 R[3]; PLAUTUS, *Merc.* 313—315; PLAUTUS, *Men.* 143—144

(108) CATO, *De Agri.* xvi
(109) BLAKE, M. E., *Ancient Roman Construction in Italy from the Prehistoric period to Augustus* (Washington 1947, pags. 310—311; 318—321)
(110) LIVY, XL. 50.3
(111) VITRUVIUS, ii.4.3; vii.2.1; ii.5.1; vii.6.1; vii.3.6
(112) VITRUVIUS, vii.3.2.—7
(113) VITRUVIUS, vii.3.7
(114) VITRUVIUS, vii.4.1—3
(115) PLINY, *Nat. Hist.* XXXV. 49
(116) PLINY, *Nat. Hist.* XXXV. 34; XXXIII, 90—91
(117) BRANZANI, L., *La pitture murali degli Etruschi, osservazioni sulla loro tecnica* (*Studi Etrusche*, Vol. VII, 1933, pags. 335, 340)
GRASSINI, R., *Esame chimico dei colori nelle pitture murali della tomba dipinta delle ficaie* (*Studi Etrusche*, Vol. VIII, 1934, pags. 327—328)
GRASSINI, R., *Esame chimico di frammenti di pitture murali di intonaci e di pavimenti* (*Studie Etrusche*, Vol. X, 1934/35, pags. 355—360)
AUGUSTI, S., *Sulla tecnica della pittura pompeiana* (*Boll. d'Arte* (*Roma*) vol. XXXV, 1950, pags. 189—191)
AUGUSTI, S., *La tecnica della pittura murale di Ercalono* (*Rend. Acc. Arch. Napoli* XXXIV, 1959, 15—19)
CAGIANO DE AZEVEDO, M., *Encausto ed encausticatura nella pittura murale romana* (*Boll. Ist. Centr. Restauro* III, 1952, 199—202)
HERMESDORF, P. F. J. M., *Muurschilderingen uit de Romeinsche villa te Vlengendaal, hunne technische opbouw* (Maasgouw, 74, 1953, 121—126)
LATNER, J., *An analysis of paints used in Roman Britain* (Paint Technol. 27, 1963, 6, 29—30; 9, 40)
PLESTERS, J., *An analysis of paints used in Roman Britain* (Paint Technol. 27, 1963, 8, 42; 11, 50)
LEHMANN, PH., *Roman wall paintings from Boscoreale* (Cambridge (Mass.), 1953
(118) SKJOLD MÜLLER, F., *Ueber die Techniken antiker Wandmalereien und Mosaiken* (*VI Int. Kongress f. Archaol.* 1939, pags. 157—162)
(119) GEILMANN, W., *Chemisch-technische Untersuchung der Wand- und Gewölbemalerei in der romanischen Kirche zu Idensen* (*Nachr. Mitt. u. Neuer. Gesch.*, Vol. II, 1936/39, pags. 71—84)
(120) FLINDERS PETRIE, W. M., *The Hawara Portefolio* (London 1913)
(121) PLINY, *Nat. Hist.* XXXV, 49 & 149
(122) PLAUTUS, *As.* 762—767
(123) PLINY, *Nat. Hist.* XXXV, 122; VITRUVIUS, 7.9.3
(124) VARRO, 3.17; SENECA, *Epist.* 121
(125) DIOSCORIDES, IV. 64—66

INDEX